Rehabilitation of the Older Adult

Rehabilitation of the Older Adult

Keith Andrews, M.D., F.R.C.P.
Medical and Research Director,
Royal Hospital and Home for Incurables,
Putney, London

Formerly Senior Lecturer in Geriatric Medicine,
University of Manchester

Edward Arnold

© Keith Andrews 1987

First published in Great Britain 1987 by
Edward Arnold (Publishers) Ltd, 41 Bedford Square, London WC1B 3DQ

Edward Arnold (Australia) Pty Ltd, 80 Waverley Road, Caulfield East,
  Victoria 3145, Australia

Edward Arnold, 3 East Read Street, Baltimore, Maryland 21202, U.S.A.

British Library Cataloguing in Publication Data

Andrews, Keith
  Rehabilitation of the older adult.
  1. Aged——Rehabilitation   2. Geriatrics
  I. Title
  618.97   RC952.5

ISBN 0-7131-4524-2

All rights reserved. No part of this publication may be reproduced, stored in a
retrieval system, or transmitted in any form or by any means, electronic,
photocopying, recording, or otherwise, without the prior permission of
Edward Arnold (Publishers) Ltd.
Whilst the advice and information in this book is believed to be true and accurate
at the date of going to press, neither the authors nor the publisher can accept any
legal responsibility or liability for any errors or omissions that may be made.

Text set in 11/12pts Times Compugraphic
by Colset Private Limited, Singapore
Printed and bound in Great Britain by
Richard Clay Ltd, Bungay, Suffolk

Preface

Rehabilitation, in its broadest sense, is a fundamental principle of geriatric medicine. It is therefore surprising that so little has been written about rehabilitation for the elderly. In searching the literature for this book I have been struck by the lack of good research into the rehabilitation component of geriatric practice. Many of the principles were described thirty or forty years ago and have not been tested against modern needs. Others have required extrapolation from studies of disability in younger people. Rehabilitation offers ideal opportunities for young research workers to make their names and advance the knowledge base without the need for expensive and high-technology trials.

This book is based on my firm belief that effective rehabilitation requires a well-integrated interdisciplinary and multiprofessional team who are prepared to work together in the interests of the disabled family. No one profession has the skill or knowledge base to be the single most important practitioner, although at any one time one professional group may be the prime worker. The role of the family is emphasized time and time again in this book, with sections on advice that can be given to families and patients on coping.

I am grateful to one of my students who helped to put into perspective the concept of rehabilitation when he said in one of our seminars 'There is no such thing as independence, only varying degrees of dependence'. This is similar in concept to the statement by Professor Wolff that 'Disability is not having found the right tool for the job'. This book aims to provide some tools to lower the level of dependency of elderly people. One of the problems is that the word 'elderly' covers an age range of 40 or 50 years and a wide range of levels of physical fitness. This book will primarily cover the problems encountered by the 'frail elderly'.

There are two prime functions of this book. The first is to provide some practical ideas for management of specific disorders. There are many views and opinions and I have tried to include as many as possible, although there is little scientific evidence to 'prove' that many of them are effective. I am sure that there will be many who will be critical that I have not included their favourite approach. I shall be only too pleased to hear their views, preferably with the research evidence to back their claims.

The second purpose of this book is to encourage further research into rehabilitation. For this reason I have included relatively detailed references as a starting point for those wishing to investigate areas in more depth.

Throughout the book I have mostly used the male sex to indicate the patient and females to indicate the carer, merely to assist the flow of the text, and I trust I will be forgiven for such an apparently sexist approach.

1987   KA

Acknowledgements

I should like to express my gratitude to the numerous people of all professional groups who have given me ideas and provided constructive criticisms for the preparation of this book. I am also indebted to the many patients and relatives who have educated me into setting appropriate and realistic goals.

The medical illustration departments of the University Hospital of South Manchester and Hope Hospital, Salford, must be thanked for their excellent contribution to the illustrations.

Finally I wish to thank my word processor for being so reliable and forgiving during the numerous redrafting sessions without which this book would never have been completed.

Contents

1

Rehabilitation of the elderly

Introduction

The purpose of this book is to investigate the concept of rehabilitation and to examine the knowledge-base of disorders that are common in the elderly and which require a rehabilitation approach. One of the major problems in attempting such a task is to know what is meant by 'rehabilitation'. A formal definition like 'the restoration of the individual to his (or her) fullest physical, mental and social capability' [1] has much to commend it, placing emphasis on social and psychological components as well as physical disability. There are, however, limitations to the definition since few 'normal' people actually ever achieve their *fullest* physical, mental and social capabilities. To expect the disabled elderly to do so seems inappropriate. It therefore seems more useful to think in terms of 'restoration of the individual to the *optimal* level of ability within the needs and desires of the individual and his or her family'. Another approach is to see rehabilitation as the orderly induction of services according to the individual's ability to benefit and recover.

The relevance of these definitions can be seen in everyday practice. A patient may respond very well to a rehabilitation programme only to return home to a lower level of activity. One reason for this may be poor goal setting; but often it is a fact that we train patients in the artificial environment of the hospital, where there is plenty of stimulation and encouragement, where floors are uncluttered in wide, open spaces which allow easy manoeuvrability with walking aids, where beds and chairs are of ideal height and where patients are confident that there is someone around to help when they get into difficulties – entirely different, in other words, from the cramped conditions of the homes of many old people, where the furniture is far from ideal and where there is lack of stimulation or purpose.

Another important component is the knowledge and attitude of the supporter or carer. In one study [2] elderly stroke patients attending a day hospital were assessed on their activities in the rehabilitation environment. They were then visited at home during the same week to assess their actual activities at home. There were quite marked differences between what the patient 'could do' and what he 'did do'. Much of this was due to a lack of knowledge on the part of the carer; but it was also due in part to the fact that carers often found it quicker, safer and less frustrating to assist the patients than to encourage independence. Under such circumstances the rehabilitation programme was ineffective.

Goal planning

It is essential right from the start of the rehabilitation programme to set both short- and long-term goals for the patient, family and rehabilitation team. Where the expectations of the patient, family and staff are different then problems can occur. This is especially true when the relationship of expectations to reality are out of line [3]. For instance, the patient who feels that he will not improve, even though there is no reason on clinical grounds why he should not, is unlikely to reach his greatest potential. On the other hand, the patient whose expectations far outstrip his actual potential may make a better recovery than the staff expect but is likely to be greatly dissatisfied and depressed by, what is to him, lack of progress. These patients frequently put great demands on staff to try harder and resist a discontinuation of the formal rehabilitation programme – a distressing problem for staff who know that their time would be more productively spent with other patients.

Similarly, when the patient's family has low expectations then there is pressure on staff to withdraw from an active rehabilitation programme which the family regards as being cruel to a frail, elderly person. They also encourage the patient to think in negative terms and try to persuade him to accept long-term care. On the other hand, families whose expectations are greater than the reality of the situation cause great distress to staff by demanding inappropriate levels of treatment.

It is also important to recognize that the therapist's view of the relevance of activities is not necessarily the same as the patient's; indeed, in one study the value of activities of daily living as perceived by stroke patients and by their therapists rarely correlated [4].

One approach to these problems is to involve the patient and the family in the early goal planning. Becker *et al.* [5] discussed 30 items of activity separately with the patient and then with the relatives. Where there were differences of opinion between the patient, relatives and staff concerning the expected goals, then compromise goals were negotiated and agreed on. These were renegotiated as the

rehabilitation programme proceeded. This approach helped to identify early conflicts of interest and improved patient – relative – staff
relationships, whilst orientating the patient and family to a rehabilitation concept.

Since each patient is different, it is part of the rehabilitation assessment to define the background of the patient, what he or she has lost
by the recent disability and what there is to be gained by recovery.
Each patient possesses a combination of assets and liabilities which
will influence the outcome. It is too easy for a rehabilitation team to
set goals for which the patient sees no relevance.

Impairment, disability and handicap

Impairment

Impairment refers to damage to or dysfunction of an organ or part of
the body. For instance, in stroke the impairment is the weakness of
one side of the body, the hemianopia or the sensory loss.

Impairment is the 'bread and butter' of the physician and, to some
extent, of the physiotherapist, for whom the emphasis of treatment is
on improving motor power, balance and range of movement.

In general, impairment is relatively easy to measure and describe.
Unfortunately the severity of the impairment has only a partial
relationship to functional ability.

Disability

Disability refers to the way in which an impairment affects the functions of an individual. For instance, in stroke the hemiplegia (the
impairment) results in a difficulty in dressing or feeding.

Many factors influence disability. A patient with a dense hemiplegia
may still be able to dress, make a cup of tea and be mobile in a wheelchair; another patient with a mild loss of motor power may be unable
to dress and be immobile, depending on a whole range of other features such a sensory involvement, cognitive function or previous
personality.

An interesting approach to the concept of rehabilitation is to start
from the recognition that *we are all disabled*. We are, for example,
unable to drill a hole in a wall with a finger or lift a car to change a
wheel. We overcome these disabilities by finding the right tool to do
the job – i.e. a drill for putting holes in walls or a jack and spanner for
removing wheels from cars. In other words, disability results from not
having found the right tool for the job. The role of rehabilitation is,
therefore, to find the correct tool, be it an aid, a drug, a technique or
social intervention.

Disability is more difficult to measure than is impairment, but a number of 'activities of daily living' scales are available.

Handicap

Handicap refers to the way in which impairment and disability influence a patient's resettlement into the community.

Consider, for example, two 78-year-old males, both of whom have had an above-knee amputation. Neither has any complicating factors such as heart disease or arthritis, both are the same weight and height, and both live in a ground-floor flat with a healthy wife. In effect the impairment and disability in these two men are identical. One of them, however, lives only for work in his garden, whereas the other enjoys writing books and reading. The gardener, therefore, has a greater handicap than the author. This is a simple example using only one variable influencing the level of handicap; in real life there are numerous potential variables, including other physical disorders, motivation, previous personality, social environment and the relationships within the family unit.

Handicap is much more difficult to measure than impairment or disability, and it is almost certain that handicap scales are unlikely to be successful unless they are tailor-made for each individual patient.

Categories of rehabilitation

Partridge [6] has described four patterns of disability applicable to the elderly, as follows:

1. Localized injuries do not usually require a multidisciplinary approach and full recovery can normally be expected. For instance, management of soft tissue injury may be by physiotherapists when the main aim is to relieve symptoms, increase the range of movement, restore muscle strength and prevent complications; or by nursing management in the case of incontinence.
2. In some conditions a return to pre-morbid levels can be expected for a large proportion of patients but the skills of several professional groups are required. Fracture of the femur and some other surgical conditions fall into this group. Quite often recovery depends as much on the management of the medical and surgical complications as on the physical therapy programme.
3. With some conditions long-standing disability is common (e.g. stroke, paraplegia or amputation) and full recovery may not be possible. Optimal recovery depends on a well-integrated multidisciplinary team approach.

4. With progressively deteriorating conditions such as parkinsonism, rheumatoid arthritis or motor neurone disease, the aim is to maintain optimal ability throughout the illness. Constant review is necessary, with reassessment of goals as the disorder progresses. A greater emphasis will be placed on maintaining the emotional, social and environmental factors than on specific rehabilitation techniques.

Rehabilitation is therefore a complex process and depends on the disability types. In this context Dasco [7] categorized elderly patients into three types:

1. Those who are not obviously ill but whose physical function is impaired;
2. Those who are chronically ill (e.g. with chronic cardiac or pulmonary disease) without manifest signs of disability;
3. Handicapped persons (e.g. those with hemiplegia, arthritis, fractures and amputation).

Another approach has been described under the acronym SPREAD [8]:

- **S**pecific control of underlying disease or impairment by medical, surgical and psychological measures. Drug therapy falls firmly into this category.
- **P**revention of secondary disability. Into this category falls the prevention of pressure sores, contractions, the painful hemiplegic shoulder and constipation.
- **RE**storative measures. These mainly involve physiotherapy or occupational therapy but may also include nursing measures for conditions such as incontinence or pressure sores.
- **AD**aptation. This includes the use of orthoses as well as environmental aids and family adjustment.

These three approaches all indicate the importance of recognizing the specific needs of the individual and the benefits of a multiprofessional team.

The size of the problem

Disablement is common in the elderly. About two-thirds of all disabled people are over the age of 65 years [9]. Not only does the prevalence of handicap increase markedly with advancing age (Fig. 1.1.), but so too does the proportion of individuals in each age group who are severely handicapped. The proportion of those 75 years and over who have severe or very severe disability is about the same as the pro-

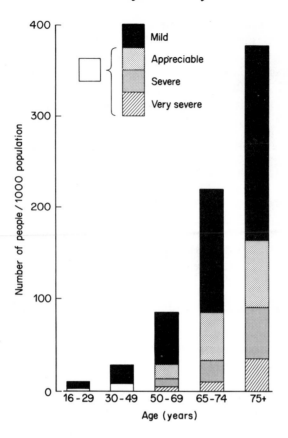

Fig. 1.1   Prevalence of handicap related to age and severity

portion of those aged 45–50 who have any degree of handicap. This has major implications for the planning of services.

Some conditions are obviously more common in the elderly than others (Fig. 1.2). For instance, 78 per cent of those with arthritis (other than rheumatoid arthritis) are over 65 years of age, compared with only 13 per cent of those with multiple sclerosis. Other conditions where the proportion of those with severe disability are predominantly elderly are stroke (78 per cent) circulatory disorders (79 per cent) and blindness (88 per cent); whereas others such as parkinsonism (47 per cent), amputation of the lower limb (46 per cent), paraplegia (51 per cent) and rheumatoid arthritis are about equally distributed between those over and those under 65 years of age [9]. Within the elderly age group, disability increases from 12 per cent in the 65–69-year sub-group to over 80 per cent of those over 80 years [10].

One of the difficulties here is lack of standardization of the terms

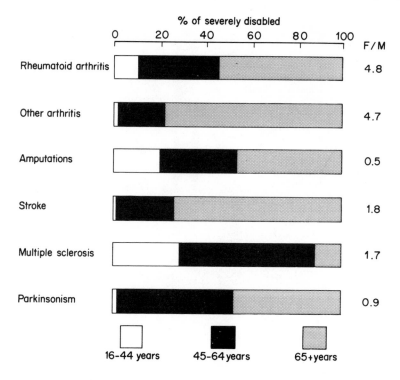

Fig. 1.2 Severe disability and age (after Harris [9])

'disability' and 'handicap', and for that matter 'severe'. Nevertheless the problems of dependency increase with advancing age.

Special problems of rehabilitating elderly people

Multiple pathology

Multiple pathology is one of the classical characteristics of advancing age. For instance, on average, elderly patients have four or more different diagnoses present at the same time [11, 12]. In one study examining the interrelationship of the 13 commonest diagnoses present in patients admitted to a geriatric unit (Fig. 1.3), as many as 42 per cent of males and 31 per cent of females had four or more of the conditions present in combination [13]. Since physical disability such as stroke or amputation increases the energy expenditure of walking [14–17], it is not surprising that cardiorespiratory disorders or anaemia are likely to complicate the rehabilitation potential. Certainly, the greater the number of disorders present the greater the mortality and the lower the discharge rate [13, 18]. Even the combination of only two con-

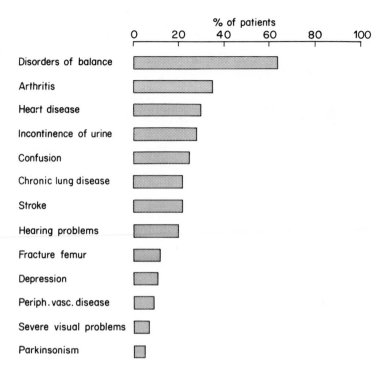

Fig. 1.3 Multiple pathology: disorders present in 184 consecutive patients admitted to a geriatric unit

ditions, such as stroke and amputation, dramatically affects the prognosis [19].

When considering multiple pathology it cannot be assumed that all conditions, even those of a degenerative nature, will automatically increase in prevalence in the same group of patients. For instance, in one study of stroke patients the proportion with associated pre-stroke balance problems increased with age; however, the proportion with arthritis of the lower limbs was less in those 75 years and over than in those 65–74 years (though both were higher than in those under 65 years [20]. On the other hand, symptomatic ischaemic heart disease was more common in those under 65 than in those in the two older age groups. This pattern of the very old not necessarily being worse than the younger elderly group will be discussed again below.

Polypharmacy

Associated with multiple pathology is polypharmacy. This can be quite a problem in rehabilitation of the elderly since so many of the drugs prescribed have a direct action on the central nervous system. It is, therefore, not surprising that falls, immobility, confusion and apathy secondary to drug side effects result in admission to rehabilitation wards. On the other hand, polypharmacy is associated with increasing poor compliance in taking the medication [21, 22]. The rehabilitation team therefore has an important role in assessing the need for the drugs, educating the patient and the family in their use, and finding appropriate techniques for improving compliance.

Mental vulnerability

The increased prevalence of dementia in the elderly has an important influence on rehabilitation potential. Since rehabilitation is an educational model of management, any condition that interferes with learning new skills will obviously limit the outcome. Indeed, intellectual impairment has been shown to be the main factor in poor functional activity [23, 24]. However, since 'rehabilitation' is a broader concept than the physiotherapy or occupational therapy approach, there is still much that can be achieved with the confused patient.

It is difficult to know how much confusion is due to inactivity or change in environment. The mental state of elderly people with mental disorders has been shown to improve following physical therapy and was associated with improvement in the physical condition [25, 26]. Clinical experience shows that many patients improve mentally on being moved to a rehabilitation environment from a general ward. This may be due to an improvement in the medical condition or due to the general rehabilitation atmosphere.

It is generally felt that the elderly are particularly likely to become confused when moved from one environment to another. The evidence for this is difficult to interpret. Most studies on this topic have described the *emergency* transfer of a large number of institutionalized patients because of fire or riots. Under these circumstances it is probably not surprising that patients become agitated and confused [27, 28], while some studies have shown an increase in mortality following such dramatic moves [27, 29]. On the other hand, where the relocation was planned there was no increase in mortality or morbidity [30, 31].

Personality traits

Another side to mental vulnerability is related to the methods of adaptation to advancing age. Reichard and Peterson [32], using cluster analysis, demonstrated in elderly men five strategies for coming to terms with old age, and these can adapted to describe rehabilitation approaches. Although these strategies were identified in men there is no reason to believe that they are not applicable to women.

Some men were of the *constructive* type. This described the well-adjusted person who is flexible, tolerant, who enjoys life and still sees a future. These individuals are a pleasure to 'rehabilitate' since they are determined, well-motivated and liked by all the staff. They usually do well wherever treated.

Some men showed *dependency*. This personality type is pleasant and popular but is perfectly happy to allow others to do things for him. The spouse tends to be the dominant partner and the patient is quite happy to allow her to look after him. This has clinical implications since this type of patient responds positively to the stimulation of the rehabilitation environment but returns home to a life of being passive and dependent. It is therefore essential to involve the family in the rehabilitation programme and to have appropriate goals. Consideration should be given to whether home rehabilitation would not be more appropriate in this situation.

Some men showed *hostility*. This type is aggressive and constantly complains; no-one seems to be able to be right in his eyes. He is habit-bound and inflexible. In the rehabilitation setting he is a difficult character who resists, almost on principle, any attempt to help him. The aggression antagonizes the staff, and there is great reluctance by community carers to accept him back and to provide support. This personality type is in danger of not receiving the optimal treatment unless his problems are fully recognized.

The fourth strategy was *defensiveness*. An individual of this type is also rather rigid, but also to some extent anxious that the professionals are going to find out something about him and pressurize him into accepting increasing levels of care. He has a fear of dependency and resists any attempt to help him. This is the classical case of the 'I'll be all right when I go home' syndrome. Again, it is important to recognize the problems otherwise there is danger of frustrated withdrawal of support. It is often easier to manage this person at home where he feels secure and confident. He is, however, suspicious of strangers. For this reason management by one person whom he trusts is often more effective than by a full rehabilitation team.

The final strategy was *self-hate*. These individuals can see no future and therefore do not make any attempt to help themselves. They are passive but at the same time resistant to the encouragement of the rehabilitation team. Even if they can be persuaded to take part in a rehabilitation programme, the benefit is short-lived. If they return home they are soon readmitted to institutional care having done absolutely nothing for themselves. It is important to recognize this personality type if unnecessary resources are not to be wasted. It is, however, also important to make sure that this pattern is due to a long-standing personality trait and not due to depression, hypothyroidism, electrolyte imbalance, anaemia, perceptual disorder or another condition requiring treatment.

These categorizations are, of course, a gross oversimplification. Nevertheless they do offer the beginnings of a recognition that different personality types will require different rehabilitation approaches.

Low expectations

The elderly are generally regarded as having lower expectations than the younger population. The high level of unreported and unrecognized illness in the elderly population has been presented as evidence for this [12, 33]. However, even in a high-risk group of patients 75 years and over in general practice, the presence of unrecognized disease was often associated with a happy and active life and involvement of a rehabilitation team was required for less than 1 per cent of the patients studied [33].

Low expectations are frequently externally induced – the 'It's just your age, dear' attitude. This is just as likely to come from professionals as from neighbours and family. 'Old age' as a diagnosis releases the professional from any obligation to investigate, treat or manage.

The nihilistic approach of professionals may be realistic if the elderly actually do have a bad prognosis. One example of this is stroke. In general, studies have shown that with advancing age there is an increase in the severity of the stroke [34, 35] and an associated worsening of the prognosis [36–38]. Other studies have not found such a direct relationship between age and functional recovery [39, 40].

The difficulty seems to be at what point the groups are compared. For instance, in one longitudinal study of stroke patients those under 65 years had significantly milder strokes (measured two weeks following onset) than those in either the 65–74 or 75 + age groups, although there was no statistically significant difference in severity between the last two groups [20]. Severe loss of function occurred in 50 per cent of those under 65, 70 per cent of those aged 65–74, and 62 per cent of those 75 years and over. When the 'maximal ability reached' was examined, those under 65 years old did significantly better than either of the two older age groups, although there was again no statistically significant difference between the latter. However, this takes no account of the time to reach that maximal recovery and includes those dying during the first few months (i.e. the time of maximal spontaneous recovery). Mortality during the first three months increased with advancing age and this would bias the results of the maximum level of recovery reached – those with severe strokes being more likely to die. When the functional ability of the *survivors* at six or twelve months was assessed there was no difference between the three age groups for recovery levels. Indeed, the trend was for a greater proportion of those 75 years and over to reach mild levels of disability than of those 65–74 years of age. When the six-month and one-year outcomes of the same three age groups who had started with severe loss of function were compared, there was again no statistical difference in the outcome; the elderly did as well (or as badly) as the younger population [41].

Expectations for recovery by the elderly can therefore be quite high. What matters seems not to be the age of the patient but the severity of the impairment. However, we must also be realistic in that the elderly are more likely to have severe disability and complications, and therefore to require longer periods of rehabilitation or have a higher incidence of admission to long-stay institutions than are younger people [42].

One of the difficulties in comparing the recovery of different age groups is that this assumes that they have similar needs, which is obviously not the case. The young person with a stroke who is trying to look after a family and continuing to work has needs that are different from those of the elderly person who may be satisfied to be able to get to the local church or social gathering. This has led to studies assessing 'potential' rather than 'performance' [43, 44]. Masterman concluded that 'older disabled people, at least from the psychological point of view, were by far the best rehabilitation prospects.'

Social liability

It has been suggested (45, 46) that there is 'a mutual withdrawal or "disengagement" between the aging person and others in the social system to which he belongs – a withdrawal initiated by the individual himself or others in the system' [45, 46]. This suggests that 'disengagement is an inevitable process in which many of the relationships between a person and other members of the society are severed, and those remaining altered in quality' [*ibid.*].

The idea that this disengagement is an inevitable part of growing old results in a nihilistic view of the rehabilitation of elderly people. The view has been challenged on the grounds that the disengagement may well be the result of chronic disease. Certainly, young chronically disabled people show disengagement which is greater than for people of their own age or even those in the older age group who are not disabled [47]. Nevertheless, in geriatric rehabilitation we are dealing with disabled elderly people who show some of the signs of disengagement – fewer contacts with other people, less desire to move out of the house, and a general lack of interest in the outside world. This has a significant influence on goal planning. The elderly person who has a great desire to be involved in local community activities has aims and needs different from those of the person who, irrespective of the level of functional recovery achieved, has no desire for involvement. This produces a level of social liability or vulnerability which many staff and relatives have difficulty in accepting.

Carers

It is generally felt that families are less caring for their elderly today than in previous decades, but there is in fact very little sociological evidence for this. A greater proportion of elderly may be in residential care in the 1980s than in the 1900s. However, there are many more elderly without children than in the days of large families, and this trend is continuing. In addition, the fact that an elderly person was still at home at the beginning of the century does not mean that the care was either good or loving. It was not uncommon for an elderly member of the family to be confined to one room and ignored by all except for the provision of basic needs.

The pressure of caring on the family can be seen in the study by Sanford [48], in which he assessed the degree of tolerance by carers of problems that were present in patients admitted to his geriatric wards. First of all it was evident that many families were attempting to cope with difficult problems such as falls, incontinence and behavioural disorders. In general, they tolerated physical conditions quite well, though falls and incontinence were less well tolerated. The least-tolerated conditions were those where there was confusion, especially when associated with sleep disturbances, wandering or aggression. This emphasizes the importance of caring for the carers as well as for the patient.

Social liability also occurs owing to the ability (or inability) of the carers to cope physically or mentally. Many elderly people live with an equally elderly spouse or sibling, while others, because of their very advanced age, are cared for by elderly children. This has implications where heavy physical support is required from a frail carer.

Another problem, not specific to the elderly, arises when the dominant partner becomes dependent and there have to be role changes. This may place an unbearable burden on family dynamics. This is also seen where there is a symbiotic relationship between two elderly people together. When one becomes ill or dies, the other is unable to cope alone. Thus social liability is not so much an environmental difficulty as a psychological dependency on a complex relationship between the patient and society.

The team concept

Much lip service is paid to the concept of the team approach. As Rubin [49] has pointed out:

> It is naive to bring together a highly diverse group of people and expect they will in fact behave like a team. It is ironic indeed to realise that a football team spends forty hours a week practising teamwork for the two hours on a Sunday afternoon, when their teamwork really counts. Teams in organisations spend two hours per year practising when their ability to function as a team counts forty hours per week.

The health care team has been defined as 'a group of persons, each possessing particular expertise, who have a common purpose and goal'. [50]. It is important to recognize that even within this definition there is a difference between 'interdisciplinary' and 'multidisciplinary' management [51]. The 'multidisciplinary' team is a group of professionals who each provide their own expertise irrespective of the techniques used, and the goals set, by other members of the team. With this approach it is possible for a physiotherapist to assist the patient to walk using one technique, the occupational therapist using another technique, a nurse yet another, and so on. In the 'interdisciplinary' team the professionals meet regularly to communicate and plan the rehabilitation programme together. Each member of the team knows the techniques being used by other members and there is overlap in the approach. Within such a team the social worker should know how the patient is walking, the occupational therapist should know the nursing problems, the physiotherapist should know the problems the patient has with dressing, and so on. The individual members of the team are, therefore, bringing their own skills to a group effort. As the patient's condition changes then the emphasis and role played by different members of the team will also change. It is relatively easy to appreciate the concept of the team when dealing with the primary members of the rehabilitation team, but it becomes more difficult when considering the input from other professional groups who see only the occasional patient and have to cover a large number of other departments.

One of the difficulties that many staff have is the fear of giving up part of their 'standing' and authority in the interests of team work. This applies as much to doctors as to other members of the team. It has been shown that in team meetings doctors do most of the talking and make most of the authoritative statements, while the other members of the team, including the patient, say little and offer few authoritative

comments [52]. This suggests either that the team meeting is concentrating excessively on the medical needs of the patient, or that the
team is lacking confidence in itself as a functioning entity. A true
interdisciplinary team [53–56], which practises a coordinated, non-
hierarchically structured, holistic approach where the patient and the
family are actively involved, is a very difficult thing to achieve in
practice.

There have been suggestions that there should be multi-purpose
rehabilitation therapists who would carry out most of the therapeutic
needs of the majority of disabled patients [57]. This would therefore
be a one-person team. Others have suggested that nurses could take on
much of the basic rehabilitation work, thereby leaving the trained
therapists free to carry out highly specialized rehabilitation techniques
[58]. Nurses are in a particularly suitable position to take on the
general rehabilitation training of patients since they are responsible
for the management of patients throughout the 24-hour period and
spend more time with patients than any other professional group.

An interdisciplinary team is more easy to achieve in a hospital,
where the members of the team are based in a relatively small area,
than in the community where large areas have to be covered by staff
whose bases may be in many different buildings, making it more difficult to meet to discuss individual patient management.

Palmer *et al.* [59] have described the following four stages of developing a psychosocial team which, although initially intended for clinical psychologists, are applicable to the general rehabilitation team:

- Stage I. *Identification* of the purpose of the intervention by the
  member of the team and the needs of the patient.
- Stage II. *Role definition*, where the skills and expertise which are
  specific or exclusive to each discipline are identified.
- Stage III. *Task assignment* to each discipline according to the skills,
  special interests and efficiency of the use of limited resources.
- Stage IV. *Integration*, where the collaboration of the team is faci-
  litated by a team coordinator.

Barriers to recovery

Some of the barriers to recovery have already been mentioned, including confusion, low expectations and general ill-health. However,
other causes for failure are common. If the goals set by the rehabilitation team are unrealistic or meaningless to the patient then success is
unlikely. This is seen in the patient who returns home having achieved
the ability to carry out activities which are of no interest to him and
therefore not carried out at home. It is also seen in the amount of
equipment that is prescribed but not used after the first few weeks.

Rehabilitation is a broad concept and involves much more than formal physiotherapy or occupational therapy. It must be based on what the patient and his carers want and on setting goals that are not only achievable but also acceptable and realistic.

References

1. Mair, A. (1972) *Report of Subcommittee of the Standing Medical Advisory Committee, Scottish Health Service Council on Medical Rehabilitation*. HMSO, Edinburgh.
2. Andrews, K. and Stewart, J. (1979) Stroke recovery: He can but does he? *Rheumatology and Rehabilitation* 18: 43-8.
3. New, P.K., Ruscio, A.T. and George, L.A. (1969) Towards an understanding of the rehabilitation system. *Rehabilitation Literature* 30: 130-9.
4. Chiou, I-I. L. and Burnett, C.N. (1985) Values of activities of daily living: a survey of stroke patients and their home therapists. *Physical Therapy* 65: 901-6.
5. Becker, M.C., Abrams, K.S. and Onder, J. (1974) Goal setting: a joint patient staff method. *Archives of Physical Medicine and Rehabilitation* 55: 87-9.
6. Partidge, C.J. (1980) The effectiveness of physiotherapy: a classification for evaluation. *Physiotherapy* 66: 153-5.
7. Dasco, M.M. (1953) Clinical problems in geriatric rehabilitation. *Geriatrics* 8: 179-84.
8. Hunt, T.E. (1980) Practical considerations in the rehabilitation of the aged. *Journal of the American Geriatrics Society* 28: 59-64.
9. Harris, A.I. (1971) *Handicapped and Impaired in Great Britain*. HMSO, London.
10. Akhtar, A.J., Broe, G.A., Crombie, A. *et al.* (1973) Disability and dependence in the elderly at home. *Age and Ageing* 2: 102-11.
11. Wilson, L.A., Lawson, I.R. and Brass, W. (1962) Multiple disorders in the elderly – a clinical and statistical study. *Lancet* ii: 841-3.
12. Williamson, J., Stokoe, I.H., Gray, S. *et al.* (1964) Old people at home: their unreported needs. *Lancet* i: 1117-20.
13. Andrews, K. Harding, M.A. and Goldstone, D. (1985) Social implications of multiple pathology. *Gerontology* 31: 325-31.
14. Bard, B. (1963) Energy expenditure of hemiplegic subjects during walking. *Archives of Physical Medicine and Rehabilitation* 44: 368-70.
15. Corcoran, P.J. and Brengelmann, G.L. (1970) Oxygen uptake in normal and handicapped subjects in relation to speed of walking beside velocity controlled cart. *Archives of Physical Medicine and Rehabilitation* 51: 78-87.
16. Ganguli, S., Datta, S.R. and Chatterjee, B.B. (1973) Performance evaluation of amputee-prosthesis system in below knee amputees. *Ergonomics* 16: 797-810.
17. Gonzalez, E.G., Corcoran, P.J. and Reyes, R.L. (1974) Energy expenditure in below knee amputees: correlation with stump length. *Archives of Physical Medicine and Rehabilitation* 55: 111-19.
18. Isaacs, B. (1969) Some characteristics of geriatric patients. *Scottish Medical Journal* 14: 243-51.
19. Varghese, G., Hinterbuchner, C.H., Monall, P.D. and Sakuma, J. (1978) Rehabilitation outcome of patients with dual disabilities of hemiplegia and amputation. *Archives of Physical Medicine and Rehabilitation* 59: 121-3.
20. Andrews, K., Brocklehurst, J.C., Richards, B. and Laycock, P.J. (1984) The influence of age on the clinical presentation and outcome of stroke. *International*

Rehabilitation Medicine **6**: 49–53.

21. Atkinson, L., Gibson, I.I.J.M. and Andrews, J. (1977) The difficulties of old people taking drugs. *Age and Ageing* **6**: 144–50.
22. Wandless, I., Mucklow, L.C., Smith, A. and Prudham, D. (1979) Compliance with prescribed medicines: a study of elderly people in the community. *Journal of the Royal College of General Practitioners* **29**: 391–6.
23. Kahn, R.L., Goldfarb, A.I., Pollack, M. and Gerber, I.E. (1960) The relationship of mental and physical status in institutionalized aged persons. *American Journal of Psychiatry* **2**: 120–4.
24. Wilson, L.A., Grant, K., Witney, P.M. and Kerridge, D.F. (1973) Mental status of elderly hospitalised patients related to occupational therapist's assessment of activities of daily living. *Gerontologia Clinica* **15**: 197–202.
25. Powell, R.R. (1974) Psychological effects of exercise therapy upon institutionalised geriatric mental patients. *Journal of Gerontology* **29**: 157–61.
26. Diesfeldt, H.F.A. and Diesfeldt-Groendijk, H. (1977) Improving cognitive performance in psychogeriatric patients: the influence of physical therapy. *Age and Ageing* **6**: 58–64.
27. Aldrich, C.K. and Mendkoff, E. (1963) Relocation of the aged and disabled: a mortality study. *Journal of the American Geriatrics Society* **11**: 185–94.
28. Roberts, G.S., Banerjee, D.K. and Mills, G.L. (1982) The emergency evacuation of a geriatric hospital in Toxteth. *Age and Ageing* **11**: 244–8.
29. Aleksandrowitz, D.R. (1961) Fire and aftermath on a geriatric ward. *Bulletin Nenninger Clinic* **25**: 23–32.
30. Borup, J.H. and Gallego, D.T. (1981) Mortality as affected by interinstitutional relocation. *Gerontologist* **21**: 8–16.
31. Watson, C.G. and Buerkle, H.R. (1976) Involuntary transfer as a cause of death and medical hospitalisation in geriatric neuropsychiatric patients. *Journal of the American Geriatrics Society* **24**: 278–82.
32. Reichard, S.L.F. and Peterson, P.G. (1962) *Aging and Personality: A Study of Eighty-Seven Older Men.* John Wiley, New York.
33. Williams, E.I., Bennett, F.M., Nixon, J.V. *et al.* (1972) Sociomedical study of patients over 75 in general practice. *British Medical Journal* **2**: 445–8.
34. Rogoff, J.B., Cooney, D.V. and Kutner, B. (1964) Hemiplegia: a study of home rehabilitation. *Journal of Chronic Disease* **17**: 539–50.
35. Wylie, C.M. (1970) The value of early rehabilitation in stroke. *Geriatrics* **25**: 107–18.
36. Shafer, S.Q., Brunn, B., Brown, R., and Richter, R.W. (1974) Stroke: early portents of functional recovery in black patients. *Archives of Physical Medicine and Rehabilitation* **55**: 264–8.
37. Haerer, A.F. and Woosley, P. (1975) Prognosis and quality survival in a hospitalised stroke population from the south. *Stroke* **6**: 543–8.
38. Richter, R.W., Bengen, B., Shafer, S.Q. *et al.* (1977) The Harlem Regional stroke program. *Archives of Physical Medicine and Rehabilitation* **58**: 224–9.
39. Anderson, T.P., Bourstom, N.C., Greenberg, F.R. and Hilyard, V.C. (1974) Predictive factors in stroke rehabilitation. *Archives of Physical Medicine and Rehabilitation* **55**: 545–53.
40. Lehmann, J.F., Delateur, B., Fowler, R.S. *et al.* (1975) Does stroke rehabilitation affect outcome? *Archives of Physical Medicine and Rehabilitation* **56**: 375–82.
41. Andrews, K., Brocklehurst, J.C., Richards, B. and Laycock, P.J. (1982) The recovery of the severely disabled stroke patient. *Rheumatology and Rehabilitation* **21**: 225–30.

42. Henriksen, J.D. (1978) Problems in rehabilitation after sixty-five. *Journal of the American Geriatrics Society* **26**: 510–12.
43. Masterman, L.E. (1958) Some psychological aspects of rehabilitation. *Journal of Rehabilitation* **24**: 4–6.
44. Reynolds, F.W., Abramson, M. and Young, A. (1959) The rehabilitation potential of patients in chronic disease institutions. *Journal of Chronic Disease* **10**: 152–9.
45. Cumming, E. and Henry, W.E. (1961) *Growing Old*. Basic Books, New York.
46. Cumming, E. (1963) Further thoughts on the theory of disengagement. *International Social Science Journal* **15**: 377–93.
47. Reed, D.L. (1970) Social disengagement in chronically ill patients. *Nursing Research* **19**: 109–14.
48. Sanford, J.R.A. (1975) Tolerance of disability in elderly dependents by supporters at home: its significance to hospital practice. *British Medical Journal* **3**: 471–3.
49. Rubin, I. (1974) In: *Making Health Teams Work* (Eds: Wise, H., Beckard, R., Rubin, I. and Kyte, A.L.). Ballinger Publ. Co., Cambridge, Mass.
50. Rothberg, J.S. (1981) The rehabilitation team: future directions *Archives of Physical Medicine and Rehabilitation* **62**: 407–10.
51. Melvin, J.L. (1980) Interdisciplinary and multidisciplinary activities and ACRM. *Archives of Physical Medicine and Rehabilitation* **61**: 379–82.
52. Rintal, D.H., Hanover, D., Alexander, J.L. *et al.* (1986) Team care: an analysis of verbal behavior during patient rounds in a rehabilitation hospital. *Archives of Physical Medicine and Rehabilitation* **67**: 118–22.
53. Keith, R.A. (1968) Need for a new model of rehabilitation. *Journal of Chronic Disease* **21**: 281–6.
54. Siller, J. (1971) On delineation of boundaries of professional practice in rehabilitation. *Archives of Physical Medicine and Rehabilitation* **52**: 410–12.
55. Wise, H., Rubin, I. and Beckart, R. (1974) Making health teams work. *American Journal of Child Health* **127**: 537–42.
56. Halstead, L.S. (1976) Team care in chronic illness: a critical review of literature of past 25 years. *Archives of Physical Medicine and Rehabilitation* **57**: 507–11.
57. Helander, E. (1977) *Towards a Multi-purpose Rehabilitation Therapist*. World Health Organisation.
58. Andrews, K. and Brocklehurst, J.C. (1984) Provision of remedial therapists in geriatric medicine. *British Medical Journal* **289**: 661.
59. Palmer, S., Conn, L., Siebens, A.A. *et al.* (1985) Psychosocial services in rehabilitation medicine: an interdisciplinary approach. *Archives of Physical Medicine and Rehabilitation* **66**: 690–2.

2

Physical modalities used in rehabilitation

Heat treatments

Heat energy is part of the electromagnetic spectrum, being a result of particulate excitation. Every atom or molecule above a temperature of 'absolute zero' (about $-273\,°C$) has excitation and is capable of transmitting energy to another particle either by direct collison or by radiation. This can only occur when the receiving particle has a lower temperature.

The human skin is a good heat reflector, a fair radiator but a poor conductor. Superficial forms of heat transmission do not penetrate very deeply into the skin (up to about 5 mm). Even when the skin temperature is raised from $32\,°C$ to $42\,°C$, tissues 2 cm below the skin surface only change temperature by about one degree, because the increased blood flow resulting from vasodilation dissipates the heat [1].

Heat can also be produced within tissues when electromagnetic waves such as shortwaves or microwaves are converted into microcurrents, or ultrasound into shearing, vibrational, frictional or mechanical compressive waves.

Physiological effects of heat

Very little hyperaemia occurs below $43\,°C$, but it increases rapidly to a maximum at $45\,°C$ [2]. There is therefore very little scope for misjudging the dose of the heat treatment.

The duration of the heat application is also a factor. Very little reaction occurs within the first five minutes of heating the skin, but the level of hyperaemia increases rapidly to reach a maximum response over the subsequent 30 minutes [2]. There is therefore little point in continuing heat treatment for longer than half an hour, after which time there is increased risk of a rise in the central core temperature, particularly in elderly patients who have poor autonomic nervous control.

19

The studies described above on the amount of heating were carried out at constant duration; and those studies on duration, at constant temperature. There is further evidence that the rate of rise of the temperature also influences the therapeutic effect – the hyperaemia being greater with a rapid rise in temperature [3,4]. Gentle heating is appropriate for sub-acute conditions, whereas rapid heating is more appropriate for chronic conditions and in the treatment of contractures.

The effect of heat also depends on a number of other factors, such as: the amount of water and fat in the subcutaneous tissues; hypothalamic and nervous control; respiratory and excretory mechanisms and efficiency; the ambient temperature and humidity; the age of the patient (the elderly tolerate heat less well than younger people); nutritional state; the level of hydration; individual sensitivity; and the presence of disease.

The effect of heat on cells

The effect of heat on cells (Fig. 2.1) is to:

1. increase metabolic and enzymatic reactions;
2. increase the requirements for oxygen, carbohydrate and protein;

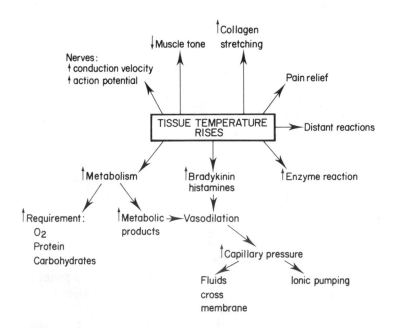

Fig. 2.1   Physiological effects of heat

3. produce vasodilatation and thus increased capilliary pressure, resulting in transudation of fluid across the endothelial membrane;
4. increase the ionic pumping of electrolytes;
5. release bradykinin and histamine-like substances;
6. produce tissue damage and inflammation, if continued for long enough and at a high enough level.

Reactions at a distance

A number of reactions also occur at a distance from the heated area.

There is relaxation of skeletal muscle when the skin is heated. The effect is largely on muscle tone, with muscle strength being variably affected: some studies showed an increase in strength [5], others a decrease [6], and yet others found no change [9]. These findings are not as contradictory as they seem since much depends on the point at which strength is tested on the heating curve – strength decreases during the early stages of heating but it increases after heating has stopped [8].

This effect is important in the elderly since the ageing muscle tends to be weaker, contracts slowly and is easily fatiguable [9] but can be improved by heating [10]. It is, therefore, important to encourage elderly people to keep warm before activity starts.

Heating one area results in an increased blood flow to another area (e.g. the contralateral limb). This effect depends on the size of the area being heated and is less than when the area is heated directly. Although blood flow in the muscles does not seem to be significantly increased by superficial heat modalities [11], there may be a reflex vasodilation, or in some circumstances a reflex vasoconstriction.

Heating of the abdominal wall results in blanching of the gastric mucosa and a decrease in gastric acidity. Along with this there is a decrease in peristalsis within the gastrointestinal tract [12]: hence the common use of a hot water bottle to settle abdominal cramps.

Finally we can mention relaxation of physical and psychological tension as another remote effect.

Clinical implications

Applied heat decreases muscle tone and spasticity [13]. This may be due partly to a direct effect on nerves by decreasing gamma fibre activity, thereby decreasing muscle spindle sensitivity to stretch, resulting in a decrease in muscle tone and spasm. However, this can also be produced by heating at a distance from the spastic muscles.

Locally applied, heat produces stretching of fibrous tissue. Although collagen length is temperature dependent [14, 15], clinically this is relatively unimportant unless a load is applied to the collagen fibres [16]. Prolonged stretching is more effective than short, intermittent stretching. This is particularly relevent when considering the effect of heat on tissue stretching in the management of contractures.

Heat may increase the extensibility of collagen in tendons and joint capsules, and can therefore be useful in the management of the 'frozen shoulder' [17].

Pain may be relieved somewhat by heat, but the reason for this is still uncertain. Several suggestions have been made (such as the release of spindle gamma afferent fibre impulses), though none is a really satisfactory explanation. Heating a nerve increases the pain threshold, but so does heating the skin away from the nerve [18]. Relief of pain in a joint may be due to an increase in the threshold to pain, to a decrease in spasm around the joint, to the effect on inflammation, or to the extensibility of collagen. However, heat has been shown to raise the threshold of pain in the normal shoulder [19], and therefore a direct effect on nerves is likely.

Abscesses can be 'ripened' by heat owing to the increased blood flow, leucocytosis and enzymatic reactions. Heat is, however, generally contraindicated in acute inflammation.

Sedation, can be mentioned, finally, as another clinical use of heat.

Contraindications to heat treatment

The following are the main contraindications:

1. acute inflammation or trauma;
2. venous obstruction;
3. haemorrhagic tendency;
4. in anaesthetic areas;
5. with caution in cardiovascular, respiratory or renal conditions, where the increase in metabolism cannot be accommodated;
6. over a malignant area since there is a possible danger of increasing the rate of tumour growth;
7. multiple sclerosis, since a rise in temperature results in an aggravation of the symptoms;
8. when conscious level is impaired.

Methods of heat delivery

There are numerous ways of delivering heat to the patient. In general, simple measures which can be used at home are as effective as the more sophisticated specialized equipment.

Superficial heat can be transmitted directly to the skin by hot water bottles, wax baths, steeping in hot water, blowing hot air or the use of infra-red radiation. To heat subcutaneous tissues, methods requiring sophisticated equipment and specialist skills are used, as in shortwave diathermy (continuous or pulsed).

Wax treatment

Paraffin wax melts at 49°C and solidifies at 40°C. Subsequent layers, produced by repeated dipping of the affected part into the wax bath, provide further insulation, thereby slowing down the heat loss. Using hot water at 45°C will damage the tissues, but wax at this higher temperature is tolerated for several reasons: the specific heat of wax baths is about 0.45 and less energy is released; the solidification of the first layer of wax produces insulation; and some air is usually trapped between the skin and the wax, adding further insulation.

The simple equipment required makes wax suitable for home use; but there is a risk of burns and it is important that a thermometer is used to monitor the wax bath temperature. The risk of fire from overheated wax must also be considered and a fire extinguisher of the carbon dioxide type should be readily available.

Infra-red radiation

This radiation can be produced from a number of sources, including infra-red bulbs. The penetration of the heat varies according to the wavelength used – the longer the wavelength the less the penetration. For instance, penetration can be as deep as 1 cm for a wavelengths of 390 nm, but only 0.05 cm for those of 12 000 nm.

Shortwave diathermy

This technique produces microcurrents in the field between two electrode plates. Muscle is heated selectively since conduction is greatest through tissues with a high water content. Heat can be generated about 3 cm below the surface. However, since the currents generated depend on a number of factors, such as the type and amount of tissues being treated, it is impossible to be sure that the correct dosage is being used. Since dosage depends on the patient's perception of heat, great care is required for use on the elderly owing to their various sensory, metabolic and structural changes.

Shortwave diathermy should not be used in the presence of metal since this concentrates the energy. (Patients should not wear metal-framed spectacles, a watch or jewellery and should not be in touch with other metal (such as zips). A *pacemaker* is an absolute contraindication – no-one with a pacemaker should be allowed within 5 metres (16 feet) of shortwave or microwave diathermy units [20].

Pulsed electromagnetic energy

There is now a tendency to use pulsed shortwave diathermy. This reduces the heat generation within tissues, allowing non-thermal effects to predominate. The reason why the treatment seems to work is uncertain but is generally thought to be related to alteration of electric potentials across cells which are usually deranged after injury.

The main use of pulsed therapy has been in soft-tissue injuries [21–23] and wound healing [21, 23–26]. There is some experimental evidence that pulsed therapy assists regeneration of nerve fibres following trauma [27, 28]; and that it increases the number of leucocytes, histiocytes and fibroblasts, accelerates the rate of oedema absorption and stimulates the rate of collagen deposition [29].

The effect of pulsed electromagnetic energy on bone healing is uncertain. In animal experiments osteogenesis is increased, with increased rate of bone repair [30, 31]; and so the technique may be useful in the treatment of non-union of bones [32–34].

Ultrasound

Ultrasound is a mechanical vibration, heat being produced by particle collisions within the tissues. To be effective it requires continuation of material, and heat is built up especially at interfaces between tissues owing to reflection and shearing forces. This means that joints can be heated specifically, even through thick layers of fat and muscle [35] – though a higher power input (wattage) is required to achieve the same effect than in a thin person [36]. It is therefore possible to produce selective heating at different levels within the tissues, which is not possible even with shortwave diathermy.

An air gap reduces transmission of the ultrasonic waves, and so an effective coupling agent (such as water or oil) is required between the generating head and the skin. This coupling agent also influences the type and depth of heating achieved [37], as will preheating the skin [38]. It is evident that skill is required in the use of ultrasound, especially for the elderly.

Thermal effects of ultrasound

The temperature of muscle, using a continuous moving ultrasonic head, rises by 1–2°C [36, 39, 40] but bone temperatures rise by about 5°C [35, 41]. Energy absorption is 10 times greater in bone than in muscle and about 25 times that of fat.

Much of the effect of ultrasound is thought to be due to an increased blood flow in skeletal muscle [42, 43], possibly from stimulation of the sympathetic nerves [44, 45]. However, in normal muscles there is no significant increase in blood flow after ultrasound [46], and in fibro-myotic muscles it may actually decrease [47].

There is increased permeability of membranes [48]; and there are variable effects on spinal reflexes, depending on dosage of the treatment [49, 50].

The effect on bone healing is debatable. The evidence suggests that it is not increased [51], though this may be because treatment was started too late. Animal experiments suggest that ultrasound increases callus formation if treatment starts during the first two weeks of fracture, producing bone repair of the juvenile type with rapid ossification but little cartilage production [52].

Non-thermal responses to ultrasound

These are said to occur when the effect is greater than could be expected from, or is different from, the direct effect of heat.

If there is tendon lengthening [14, 16] this is probably due to changes in the polypeptide bonds following ultrasound absorption [54]. There is evidence that collagen itself increases the ultrasound attentuation [54]. This may be relevant in the elderly since there is an age-dependent variation in collagen.

There may be haemolysis in extreme conditions [2]. Blood coagulation occurs if the ultrasound wave is stationary [55, 56] but does not occur if the ultrasound head is moved around the area or if pulsed ultrasound is used. This effect can certainly be demonstrated *in vitro* [57, 58] but does not seem to occur with modern therapeutic techniques.

Stimulation of tissue regeneration has been observed owing to increased protein synthesis in fibroblasts [59–62].

There are variable reports of the effect of ultrasound on nerve conduction, with some [63–65] showing an increase and others [63, 66] a decrease in nerve conduction rates. This is probably because responses depend on dosage being decreased when the ultrasonic intensity is between 0.5 and 1.5 W/cm^2 but increased when above 2 W/cm^2 or below 0.5 W/cm^2 [67]. It is debatable whether these effects are thermal or non-thermal, though similar results are obtained when tissue temperatures are raised by means other than ultrasound [69], suggesting that it is largely a thermal response.

Cavitation is a possibility. Bubbles are generated in liquids by sound waves, and if they continue to vibrate they can disrupt cells [69–71].

For this reason ultrasound should not be used over areas with a high fluid content, such as the eye, the spinal cord or the brain.

Contraindications to ultrasound treatment

The contraindications are similar to those for heat in general, but in addition include the following:

1. over oedema, wet dressings or boney prominences where excessive heat may be generated;
2. where metal is near to the skin surface since this tends to generate high levels of heat which cannot be transmitted away. (Deeper metal implants are not affected since the metal is a good conductor of heat which is rapidly transmitted away [72, 73], and there is little or no rise in temperature in front of the metal [4, 53]. However, there may be problems with the surrounding cement, especially if air bubbles are trapped during its mixing; this will result in overheating [74].);
3. over malignant areas;
4. when the patient is wearing a cardiac pacemaker [75], since this can cause interference with its function;
5. over the eye, since there is a high risk of cavitation within the vitreous;
6. directly over the heart, since this can produce cardiac dysfunction [76]. At least one patient with heart disease is thought to have developed cardiogenic shock due to ultrasound therapy [71];
7. peripheral vascular disease, owing to the increase in metabolism;
8. thrombophlebitis, since there is a theoretical possibility of emboli;
9. acute bone or tissue sepsis;
10. during or for six months after radiotherapy, since there is a theoretical possibility of activating the tumour (though this is still unproven);
11. with caution in diabetics, since it is reported [77] that they may become hypoglycaemic (presumably owing to the increased metabolic demands).

Some therapeutic uses of ultrasound

Joint pain

The main use for ultrasound is in the treatment of joint pain in chronic arthritis or periarticular disorders [17, 78–82]. As has been indicated in the foregoing, the temperature rise is quite high at the level of bone. Since the periosteum is rich in sensory receptors there is a damping effect on the pain. This approach is probably best for larger joints such as the hip and shoulder. There is little evidence that ultrasound is any more effective than superficial heat for joints of the hand in rheumatoid arthritis [83].

Scar tissue and contractures

Pain due to scar tissue can be decreased [84, 85], probably owing to softening and lengthening of the collagen fibres. Ultrasound helps to increase the range of movement in hypertrophic scar tissue, but is less effective in keloid tissue [86, 87]. The effect can be used for contracture of the hip following internal fixation [88], or in the treatment of periarthritis of the shoulder [17]. Early cases of Dupuytren's contraction also respond to ultrasound, and even severe cases can be improved to some degree [89].

Wound healing

This is helped by stimulation of tissue regeneration [61, 90] and can be particularly useful for pressure sores [91] or varicose ulceration [61].

Neuroma pain

Pain in neuromas can sometimes be diminished, and ultrasound is therefore of value in the management of pain following amputation [84].

Haematomas

Ultrasound can help to speed the resorption of the clot. In view of the laboratory evidence that clotting time can be increased by ultrasound, it is wise to wait until the bleeding into the haematoma has ceased.

Cold therapy

Ice and other coolants have been widely used in the management of a number of conditions in rehabilitation. Cold results in a decrease in metabolism and produces vasoconstriction. It`is difficult to cool muscles by external cooling since, although the skin temperature falls rapidly (by about 15°C) within a few minutes of applying cold therapy, the temperature in the muscle falls by only 3–5 degrees even after a prolonged period [92–94]. However, skin cooling can persist for up to one and a half hours following ice treatment [95].

Clinical indications

Inflammation

The anti-inflammatory response to cold is generally thought to be due to vasoconstriction, a decrease in metabolism, decrease in the normal responses such a leucocytosis, enzymatic reactions and a decrease in tissue swelling associated with vasoconstriction. The effect on pain may be related to these changes or to direct action on sensory nerves. Cold therapy is of value in acute injuries such as sprains and soft-tissue trauma or for acute local infections and inflammation.

Oedema

Cold compresses, as traditionally used in the oedema of acute trauma, seem to be effective in a wide range of traumatic and surgical injuries [96–98]. There is no evidence that it is of any value in chronic oedema.

Pain

Analgesia is achieved partly by a reflex nervous response, but it is also partly due to the damping down of inflammation or muscle spasm. Cold is more effective than heat in increasing the threshold to pressure in normal shoulders [19] and improving the range of joint movement in painful hemipegic shoulders [99]. Ice treatment can help to decrease the pain due to muscle spasm [100–102].

The techniques used vary, from the applications used in the treatment of spasticity (see below), to massaging the skin with an ice cube until the skin is numb (about five minutes) [100].

Arthritis

Cold therapy is useful in the acute stage of rheumatoid arthritis because it decreases the inflammatory response and has an effect on pain thresholds. There also seems to be an inhibiting effect on enzymatic activity, thus preventing further damage [103].

Although cold therapy is primarily used for the acute arthritides, it has also been shown to be effective in chronic arthritis [104, 105], though it does tend to make joint stiffness worse [106, 107].

Spasticity

A number of studies have shown that cooling a spastic limb in cold water or an ice bath, or wrapping it in cold towels, reduces spasticity and hyperclonus [95, 104, 108–111]. Application must be for about

15–20 minutes to have a clinically significant effect [111]. There is often an increase in tone during the first few minutes of treatment [95]. The decrease in tone lasts for up to two hours [109, 111], which allows the opportunity to carry out physiotherapy techniques.

The mechanism of the effect of cold therapy on increased muscle tone is uncertain. There may be decreased sensory input from the skin receptors; but most work indicates that the effect is due to a decrease in muscle spindle discharge associated with cooling of the muscle [112–114], and clonus does not disappear unless this is achieved [109]. From animal experiments it is known that the rate of discharge from muscle spindles has a direct linear correlation with the fall in temperature [115, 116].

The effect on spasticity is unlikely to be due to the cooling of the muscles since this is difficult to achieve. Although small changes in temperature may be expected to have clinically significant effects, there does not seem to be a change in the H-reflex even when the temperature of the muscle falls by 4–5 degrees Celsius [109, 117]. There is also a clinically detectable decrease in spasticity during cold therapy while the muscle temperature is still normal [95].

One approach has been to cool the tissues over the affected muscles whilst warming uninvolved parts of the body; the combined method being more effective than single modality treatment [118, 119].

The technique normally used is to put the cooling pack over the equivalent dermatome of the affected muscles. In view of the danger of hypothermia in the elderly the room must be kept warm and the rest of the body well covered. The longer the patient can tolerate the cold the longer will be the effect on the spasticity. Usually half an hour of cooling is sufficient to produce the required effect.

Hypotonicity

It seems contradictory that cold therapy should be beneficial for hypo- as well as hyper-tonicity. It has already been mentioned that for the first few minutes of applying cold to the skin there is an increase in muscle tone. This can be used to assist the increase in tone of hypotonic muscles.

There are two techniques. One uses short periods of cold application to the skin to stimulate the sensory nerve endings [120]; the other is to stroke or brush the skin over the dermatomes of the affected group of muscles [121].

Contraindications to cooling

The following are the main contraindications to cooling:

1. peripheral vascular disease: obvious are Raynaud's disease, angiopathies or artherioscierotic peripheral vascular disease;
2. sensory abnormalities, since the patient is unaware when adverse symptoms are being produced;
3. autonomic disorders, which may make the patient vulnerable to hypothermia;
4. chronic wounds or inflammation, which may be made worse by damping down an already compromised healing reaction;
5. ischaemic heart disease.

Some patients with ischaemic heart disease develop angina when exposed to cold. This is less likely to occur when the area of cold application is localized. In one study of 25 stroke patients with ischaemic heart disease, only one developed ECG changes when the shoulder was treated with cold packs for 10 minutes [99]. A slight rise in blood pressure is recorded with local cold therapy [99, 122], though quite significant rises can occur if the whole arm is immersed in water at 0°C [23].

Methods of cooling

Cooling can be produced by ice packs. This can be crushed ice in a plastic bag or, as often used by community therapists, a bag of frozen peas. It must be emphasized that the ice should be crushed to avoid local pressure areas.

An alternative is terry towelling that has been soaked in water containing crushed ice and wrung out. The towels need changing every few minutes, so this is not a popular method.

Immersion of the limb in cold water is also possible, but this is not recommended for the elderly since the area covered is too large and the patient is at risk of hypothermia.

Evaporation of liquids, such as ethyl chloride, sprayed on to the skin raises pain thresholds [124,125]. This has been shown in a controlled trial to increase the pain threshold in normal subjects [126] and to relieve neck stiffness [127]. Ethyl chloride is highly inflammable, and so other agents such as the chlorofluoromethanes, though producing less cooling, are probably preferable. The effect is sufficient to allow an increase in passive stretch in normal subjects [128, 129].

Ultra-violet irradiation

Ultra-violet light is a high-energy form of electromagnetic waves. It can only penetrate to the capillaries of the dermis (i.e. about 0.1 mm), although this is dependent on the thickness of the skin and the amount of pigmentation. Ultra-violet energy is capable of producing chemical changes, as opposed to the mechanical changes of infra-red irradiation.

A bacteriocidal effect is produced by inhibition of bacterial mitosis. This seems to be due to dimerization of the thiamine part of DNA [130]. For this reason ultra-violet light is used in the treatment of ulcers where the bacteria are superficial in the wound. It must be noted in this context that high doses of ultra-violet light delay wound healing.

An increase in vitamin D synthesis is produced from the chemical reaction between ultra-violet light and 7-hydrocholesterol in the tissues, so there is a place for ultra-violet treatment in the prevention of osteomalacia in long-stay institutions [131, 132].

The eye is particularly susceptible to inflammation, with the production of conjuctivitis and keratitis. For this reason protective spectacles should be worn during treatment.

Some of the side effects from exposure to ultra-violet light may be undesirable. For example, erythema occurs several hours after exposure, as seen in sunburn. The longer-waved ultra-violet light UVA, which is predominant in commercial 'sunbeds', does not produce the erythema as much as does UVB light. Much will depend on skin colouring, with fair-skinned people being more susceptible to develop erythema. Tanning is a protective attempt to decrease the effect of ultra-violet light, and this inhibits the production of erythema. It usually develops two or three days after exposure and fades as the melanin-containing superficial layers are discarded.

Epithelialization is due to an increased rate of epidermal cell division. This is partly responsible for premature ageing and skin cancers and is associated with the UVB component.

Other side effects from overexposure to ultra-violet light are more serious. They include acute inflammation with pain and oedema, blister formation and skin peeling (as in sunburn), fever, and in extreme cases shock. Certain infections, especially herpes simplex, may be activated. In certain individuals these effects can be produced early in the presence of a photosensitizer, which may be an underlying condition such as porphyria, an autoimmune disorder (scleroderma, systemic lupus, polyarteritis nodosa), infection (tuberculosis) or a dermatological disease. Drugs (tetracyclines, methotrexate, sulphonamides, chlorpromazine or barbiturates) or chemicals found in some perfumes and soap can also act as photosensitizers.

References

1. Lehmann, J.F., Silverman, D.R., Baum, B.A. *et al.* (1966) Temperature distributions in the human thigh, produced by infrared, hot pack and microwave applications. *Archives of Physical Medicine and Rehabilitation* **47**: 291-9.
2. Lehmann, J.F. (1953) The biophysical basis of biologic ultrasonic reactions with special reference to ultrasonic therapy. *Archives of Physical Medicine and Rehabilitation* **34**: 139-52.
3. Dodt, E. and Zotterman, Y. (1952) Mode of action of warm receptors. *Acta Physiologica Scandinavica* **26**: 345-7.
4. Lehmann, J.F., Brunner, G.D. and McMillan, J.A. (1958) Influence of surgical metal implants on temperature distribution in thigh specimens exposed to ultrasound. *Archives of Physical Medicine* **39**: 692-5.
5. King, P.G., Mendryk, S., Reid, D.C. and Kelley, R. (1970) The effect of actively increased muscle temperature on grip strength. *Medicine and Science in Sport* **2**: 172-5.
6. Clarke, R. and Stelmach, G.E. (1966) Muscular fatigue and recovery curve parameters at various temperatures. *Research Quarterly* **37**: 468-79.
7. Grose, J.E. (1958) Depression of muscle fatigue curves by heat and cold. *Research Quarterly* **29**: 19-31.
8. Barnes, W.S. and Larson, M.R. (1985) Effects of localised hyper- and hypothermia on maximal isometric grip strength. *American Journal of Physical Medicine* **64**: 305-14.
9. Davies, C.T.M. and White, M.J. (1983) Contractile properties of elderly human triceps surae. *Gerontology* **29**: 19-25.
10. Davies, C.T.M. and Young, K. (1985) Effect of heating on the contractile properties of triceps surae and maximal power output during jumping in elderly men. *Gerontology* **31**: 1-5.
11. Wyper, D.J. and McNiven, D.R. (1976) Effects of some physiotherapeutic agents on skeletal muscle blood flow. *Physiotherapy* **62**: 83-5.
12. Bisgard, J.D. and Nye, D. (1940) The influence of hot and cold application upon gastric and intestinal motor activity. *Surgery Gynaecology and Obstetrics* **71**: 172-80.
13. Fountain, F.P., Gersten, J.W. and Sengir, O. (1960) Decrease in muscle spasm produced by ultrasound, hot packs and infra-red radiation. *Archives of Physical Medicine* **41**: 293-8.
14. Gersten, J.W. (1955) Effect of ultrasound on tendon extensibility. *Journal of Physical Medicine* **34**: 362-9.
15. Castor, C.W. (1976) Connective tissue activation: the effects of temperature studied in vitro. *Archives of Physical Medicine and Rehabilitation* **57**: 5-11.
16. Lehmann, J.F., Masock, A.J., Warren, C.G. and Koblanski, J.N. (1970) Effect of therapeutic temperatures on tendon extensibility. *Archives of Physical Medicine and Rehabilitation* **51**: 481-7.
17. Lehmann, J.F., Erickson, D.J., Martin, G.M. and Krusen, F.H. (1954) Comparison of ultrasound and microwave diathermy in the physical treatment of periarthritis of the shoulder. *Archives of Physical Medicine and Rehabilitation* **35**: 627-38.
18. Lehmann, J.F., Brunner, G.D. and Stow, R.W. (1958) Pain threshold measurements after therapeutic application of ultrasound, microwaves, and infrared. *Archives of Physical Medicine and Rehabilitation* **39**: 560-5.
19. Benson, T.B. and Copp, E.P. (1974) The effects of therapeutic forms of heat and ice on pain threshold of the normal shoulder. *Rheumatology and Rehabilitation* **13**: 101-4.
20. Jones, S.L. (1976) Electromagnetic field interference and cardiac pacemakers. *Physical Therapy* **56**: 1013-18.

21. Wilson, D.H. (1972) Treatment of soft tissue injuries by pulsed electrical energy. *British Medical Journal* 2: 269-70.
22. Kaplan, E.G. and Weinstock, E.F. (1968) Clinical evaluation of Diapulse as adjunctive therapy following foot surgery. *Journal of the American Podiatry Association* 58: 218-21.
23. Wilson, D.H. (1974) Comparison of short wave diathermy and pulsed electromagnetic energy in the treatment of soft tissue injuries. *Physiotherapy* 60: 309-10.
24. Cameron, B.M. (1964) A three phase evaluation of pulsed high frequency radio short waves. *American Journal of Orthopaedics* 6: 72-8.
25. Goldin, J.H., Broadbent, N.R.G., Nancarrow, J.D. and Marshall, T. (1981) The effects of Diapulse on the healing of wounds: a double blind randomised controlled trial in man. *British Journal of Plastic Surgery* 34: 267-70.
26. Pasila, M., Visuri, T. and Sundholm, A. (1978) Pulsating shortwave diathermy value in treatment of recent ankle and foot sprains. *Archives of Physical Medicine and Rehabilitation* 59: 383-6.
27. Wilson, D.H., Jagadeesh, P., Newman, P.P. and Harriman, D.G.F. (1974) The effects of pulsed electromagnetic energy on peripheral nerve regeneration. *Annals of New York Academy of Sciences* 238: 575-8.
28. Wilson, D.H. and Jagadeesh, P. (1976) Experimental regeneration in peripheral nerves and the spinal cord in laboratory animals exposed to a pulsed electromagnetic field. *Paraplegia* 14: 12-20.
29. Cameron, B.M. (1961) Experimental acceleration of wound healing. *American Journal of Orthopaedics* 3: 196-9.
30. Bassett, A., Pawluk, R.J. and Pilla, A.A. (1974) Augmentation of bone repair by inductively coupled electromagnetic fields. *Science* 184: 575-7.
31. Nixon, J. (1985) Electromagnetic induction of bone? *British Medical Journal* 290: 490-1.
32. Brighton, C.T. (1981) The treatment of non-unions with electricity. *Journal of Bone and Joint Surgery* 63-A: 847-51.
33. Bassett, C.A.L., Mitchell, S.N. and Gaston, S.R. (1981) Treatment of ununited tibial diaphyseal fractures with pulsing electromagnetic fields. *Journal of Bone and Joint Surgery* 63-A: 511-23.
34. Sutcliffe, M.L., Sharrard, W.J.W. and McEachern, A.G. (1980) The treatment of fracture non-union by electro-magnetic induction. *Journal of Bone and Joint Surgery* 63-B: 123.
35. Lehmann, J.F., McMillan, J.A., Brunner, G.D. and Blumberg, J.B. (1959) Comparative study of the efficiency of shortwave, microwave and ultrasonic diathermy in heating the hip joint. *Archives of Physical Medicine and Rehabilitation* 40: 510-12.
36. Lehmann, J.F., de Lateur, B.J., Stonebridge, J.B. and Warren, C.G. (1967) Therapeutic temperature distribution produced by ultrasound as modified by doseage and volume of tissue exposed. *Archives of Physical Medicine and Rehabilitation* 48: 662-6.
37. Lehmann, J.F., de Lateur, B.J. and Silverman, D.R. (1966) Selective heating effects of ultrasound on human beings. *Archives of Physical Medicine and Rehabilitation* 47: 331-9.
38. Lehmann, J.F., Stonebridge, J.B., De Lateur, B.J., Warren, C.G. and Halar, E. (1978) Temperatures in human thighs after hot pack treatment followed by ultrasound. *Archives of Physical Medicine and Rehabilitation* 59: 472-6.
39. Lota, M.J. (1965) Electronic plethysmographic and tissue temperature studies of the effects of ultrasound on blood flow. *Archives of Physical Medicine and Rehabilitation* 46: 315-22.
40. Abramson, D.I., Burnett, C., Bell, V. *et al.* (1960) Changes in blood flow,

oxygen uptake and tissue temperature produced by therapeutic physical agents. I: The effect of ultrasound. *American Journal of Physical Medicine* **39**: 51–62.

41. Lehmann, J.F., De Lateur, B.J., Warren, C.G. and Stonebridge, J.B. (1968) Heating of joint structures by ultrasound. *Archives of Physical Medicine and Rehabilitation* **49**: 28–30.

42. Paul, W.D. and Imig, C.J. (1955) Temperature and blood flow studies after ultrasonic irradiation. *American Journal of Physical Medicine* **34**: 370–5.

43. Abramson, D.I. (1965) Physiologic basis for the use of physical agents in peripheral vascular disorders. *Archives of Physical Medicine and Rehabilitation* **46**: 216–44.

44. Schroeder, K.P. (1962) Effect of ultrasound on the lumbar sympathetic nerves. *Archives of Physical Medicine and Rehabilitation* **43**: 182–5.

45. Stuhlfauth, K. (1952) Neurological effects of ultrasonic waves. *British Journal of Physical Medicine* **15**: 10.

46. Hansen, T.I. and Kristensen, J.H. (1973) Effect of massage, short wave diathermy and ultrasound upon ^{133}Xe disappearance rate from muscle and subcutaneous tissue in the human calf. *Scandinavian Journal of Rehabilitation Medicine* **5**: 179–82.

47. Klemp, P., Staberg, B., Korsgard, J. *et al.* (1982) Reduced blood flow in fibromyotic muscle during ultrasound therapy. *Scandinavian Journal of Rehabilitation Medicine* **15**: 21–3.

48. Lehmann, J.F. and Biegler, R. (1954) Changes of potentials and temperature gradients in membranes caused by ultrasound. *Archives of Physical Medicine and Rehabilitation* **35**: 287–95.

49. Anderson, T.P., Wakim, K.G., Herrick, J.F. *et al.* (1951) An experimental study of the effects of ultrasonic energy on the lower part of the spinal cord and peripheral nerves. *Archives of Physical Medicine* **32**: 71–83.

50. Shealy, C.N. and Henneman, E. (1962) Reversible effects of ultrasound on spinal reflexes. *Archives of Neurology* **6**: 374–86.

51. Ardan, N.I., Janes, J.M. and Herrick, J.F. (1957) Ultrasonic energy and surgically produced defects in bone. *Journal of Bone and Joint Surgery* **39-A**: 394–502.

52. Brookes, M. and Dyson, M. (1985) Stimulation of bone repair by ultrasound. *International Journal of Rehabilitation Research* **8** (Suppl. 4): 73.

53. Gersten, J.W. (1958) Effect of metallic objects on temperature rises produced in tissue by ultrasound. *American Journal of Physical Medicine* **37**: 75–82.

54. Goss, S.A. and Dunn, F. (1980) Ultrasonic properties of collagen. *Physics in Medicine and Biology* **25**: 827–37.

55. Dyson, M., Woodward, B. and Pond, J.B. (1971) Flow of red blood cells stopped by ultrasound. *Nature* **232**: 572–3.

56. Zarod, I. and Hardy, J.D. (1958) Influence of cold exposure on thermal burns in the rat. *Journal of Applied Physiology* **12**: 147–54.

57. Chater, B.V. and Williams, A.R. (1977) Platelet aggregation induced in vitro by therapeutic ultrasound. *Thrombosis and Haemostasis* **38**: 640–51.

58. Williams, A.R., Chater, B.V., Allen, K.A. *et al.* (1978) Release of beta-thromboglobulin from human platelets by therapeutic intensities of ultrasound. *British Journal of Haematology* **40**: 133–42.

59. Dyson, M., Pond, J.B., Joseph, J. and Warwick, R. (1968) The stimulation of tissue regeneration by means of ultrasound. *Clinical Science* **35**: 273–85.

60. Dyson, M. and Pond, J.B. (1970) The effect of pulsed ultrasound on tissue regeneration. *Physiotherapy* **56**: 136–42.

61. Dyson, M. and Suckling, J. (1978) Stimulation of tissue repair by ultrasound: a survey of the mechanisms involved. *Physiotherapy* **64**: 105–8.

62. Harvey, W., Dyson, M., Pond, J.B. and Grahame, R. (1975) The stimulation of protein synthesis in human fibroblasts by therapeutic ultrasound. *Rheumatology and Rehabilitation* **14**: 273.

63. Madsen, P.W. and Gersten, J.W. (1961) Effect of ultrasound on conduction velocity of peripheral nerve. *Archives of Physical Medicine and Rehabilitation* **42**: 645–9.

64. Currier, D.P., Greathouse, D. and Swift, T. (1978) Sensory nerve conduction: effect of ultrasound. *Archives of Physical Medicine and Rehabilitation* **59**: 181–5.

65. Hall, J.S., Scoville, C.R. and Greathouse, D.G. (1981) Ultrasound's effect on the conduction latency of the superficial radial nerve in man. *Physical Therapy* **61**: 345–50.

66. Zankel, H.T. (1966) Effect of physical agents on motor conduction velocity of the ulnar nerve *Archives of Physical Medicine and Rehabilitation* **47**: 787–92.

67. Farmer, W.C. (1968) Effect of intensity of ultrasound on conduction velocity of motor axons. *Physical Therapy* **48**: 1233–7.

68. Currier, D.P. and Kramer, J.F. (1982) Senory nerve conduction: heating effects of ultrasound and infrared. *Physiotherapy Canada* **34**: 241–6.

69. Baker, M.L. and Dalrymple, G.V. (1978) Biological effects of diagnostic ultrasound: a review. *Radiology* **126**: 479–83.

70. Coakley, W.T. (1978) Biophysical effects of ultrasound at therapeutic intensities. *Physiotherapy* **64**: 166–9.

71. Wakim, K.G. (1953) Ultrasonic energy as applied to medicine. *American Journal of Physical Medicine* **32**: 32–46.

72. Lehmann, J.F., Brunner, G.D., Matinis, A.J. and McMillan, J.A. (1959) Ultrasonic effects as demonstrated in live pigs with surgical metallic implants. *Archives of Physical Medicine* **40**: 483–8.

73. Lehmann, J.F. (1965) Ultrasound therapy. In: *Therapeutic Heat* (Eds: Licht, S. and Licht, E.), pp. 321–86. Waverly Press, Baltimore.

74. Lehmann, J.F., Stonebridge, J.B., Wallace, J.E. *et al.* (1979) Microwave therapy: stray radiation, safety and effectiveness. *Archives of Physical Medicine and Rehabilitation* **60**: 578–84.

75. Bryan, P., Furman, S. and Escher, D.J. (1969) Input signals to pacemakers in a hospital environment. *Annals of New York Academy of Science* **167**: 823–4.

76. Mortimer, A.J., Roy, O.Z., Taichman, T. *et al.* (1978) The effect of ultrasound on the mechanical properties of rat cardiac muscle. *Ultrasonics* **16**: 179–82.

77. Oakley, E.M. (1978) Dangers and contra-indications of therapeutic ultrasound. *Physiotherapy* **64**: 173–4.

78. Munting, E. (1978) Ultrasonic therapy for painful shoulders. *Physiotherapy* **64**: 180–1.

79. Buchan, J.F. (1970) Use of ultrasonics in physical medicine. *The Practitioner* **205**: 319–26.

80. Echternach, M.S. (1965) Ultrasound an adjunct treatment for shoulder disabilities. *Journal of the American Physical Therapy Association* **4**: 865–9.

81. Flax, H.J. (1964) Ultrasound treatment of peritendinitis calcarea of the shoulder. *American Journal of Physical Medicine* **43**: 117–24.

82. Binder, A., Hodge, G., Greenwood, A.M., Hazleman, B.L. and Thomas, D.P.P. (1985) Is therapeutic ultrasound effective in treating soft tissue lesions? *British Medical Journal* **290**: 512–14.

83. Hawkes, J., Care, G., Dixon, J.S., Bird, H.A. and Wright, V. (1985) Comparison of three physiotherapy regimes for hands with rheumatoid arthritis. *British Medical Journal* **291**: 1016.

84. Rubin, D. and Kuitert, J. (1955) Use of ultrasound vibration energy in the

treatment of pain arising from phantom limbs, scars and neuromas. *Archives of Physical Medicine and Rehabilitation* **36**: 445–52.
85. Bierman, W. (1954) Ultrasound in the treatment of scars. *Archives of Physical Medicine and Rehabilitation* **34**: 209–14.
86. Wright, E.T. and Haase, K.H. (1971) Treatment of keloids with ultrasound. *Archives of Physical Medicine and Rehabilitation* **52**: 280–1.
87. Inalsingh, C.H. (1974) An experience of treating five hundred and one patients with keloids. *John Hookins Medical Journal* **134**: 284–90.
88. Lehmann, J.F., Fordyce, W.E., Rathburn, L.A. *et al.* (1961) Clinical evaluation of a new approach in the treatment of contractures associated with hip fractures after internal fixation. *Archives of Physical Medicine and Rehabilitation* **42**: 95–100.
89. Markham, D.E. and Wood, M.R. (1980) Ultrasound for Dupuytren's contracture. *Physiotherapy* **66**: 55–8.
90. Webster, D.F., Harvey, W., Dyson, M. and Pond, J.B. (1980) The role of ultrasound induced cavitation in the 'in vitro' stimulation of collagen synthesis in human fibroblasts. *Ultrasonics* **18**: 33–7.
91. Paul, B.J., La Fratta, C.W., Dawson, A.R. *et al.* (1960) Use of ultrasound in the treatment of pressure sores in patients with spinal cord injury. *Archives of Physical Medicine and Rehabilitation* **41**: 438–40.
92. Lightfoot, E., Verrier, M. and Ashby, P. (1975) Neurophysiological effects of prolonged cooling of the calf in patients with complete spinal transection. *Physical Therapy* **55**: 251–8.
93. Urbscheit, N., Johnston, R. and Bishop, B. (1971) Effects of cooling on the ankle jerk and H-response in hemiplegic patients. *Physical Therapy* **51**: 983–88.
94. Abramson, D.I., Chu, L.S.W. and Tuck (1966) Effect of tissue temperature and blood flow on nerve conduction velocity. *Journal of the American Medical Association* **198**: 156–62.
95. Hartviksen, K. (1962) Ice therapy in spasticity. *Acta Neurologica Scandinavica* **38** (Suppl. 3): 79–84.
96. Schmidt, K.L., Ott, V.R., Rocher, G. *et al.* (1979) Heat, cold and inflammation. *Rheumatology* **38**: 391–404.
97. Basur, R.L., Shepherd, E. and Mouzas, G.L. (1976) A cooling method in the treatment of ankle sprains. *Practitioner* **216**: 708–11.
98. Moore, C.D. and Cardea, J.A. (1977) Vascular changes in leg trauma. *Southern Medical Journal* **70**: 1285–6.
99. Lorenze, E.J., Carantonis, G. and DeRosa, A.J. (1960) Effect on coronary circulation of cold packs to hemiplegic shoulders. *Archives of Physical Medicine and Rehabilitation* **41**: 394–9.
100. Grant, A.E. (1964) Massage with ice (cryokinetics) in the treatment of painful conditions of the musculoskeletal system. *Archives of Physical Medicine and Rehabilitation* **45**: 233–8.
101. Hayden, C.A. (1964) Cryokinetics in an early treatment programme. *Physical Therapy* **44**: 990–3.
102. Lane, L.E. (1971) Localised hypothermia for the relief of pain in musculoskeletal injuries. *Physical Therapy* **51**: 182–3.
103. Harris, E. and McCroskery, P.A. (1974) The influence of temperature and fibril stability on degredation of cartilage collagen by rheumatoid synovial collagenase. *New England Journal of Medicine* **290**: 1–6.
104. Kirk, J.A. and Kersley, G.D. (1968) Heat and cold in the physical treatment of rheumatoid arthritis of the knee. *Archives of Physical Medicine* **9**: 270–4.
105. Pegg, S.M.H., Littler, T.R. and Littler, E.N. (1969) A trial of ice therapy and exercise in chronic arthritis. *Physiotherapy* **55**: 51–6.

106. Wright, V. and Johns, R.J. (1961) Quantitative and qualitative analysis of joint stiffness in normal subjects and in patients with connective tissue diseases. *Annals of Rheumatic Diseases* **20**: 36–46.
107. Backlund, L. and Tiselius, P. (1967) Objective measurement of joint stiffness in rheumatoid arthritis. *Acta Rheumatica Scandinavica* **13**: 275–88.
108. Petejan, J.H. and Watts, N. (1962) Effects of cooling on the triceps surae reflex. *American Journal of Physical Therapy* **61**: 240–51.
109. Miglietta, O. (1962) Evaluation of cold in spasticity. *American Journal of Physical Medicine* **52**: 198–205.
110. Miglietta, O. (1973) Action of cold on spasticity. *American Journal of Physical Medicine* **52**: 198–205.
111. Lee, J.M. and Warren, M.P. (1974) Ice, relaxation and exercise in reduction of muscle spasticity. *Physiotherapy* **60**: 296–302.
112. Lippold, O.C.J., Nicholls, J.G. and Redfearn, J.W.T. (1960) A study of the afferent discharge produced by cooling a mammalian muscle spindle. *Journal of Physiology* **153**: 218–31.
113. Michalski, W.J. and Sequin, J.J. (1975) The effect of muscle cooling and stretch on muscle spindle secondary endings in the cat. *Journal of Physiology* **253**: 341–56.
114. Ottoson, D. (1965) The effects of temperature on the isolated muscle spindle. *Journal of Physiology* **180**: 636–48.
115. Matthews, P.B.C. (1964) Muscle spindles and their motor control. *Physiological Review* **44**: 219–88.
116. Eldred, E., Lindsley, D.F. and Buchwald, J.S. (1960) The effect of cooling on mammalian muscle spindles. *Experimental Neurology* **2**: 144–57.
117. Knutsson, E. and Mattsson, E. (1968) Effects of local cooling on monosynaptic reflexes in man. *Scandinavian Journal of Rehabilitation Medicine* **1**: 126–32.
118. Don Tigny, R.C. and Sheldon, K.W. (1962) Simultaneous use of heat and cold in treatment of muscle spasm. *Archives of Physical Medicine* **43**: 235–7.
119. Newton, M.J. and Lehmkuhl, D. (1965) Muscle spindle response to body heating and cooling. *American Journal of Physical Therapy* **45**: 91–105.
120. Clendenin, A. and Szumski, A.J. (1971) Influence of cutaneous ice application on single motor units in humans. *Physical Therapy* **51**: 166–75.
121. Weisberg, J. (1976) Influence of icing and brushing on the Achilles tendon reflex in adult human subjects. *Canadian Journal of Physiotherapy* **28**: 21–3.
122. Waylonis, G.W. (1967) The physiologic effects of ice massage. *Archives of Physical Medicine and Rehabilitation* **48**: 37–42.
123. Clarke, R.S.J., Hellon, R.F. and Lind, A.R. (1958) Vascular reactions of the human forearm to cold. *Clinical Science* **17**: 165–78.
124. Ellis, M. (1961) Relief of pain by cooling the skin. *British Medical Journal* **1**: 250–2.
125. Satran, R. and Goldstein, M.N. (1973) Pain perception: modification of threshold intolerance and cortical potentials by cutaneous stimulation. *Science* **180**: 1201–2.
126. Parsons, C.M. and Goetzl, F.R. (1945) Effect of induced pain on pain threshold. *Proceedings of the Society of Experimental and Biological Medicine* **60**: 327–9.
127. Travell, J. (1949) Rapid relief of acute 'stiff neck' by ethyl chloride spray. *Journal of the American Women's Association* **4**: 89–95.
128. Halkovich, L.R., Personius, W.J., Clamann, H.P. *et al.* (1981) Effect of Fluori-Methane spray on passive hip flexion. *Physical Therapy* **61**: 185–9.
129. Newton, R.A. (1985) Effects of vapocoolants on passive hip flexion in healthy subjects. *Physical Therapy* **65**: 1034–6.

130. Giese, A. (1970) *Photophysiology*, Vol. 5, Chapters 6 and 7 (Ed. Giese, A.). Academic Press, New York.
131. Neer, R.M., Davies, T.R.A., Walcott, A. *et al.* (1971) Stimulation by artificial lighting of calcium absorption in elderly human subjects. *Nature* **229**: 255–7.
132. Snell, A.P., MacLennan, W.J. and Hamilton, J.C. (1978) Ultra-violet irradiation and 25-hydroxy-vitamin D levels in sick old people. *Age and Ageing* **7**: 225–8.

3

Some equipment for rehabilitation of the elderly

The equipment available to help the elderly is too numerous to cover fully in this book. It is, however, worthwhile to consider some of the more useful and less well-known pieces of equipment which have uses in a number of the disorders discussed in later chapters.

The bead pillow mattress

This is an effective and inexpensive form of equipment with a number of uses. It consists of a series of ten pillows (Fig. 3.1) filled with small polystyrene beads. The pillows are attached to a plastic cover by Velcro tape and the cover fits over the mattress of a bed. The pillows allow a redistribution of a person's weight by moulding around that part of the body they are supporting. The distance between the pillows determines the firmness of the supporting surface. For instance, for patients with backache the pillows are placed close together to provide a firm support in the lumbar region. Where weight needs to be distributed more widely the pillows are placed further apart.

The prime use of the bead pillow mattress is in the prevention and treatment of pressure sores, since the body's weight is distributed over a wide area. In one randomly allocated controlled trial, this mattress, in conjunction with vacuum packs (see below), significantly reduced

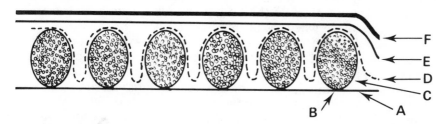

Fig. 3.1 Bead pillow mattress: A = plastic cover over mattress; B = Velcro fitting; C = bead pillow; D = thin plastic cover; E = nylon sheet; F = bed sheet

39

pressure sores in patients with fracture of the femur on orthopaedic wards [1]. Other uses include providing firm lumbar support for those with backache, and maintaining the correct positioning of stroke patients in bed.

There are no mechanical moving parts to go wrong. The pillows can be washed, and when they need replacing they can be replaced individually at relatively low cost.

The bedsheet on the surface of the mattress allows the patient to be turned easily by one nurse with very little effort and without producing shearing forces on the skin. It lies on a nylon-type sheet which allows it to move with little resistance when pulled towards the nurse in an upward and outward direction. Since the patient is not being pulled across the bed, but is being rolled on to his side, no friction occurs on the skin – the sheet is acting as a conveyor belt.

The mattress is ideal for incontinent patients because there is a thin plastic sheet fitting loosely over the pillows and tucked down into the crevices. This plastic sheet does not interfere with the effectiveness of the pillows; but urine can collect in the crevices, and the patient remains relatively dry. The plastic sheet may be carefully removed to carry the urine away for disposal and the sheet easily disinfected.

It is essential that the bedsheet covering the pillows is not tucked in under the mattress, otherwise the pillows are held firm and the equipment becomes ineffective.

Although most patients seem to find the bed comfortable, some do not like it. This usually means that it has not been set up correctly or that it is being misused. One problem is that the bed always looks untidy, and well-meaning attendants attempt to make it look neater by tucking in the bedsheet.

The vacuum pack

The vacuum pack is a bag containing polystyrene beads which can be set hard by extracting the air from the pack. The pack can therefore be positioned around parts of the body to provide a snug fit and will maintain this shape when the air is extracted.

The pack is particularly useful for patients with poor sitting balance, such as in stroke. The patient can be placed in the optimal management position while sitting on the pack and the air extracted. The patient's position can be changed at regular intervals simply by re-inflating the pack, repositioning the patient and re-extracting the air.

The pack can also be used to redistribute the body weight over a larger area when, for instance, sitting a patient with sacral pressure sores. The technique is to place a gauze pack over the pressure area before positioning the patient and extracting the air from the bag; when the vacuum pack has 'set', the gauze pack is removed and there is then no pressure at the site of the sore.

Another use for the pack is to provide the optimal degree of lumbar support whilst sitting or lying for those patients with back pains, especially for those who tend to 'slump' in their chairs.

Pressure sores are a problem when a patient is lying for a long period. The pack has been shown to make a valuable contribution to the prevention of pressure sores in elderly patients presenting with fracture of the femur when used on theatre trolleys and operating tables, which are particularly firm surfaces [1].

Flexistand

The Flexistand Major (Fig. 3.2) is a standing frame which provides a three-point splinting of the patient in the standing position. The

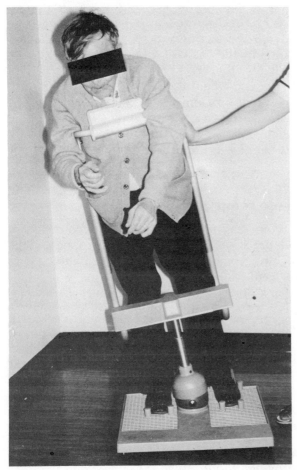

Fig. 3.2 The Flexistand Major dynamic standing frame

equipment is adjustable to provide optimal splinting at the knees, buttocks and chest.

The major advantage of this equipment over other static standing frames is that it allows variable and controllable degrees of movement in the lateral and anteroposterior directions by alteration of a simple blocking mechanism in the base. It can also be set to provide a fixed degree of leaning in one of several directions. A tall, adaptable table is available so that the patient can carry out activities, such as reading or handicrafts, while standing. There is also an electronic hoist adaptor to assist in standing the patient into the frame.

The equipment can provide static balance training by simply splinting the patient in the standing position. It can also be used to increase dynamic standing balance by creating movement in the lateral and/or anteroposterior directions while the patient is held securely in the standing position.

Patients with a persistent backwards lean seem to benefit from standing in the frame with the mechanism set at a slight leaning-forward position: presumably the postural reflexes are 'reset'.

Some patients, following hip surgery, are frightened to place weight on the affected leg. This can hold back the rehabilitation programme for some time and often results in an unnecessarily abnormal gait. The Flexistand helps the patient to gain confidence by (i) ensuring that when he is standing weight can be placed through both legs, and (ii) that controlled weight-bearing through the affected leg can be encouraged.

Intermittent pneumatic compression

Intermittent pneumatic compression (IPC) is a technique consisting of alternate inflation and deflation of a bag placed around a limb (Fig. 3.3). There are two components to the available equipment – the pressure garment (sleeve) and the pump.

The sleeve can be either a single-chamber [2] or a multi-chamber [3] garment. The latter has a series of compartments which encircle the limb and which are sequentially inflated from the periphery proximally until the whole sleeve is inflated, and then the cells deflate together. This action is said to be more effective for improving venous return.

The second component is the pump, which can have either a fixed inflation – deflation cycle with a variable pressure, or variable pressure and cycle times [4]. It is important to recognize that the power of the pump influences the speed at which the sleeve can be inflated; many pumps are unable to provide optimal pressures in the times recommended for improving venous return [5].

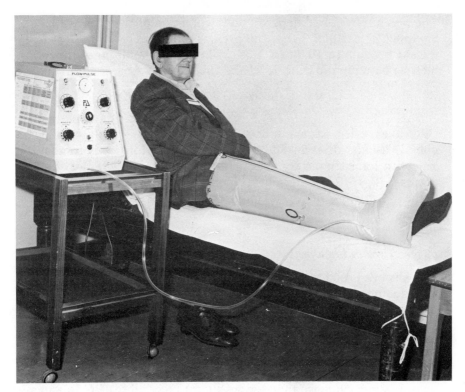

Fig. 3.3 Intermittent pneumatic compression

Prevention of deep-vein thrombosis

It is generally recognized that activity of the calf muscle pump mechanism is a major factor in improving venous stasis. There is evidence that IPC can produce a similar effect, lowering the incidence of deep-vein thrombosis and pulmonary emboli [6–9]. This effect may be due to a combination of factors, such as improving the peak blood flow [10–14], increasing the volume of blood flow [10, 15], and increasing fibrinolysis [10, 16] probably by releasing fibrinolytic activator from the walls of blood vessels [17, 18]. The latter has interesting possibilities in that thrombosis can be prevented by using IPC on other limbs [9, 19]. This is particularly important since IPC is contraindicated on a limb where deep-vein thrombosis is present or suspected.

Management of oedema and lymphoedema

IPC has been shown to assist the removal of fluid of venous [20], lymphatic [20], post mastectomy [21, 22] and rheumatoid [23] origin.

The pressure required depends on the position of the patient [2, 24]. Sayegh [24] calculates that the pressure (in mmHg) in the garment should become to $10 + (d/1.35)$, where d is the distance (in centimetres) between the heart level and the feet.

Improving circulation

Clinical experience suggests that IPC improves the symptoms of peripheral vascular disease. The scientific evidence for this is controversial, with some studies showing an improvement [10, 15] and others a decrease [2, 16, 25] in peripheral blood flow. This is probably related to the cycle time – fast cycles improve the flow [10, 15] but slow cycles decrease it [10, 13, 16].

Surgical wound healing

IPC has been used to assist the healing of surgical wounds, probably by reducing oedema [27–29], removing fluid that has accumulated in the wound [28, 29] and preventing haematoma formation [29].

Leg ulcers

Leg ulcers that are slow to heal are often associated with oedema, and there is some evidence that venous ulcers respond to IPC treatment [30].

Contractures

Clinical experience shows that IPC used at high pressure and slow cycles can be an alternative to serial splinting of contractures at the knee. It has the advantage of avoiding the need to splint the leg continually in positions that prevent ambulation.

Stroke

Very slow cycles and low-pressure IPC can assist in decreasing spasticity following stroke. Fast cycles at high pressure, on the other hand, can assist the management of the flaccid limb by increasing stimulation. Neither of these approaches is ideal since it is difficult to provide the best joint positions; but they are useful adjuncts when little therapy time is available. High pressure and fast cycles are also useful in the management of unilateral neglect, partly by providing tactile/pressure stimulation but also by providing an increased amount of attention to the affected side.

References

1. O'Reilly, M., Whyte, J. and Goldstone, L. (1981) A pressure sore survey. *Nursing Times* Theatre Nursing Supplement, 30th Sept.: 10–17.
2. Johnson, H.D. and Pflugg, J. (1975) In: *The Swollen Leg*. Heinemann, London.
3. Zelikovski, A., Manoach, M., Giler, S. and Urca, I. (1980) Lymphapress: a new pneumatic device for the treatment of lymphoedema of the limbs. *Lymphology* **13**: 68–73.
4. Rithalia, S.V.S., Sayegh, A. and Edwards, J. (1987) Consumer report on intermittent pneumatic compression devices. *Clinical Rehabilitation* **1**: 67–72.
5. Sayegh, A., Rithalia, S. and Andrews, K. (1987) Performance characteristics of intermittent pneumatic compression systems. *Clinical Rehabilitation* **1**: 73–7.
6. Sabri, S., Roberts, V.C. and Cotton, L.T. (1971) Prevention of early postoperative deep vein thrombosis by intermittent compression of the leg during surgery. *British Medical Journal* **4**: 394–6.
7. Hills, N.H., Pflug, J.J., Jeyasingh, K., Boardman, L. and Calnan, J.S. (1972) Prevention of deep vein thrombosis by intermittent pneumatic compression of the calf. *British Medical Journal* **1**: 131–5.
8. Clark, W.B., Prescott, P.R., McGregor, A.B. and Ruckley, C.V. (1974) Pneumatic compression of the calf and postoperative deep-vein thrombosis. *Lancet* **2**: 5–7.
9. Tarnay, T.J., Rohr, P.R., Davidson, B.A. *et al.* (1980) Pneumatic calf compression, fibrinolysis and the prevention of deep venous thrombosis. *Surgery* **88**: 489–95.
10. Ah-See, A.K., Arfors, K.E., Bergovist, D. and Dahlgren, S. (1976) The haemodynamic and antithrombotic effects of intermittent pneumatic calf compression on femoral vein blood flow. *Acta Chirguria Scandinavica* **142**: 381–5.
11. Roberts, V.C. (1971) External pressure and femoral-vein flow. *Lancet* **1**: 136–7.
12. Roberts, V.C., Sabri, S., Beeley, A.H. and Cotton, L.T. (1972) The effects of intermittently applied external pressure on the haemodynamics of the lower limb in man. *British Journal of Surgery* **59**: 223–6.
13. Sabri, S., Roberts, V.C. and Cotton, L.T. (1971) Effects of externally applied pressure on the haemodynamics of the lower limb. *British Medical Journal* **3**: 503–8.
14. Hopkins, G.R. and Tarnay, T.J. (1974) Performance of pneumatic lower limb circulatory assist device. *Medical Instrumentation* **8**: 135–6.
15. Allwood, M.J. (1957) The effect of an increased local pressure gradient on blood flow in the foot. *Clinical Science* **16**: 231–9.
16. Allenby, F., Boardman, L., Pflug, J.J. and Calnan, J.S. (1973) Effects of external pneumatic intermittent compression on fibrinolysis in man. *Lancet* **2**: 1412–4.
17. Chakrabarti, R., Birks, P.M. and Fearnley, G.R. (1963) Origin of blood fibrinolytic activity from vein walls and its bearing on the fate of venous thrombi. *Lancet* **1**: 1288–90.
18. Kernoff, P.B.A. and McNichol, G.P. (1977) Normal and abnormal fibrinolysis. *British Medical Bulletin* **33**: 239–44.
19. Knight, M.T.N. and Dawson, R. (1976) Effect of intermittent compression of the arms on deep venous thrombosis in the legs. *Lancet* **2**: 1265–8.
20. Pflug, J.J. (1975) intermittent compression in the management of swollen legs in general practice. *Practitioner* **215**: 69–76.
21. Stilwell, G.K. (1958) Physical medicine in the management of patients with post-

mastectomy lymphoedema. *Journal of the American Medical Association* **171**: 2285–91.
22. McNair, T.J., Martin, I.J. and Orr, J.D. (1976) Intermittent compression for lymphoedema of the arm. *Clinical Oncology* **2**: 339–42.
23. Holt, P.J.L. and Bennet, R.M. (1972) Pneumatic stockings to treat 'rheumatic oedema'. *Lancet* **2**: 688–9.
24. Sayegh, A. (1987) Intermittent pneumatic compression: past, present and future. *Clinical Rehabilitation* **1**: 61–6.
25. Halperin, M.H., Friedland, M.D. and Wilkins, R.W. (1948) The effect of local compression upon blood flow in the extremities of man. *American Heart Journal* **35**: 221–37.
26. Spiro, M., Roberts, V.C. and Richards, J.B. (1970) Effect of externally applied pressure on femoral vein blood flow. *British Medical Journal* **1**: 719–23.
27. Pflug, J.J. (1974) Intermittent compression: a new principle in treatment of wounds? *Lancet* **2**: 355–6.
28. Melrose, D.G., Knight, M.T.N. and Simandl, E. (1979) The stripping of varicose veins: a clinical trial of intermittent compression dressing. *British Journal of Surgery* **66**: 53–5.
29. Hazarika, E.Z., Knight, M.T.N. and Frazer-Moodie, A. (1979) The effect of intermittent pneumatic compression on the hand after fasciectomy. *The Hand* **2**: 309–14.
30. Hazarika, E.Z. and Wright, D.E. (1981) Chronic leg ulcers: the effect of pneumatic intermittent compression. *Practitioner* **225**: 189–92.

4

Arthritis

General features of the arthritic condition

There are great difficulties in making an accurate diagnosis between the types of arthritis in the elderly [1, 2], the diagnosis being complicated by the high incidence (42 per cent) of rheumatoid factor without evidence of an arthropathy [3].

Rheumatoid arthritis

The prevalence of rheumatoid arthritis rises with age and is more common in females. It is estimated that about 24 per cent of women and 14 per cent of men over 75 years of age have some degree of rheumatoid arthritis [4]. In men especially, pain becomes a less predominant feature as the disease progresses. Rheumatoid arthritis in the elderly may occur for the first time or may be long-standing (either active or inactive).

Although the clinical features are similar in the elderly and in younger patients [2], the disease onset may be more fulminant [2, 5] but often tends to be milder and result in less deformity in the elderly [6–8]. Subcutaneous nodules are found less frequently [9], although the shoulder is more likely to be involved [6] and the shoulder-hand syndrome more common [6, 7] in the elderly. Synovitis of the ankles and wrists is less common in the elderly and does not involve the hip as frequently in elderly males [6]. Ulnar deviation is more common in the elderly rheumatoid arthritic [10–12], although it sometimes occurs without other evidence of rheumatoid arthritis [13]. The reason for the abnormility is unknown. It does not seem to be due to previous occupational trauma [11, 13], muscle wasting [14] or nerve lesions [11]. The most consistent association is widening of the joint space [15], which is possibly due to stretching of the ligaments.

Studies of the effectiveness of rehabilitation in rheumatoid arthritis are few. Elderly patients with rheumatoid arthritis seem to benefit from a rehabilitation programme as much as [16] or better than [6] do

47

younger patients. In uncontrolled trials, hospital admission for rheumatoid arthritis resulted in improvement, which was maintained in about three-quarters of the patients following discharge, even for severely disabled patients. [17–20].

There has also been very little research into the benefits of different types of rehabilitation in arthritis. In one study, three forms of heat treatment were compared: (a) wax bath treatment to the hands followed by exercises; (b) ultrasound followed by exercises; and (c) ultrasound plus faradic hand baths followed by standard exercises [21]. No differences were found between the outcomes of the three types with regard to grip strength, pain, swelling, range of movements or ability to carry out activities. This is obviously important since ultrasound and faradic treatments require the skills of a physiotherapist, usually in a hospital, whereas wax baths can be used unsupervised at home once the technique has been taught.

Oesteoarthrosis

There is a very marked correlation of osteoarthrosis with advancing age [22, 23]. About 20 per cent of people over 60 years of age suffer from symptomatic joint disease [23], over 80 per cent have radiological evidence of osteoarthrosis [24], and probably all have some early pathological changes.

Osteoarthrosis of the hand is common in elderly people, with a tendency to increase in severity with advancing age [25], and is more marked in females. The pattern of joint involvement is greatest in the distal interphalangeal joints, especially of the index and middle fingers [25, 26]. It seems that functional disability from involvement of the hand is related more to the severity of the disease than to the number of joints involved and, in general, is relatively benign [27].

As with rheumatoid arthritis, pain and stiffness are the main symptoms. However, in osteoarthrosis the pain is often relieved by exercise, and many patients comment that as long as the they can keep going the pain settles and that it seems to be worst when they are relaxing after a period of exercise. The stiffness, too, may differ from that of rheumatoid arthritis in not being worse in the morning but appearing at any time throughout the day, especially after being in one position for a period of time.

Management of rheumatoid arthritis in the acute phase

The role of bed rest in the treatment of rheumatoid arthritis is uncertain, although it is generally regarded as being important during acute exacerbations [28–30]. The main concern is that inactivity produces

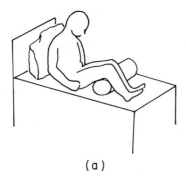

(a)

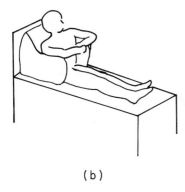

(b)

Fig. 4.1 Position of the patient with rheumatoid arthritis: (a) bad positioning; (b) correct positioning

muscle atrophy, with about 5 per cent loss of strength per day [31]. However, drug therapy and short-term immobilization in a cylinder splint is thought to reduce the pain and swelling without significantly reducing muscle strength [32].

The basis of rehabilitation in the acute phase is protection of the joints. The patient should *not* be nursed with pillows under the knees (Fig. 4.1a) since this results in fixed flexion deformities. Similarly, a soft bed produces abnormal positioning and exacerbates the tendency to deformity. The bed should be firm and a bed cradle used to protect the legs from the weight of bed clothes. A full-length backslab may be required to maintain the legs in the optimal position: it should preferably be cast with the patient in the prone position to provide optimal correction of the deformity. In addition, the patient should lie prone for 20–30 minutes two or three times a day.

Correct nursing (Fig. 4.1b) ensures that the patient's back is kept straight (as opposed to being flexed), the legs are supported laterally by pillows, the arms supported on pillows and the feet prevented from plantar flexion by supports. If the ankle joint is involve a footpiece can be incorporated in the backslab.

Where there is already a flexion deformity of the hip it is important to avoid secondary contraction of the knee. Therefore, the patient should not be allowed to lie with the knee flexed. The knee can be kept extended in spite of the hip flexion by supporting the lower part of the leg on pillows. Similarly, if the knee is flexed, secondary contracture of the hip can be prevented by elevating the upper leg and buttock on an extra supporting mattress.

Local splinting helps to control acute inflammation [33–37]. It is generally felt that even passive movement of the joints is unnecessary in the acute phase. Indeed, it seems from animal experiments that passive or active exercise increases joint inflammation [36]. Pain usually indicates that there is intra-articular pressure, which is further increased by movement. As the swelling subsides the joint can then be moved gently through a range of movement. Meanwhile the aim is to hold the joint in a neutral position – the splint extending over an area large enough to allow the stability of the joint to be maintained with comfort.

When splinting the hand, the wrist is held at 10–25° of extension, the ulnar deviation corrected and the metacarpophalangeal joints held in slight flexion (note *not* extension). As the inflammation settles the patient will only need to wear the splint at night or when in vulnerable situations, such as when travelling. Indeed, patients tend to stop using the splints when the pain settles [37] and are more likely to wear them for activities requiring strength rather than dexterity [38]. Non-compliance is more frequent in the elderly (38) than in middle-aged patients [38], although others have found that the elderly, especially women [37, 39], are more likely to use their splints.

There is evidence that some finger stiffness is due to accumulation of extracellular fluid [40, 41]. This may explain why elasticated gloves [42, 45] or pneumatic splints [46] improve mobility, and decrease morning stiffness or pain, in rheumatoid arthritic hands.

In pneumatic splinting the sleeve (at a pressure of 40 mmHg for 20 minutes) is placed over the hand with the wrist in the neutral position and the fingers extended; and then this is repeated with the hand closed into a fist.

There is no urgent need for mobilization of the joints during the first three weeks, or until the inflammation is showing signs of settling down. After this, passive exercises can start followed by active and then resistive exercises (see later). If pain and stiffness increase then the programme needs to altered and activity decreased.

During the acute phase ice packs may help to relieve the pain and swelling, but as the inflammation resolves heat can be introduced.

Activity is gradually introduced, but weight bearing is encouraged only when the muscles are strong enough, otherwise there is a danger of producing permanent damage to unsupported joints.

Management of chronic osteoarthrosis and rheumatoid arthritis in the non-acute phase

Rehabilitation in arthritis is basically prophylactic: damage is largely irreversible, and so further deterioration is to be prevented or slowed down.

One of the major problems is that 'therapy' should be continued daily for the rest of the patient's life and this is extremely difficult for the average person to maintain.

The aims of management are to relieve pain, prevent further deformities, mobilize the joints, strengthen the muscles and retrain function.

Pain

Pain is the most distressing symptom of arthritis. Unfortunately it is notoriously difficult to assess since pain thresholds vary between individuals and within the same individual at different times depending on the pathological disorder, the psychological response and other external factors. This is relevant since ultrasound may be effective in damping down pain from a pathological lesion, but it will have little effect if there is a strong psychological element.

The first step is to find the source of the pain. It is usually difficult for patients to differentiate pain arising from bone, joints, tendons or muscle, and some pain may be referred from other areas. For example, a hip disorder may produce pain in the knee, or shoulder pain may result from a cardiac source. Pain felt over the iliac crest may be spinal or renal in origin. Pain from the shoulder radiating down the outer side of the arm often indicates disorders of the scapulohumeral joint or subacromial bursa, whereas pain spreading to the trapezius ridge usually indicates the source is in the shoulder girdle.

It is helpful to ask the patient to point to the area of the pain rather than to name the area. It is then necessary to find which movements produce the pain and to detect areas of tenderness, though the latter may also occur with referred pain. In some cases injected local anaesthetic can be used as a diagnostic aid.

Pain is an important clue to the amount of activity that can be allowed. There is a danger that strong analgesia removes the pain, allowing the joint to be damaged during exercise. When joint pain is felt at rest in rheumatoid arthritis this usually implies that there is acute synovitis; when it occurs with movement the inflammation is likely to be less severe; and when it is only produced by specific movements the synovitis is likely to be mild [47]. In osteoarthrosis the pain on movement is usually associated with osteophyte formation and mechanical damage, though this cannot be the full explanation since many people develop marked deformity without pain.

Heat treatment

Although the formal evidence for the value of heat therapy is limited, there is no doubt that many patients benefit, even if only in the short term. This then allows an exercise programme to be carried out to strengthen muscles and improve the range of movement, which in turn improves function over the longer term. In addition it helps to break the pain–anxiety–pain cycle.

Heat produced by specialist physiotherapy equipment is probably no better in this context than a soak in a warm bath, and there is little difference between the various heat modalities.

Cold therapy

Ice therapy is effective in decreasing pain in chronic as well as in acute arthritis [48].

Electrical stimulation

Transcutaneous electrical nerve stimulation (TENS) relieves joint pain [49–51], especially when it is chronic. High doses are most effective [47]. TENS can also relieve some of the morning stiffness and is therefore useful for self-administration, allowing the patient to start activities earlier in the day.

How TENS works is unknown. It has been suggested that it works through the gate control of pain by stimulating nerve fibres not carrying pain sensation, thereby blocking the pain fibres. The main action is on C-fibre mediated pain, though there also seems to be some effect on acute pain mediated by A-delta fibres. Its effect does not seem to be due to a placebo response [49, 51], and it has been suggested that there is an associated release of endorphines which may account for some of the pain relief [52].

There are few contraindications to the use of TENS, though pain may return in greater intensity when the TENS-induced analgesia has worn off [49, 53]. It has also been suggested that some patients with good pain relief may then stress the joint, resulting in further damage [51]. The most frequent side effect is unpleasant sensations and skin irritation under the electrode [54]. Cardiac dysrhythmias [55] and interference with cardiac pacemakers [56] have also been reported.

Joint protection

It is essential to prevent further damage to joints. Resting splints at night time and supportive splints during activity help to achieve this (see below). For the hand, lightweight splints are preferable to plaster of Paris, and the modern heat-mouldable plastics or fibreglass are durable and comfortable [57].

There are a number of possibilities for management of the knee joint. A long leg brace provides excellent support and optimal alignment of the joint [58, 59], but because it prevents bending at the knee it can immobilize the elderly patient. For this reason some form of hinged knee brace is preferred. Some elderly people find a simple elasticated bandage gives sufficient support for their very limited activities.

Joints should be protected from developing abnormal positions during daily activities. This may mean carrying out activities in a way that is slightly unsual. Brattstrom [60] has described these in great detail. The following list gives some ideas:

1. When sitting, avoid resting the chin on the hand since this tends to produce ulnar deviation. Avoid lying in bed holding a book since this also encourages ulnar deviation. A more appropriate way is to use a book rest.
2. When slicing food avoid the pressure of the knife handle pressing the fingers into ulnar deviation. There are several ways of overcoming this: (a) hold the knife so that the pressure is taken by the metacarpophalangeal joints transmitting the force in a radial direction, or (b) use a slicing machine, or (c) use a knife with a vertical grip.
3. For tin opening avoid the small openers with butterfly knobs, which require a lot of pressure. A wall-mounted tin opener with a large handle or one that is electrically controlled is better.
4. Avoid lifting a heavy cup by: (a) only half filling the cup, or (b) using a lightweight cup, or (c) using a cup with two handles, or (d) fitting an extension to the handle.
5. Avoid lifting heavy pans by ladling out the contents into smaller containers, and avoid lifting a heavy teapot by using a tilting teapot support.
6. When using a turning or twisting wrist action (e.g. taking off a jar top or turning on a tap), twist the object towards the ulnar side of the hand so that the pressure is transmitted to the radial side. For instance, when screwing a jar top remove the top with the left hand

and replace it with the right hand (turn to produce pressure in a radial direction). Alternatively use an aid to remove the top.

7. When carrying a heavy object avoid using only the fingers. Instead hold it underneath with both palms. Alternatively avoid carrying heavy objects by using a small trolley and use lightweight (either plastic or aluminium) equipment.
8. When closing drawers avoid pressure on the hands by using the buttock.
9. During activity, wherever possible, keep the fingers in extension. When washing or dusting a surface keep the hand flat on that surface.

Joints can be further protected by finding the appropriate aid. Since a greater degree of grip is required for a small object than for a large one, thicken the handles of cutlery, combs or any object with a handle. Similarly, the torque on a lever can be achieved with less effort by simply increasing the length of the handle – as, for instance, in aids for turning taps, keys, door handles or opening bottles.

Much of the joint protection of the hip involves relief of weight bearing stresses by using a walking stick or frame. Since walking produces a force three times that of body weight on the tibial plateau [61], weight reduction in the obese patient also has an important contribution to make. Well-fitting shoes with shock-absorbing soles also help to protect joints.

Splinting

Orthotic devices are used to provide symptomatic relief of pain; decrease local inflammation; prevent deformities; correct deformities; prevent trauma in unstable joints; and improve function.

The choice of material used in splinting depends on the degree of strength required, the durability of the material, the ease of use and patient acceptance. For elderly people the modern lightweight thermoplastic materials are usually preferable to plaster of Paris, since it is rare to require the splint to withstand heavy stresses and the weight may be so great in relation to strength that activity is markedly inhibited.

Prevention of joint deformities

In the non-acute inflammatory phase, dynamic splinting is used to prevent worsening of the deformity. The ideal splint should permit the normal planes of motion necessary for essential function, but block all faulty planes that result in significant deformity [62]. Although dynamic splints are theoretically correct the evidence suggests that they are less successful in practice [63].

Correction of deformities

Joint deformities may be due to contractures or to physical distruction of bone. A contracture is usually due to fibrosis of the capsule or the ligaments. Contributing factors include chronic synovitis, ineffective tendon motion during tenosynovitis, shortening of the collateral ligaments owing to poor positioning, periarticular oedema, subluxation and muscle weakness [64].

In the early stages where the contracture is due to soft-tissue shortening, physiotherapy can correct the deformity by producing continuous stretching [65], preferably while the tissues are heated [66]. In the later stages, and where there is a flexion deformity greater than 15° of stretching, physiotherapy is less effective and splinting is required. Much of this can be achieved by specific exercises, but again the elderly tolerate these relatively poorly. The use of pneumatic intermitten compression (see Chapter 3) with cycle times of one or two minutes is often a more realistic approach.

Long leg braces have been used for many years in the management of lower-limb rheumatoid arthritis. In the elderly, unfortunately, when a fixed deformity has occurred with shortening of the muscles and capsular changes it is rarely possible to correct the deformity, even with progressive splinting [33, 65]. Attempts to do so causes great pain and anxiety without achieving a practical outcome. At this stage it is essential to prevent further deformity and support the disordered joint rather than to be over-zealous in trying to straighten the deformity.

Exercises

Range-of-movement exercises

Since the range and type of movement at each joint is different, the patient should be taught the limits and directions of movement to practise. Exercises should be carried out at least once a day, but few patients are persistent in doing so. The decrease in the range of motion starts at the extremes of the movement, and therefore it is not surprising that limitation of joint action can arise insidiously in spite of daily exercises. It is therefore important to stress that simply moving each joint is insufficient to prevent deterioration unless the exercise involves the extremes of joint action.

Elderly people often do not carry out daily exercises, so they should ensure that those activities they *do* perform include a wide range of movement. For instance, when ironing or dusting they should perform the activity with wide sweeps to include as much range of movement as possible.

Since activity is more likely to be effective if the joints are in the optimal condition, washing hands in warm water before starting hand activities may be a simple but effective procedure.

Leg muscle power

Exercises against progressively increasing levels of resistance are used to maintain muscle power. Ideally these should be carried out in a non-weight-bearing position.

Disorders of the knee are frequently associated with weakness of the quadriceps muscle, which may be partly due to mechanical derangement. For instance, injecting plasma into the knee results in difficulty contracting the quadriceps [67]. Since the pressure within the knee is less with the knee flexed this encourages the development of flexion deformities. In one sense weakness may be protective, being secondary to reflex inhibition from pain in the knee; the facilitation of the hamstring muscles produces flexor withdrawal to avoid weight bearing, and the abnormal distribution of muscle tone produces further derangement of the joint on attempting to walk.

Rehabilitation of the 'orthopaedic knee' must therefore be thought of in terms of *neuromuscular* management. In the early stages it is important to inhibit the protective reactions to allow correct movement in the opposing muscle groups. The following neuromuscular approach is taken from Vasey and Crozier [68]:

1. *A good starting position* is required to provide postural control. The head is extended upwards, which results in controlled contraction of the spinal muscles with the minimum of effort. Further support is derived by gaining scapular 'adhesion' to the supporting surface: this is achieved by protracting the shoulder and then elevating and retracting it. Each buttock in turn is then lifted slightly and moved forward on the plinth. This helps to decrease the stretch reflex during subsequent exercises.
2. *Movements begin proximally and progress distally.* The emphasis is on slow and gentle movements, with the dual aims of achieving movement with minimum muscle effort and controlling reflex protective reactions. With the therapist's hand on the greater trochanter, the patient is asked to gently and slowly push the hip of the affected side away, to hold the position, and then to relax. Movement is actually produced by contraction of the muscles on the opposite side of the body, which results in reciprocal inhibition of the muscles of the affected side. This is continued until maximal

control is obtained, resulting in limited gentle stretching of the hamstrings. The exercises progress to similar activity at the level of the knee and ankle, and then dorsiflexion of the foot.

Shoulder problems

The shoulder may be affected in rheumatoid arthritis. In the early stages a synovitis may produce pain, though there will be few X-ray abnormalities unless arthrography is carried out. In more advanced forms there is narrowing of the joint space, possibly capsular fibrosis and rupture of the rotator cuff. In the very severe form there is joint damage and the shoulder is fixed in its range of movement.

The rehabilitation approach is to maintain a good range of movement. There is a danger that the patient will keep the arms immobile in the most comfortable position, with resulting fixed contractures developing. Splinting is very difficult, and so the patient should be nursed with the arms supported with the shoulder abducted in bed and when sitting (Fig. 4.1b). Isometric contractions to improve deltoid, pectoralis major and internal rotator muscles are important.

One simple but useful exercise to improve shoulder function is to stand and lean forward with the arm and hand hanging vertically. Rotating the arm in increasing circles allows a good range of movement to be built up. This action seems to be effective in that it helps to relieve the secondary spasticity and uses the effect of gravity to assist the action.

The occupational therapist has an important role in finding appropriate aids to overcome the limited movement of the shoulder. These will include long-handled brushes and combs, sponges on a curved stick to wash the neck, and the use of Velcro fastenings on clothing. Appropriate dressing techniques can be taught to the patient. For instance, a coat can be hung by a loop from a hook on a door or the wall: this enables the patient to slide the arm into the coat and then release the hook by standing up.

Hydrotherapy

Although hydrotherapy is generally regarded as being helpful in rheumatoid arthritis, few patients have access to a pool. The buoyancy of the water along with its warmth relaxes the muscle groups around painful joints. The buoyancy allows limbs to move in a supportive environment and the exercises are effective in improving muscle strength. However, many frail elderly people dislike being submerged in water or are frightened of hoists, and have difficulty in climbing into the pool.

Some convenient aids to independence

Mobility aids

Younger patients with arthritis can often manage with crutches of one form or another, but they are less helpful to the elderly.

If a walking stick is used it should have a flat, straight handgrip – curved ones can produce damage to the arthritic hand. More practical is a stick with a handgrip moulded to the shape of the palm; these are available for both the right and left hand (i.e. one stick

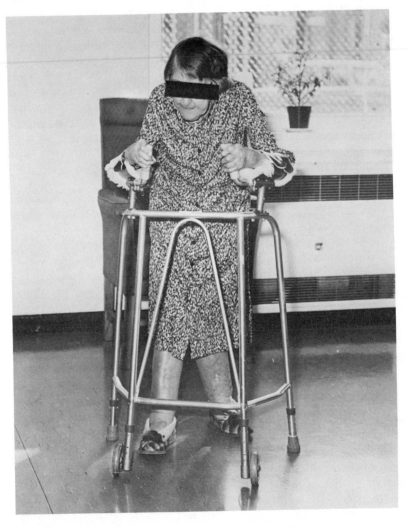

Fig. 4.2   Gutter frame for rheumatoid arthritic patients

cannot be used for either hand). Whatever type of stick is used it should be used in the least affected hand.

Where a walking frame is required then one with gutter forearm supports is usually the most practical for a frail elderly person (Fig. 4.2). This is especially the case where the hands are affected because weight can be taken through the forearms.

Chairs

The chair is one of the most important pieces of furniture for an elderly person with arthritis since he or she is likely to spend a large amount of time sitting. 'Easy chairs' usually are not easy – the most comfortable chair can be the most difficult.

The chair should be comfortable and sufficiently high to allow ease of transferring. It should provide support for the back and other joints [69], and the feet should be well supported on the ground to avoid contractures. However, since prolonged sitting with the knees bent is likely to lead to flexion contractures of the knees, the patient should ideally sit with the legs extended, preferably with the feet supported on a small rocking stool which keeps the ankles at right angles.

As for many conditions which affect transferring from a chair, raising the height of the seat by about 10–15 cm can relieve much of the strain of standing up. Where there is a stiff knee the chair can have a divided front section; and where the hips are stiff benefit may be had from a working chair consisting of a bicycle saddle with a firm backrest [60]. Where the knees are weak, a spring-loaded seat (Fig. 4.3) can be helpful, though these should be used with caution.

When standing the patient should avoid pressing down on the arms of the chair with the fingers. Many patients find it easier to stand by ensuring that the feet are under the front edge of the seat and by putting both hands on the knees, bending forwards to bring the body weight over the knees.

There are several guidelines to the selection of an armchair [70]. The floor-to-seat height is the most important parameter. A chair which can support the legs with the knees at right angles and the feet flat on the ground is preferred, but it should not be so high that the feet are suspended above the floor. The seat should be horizontal or only very slightly sloping backwards, and the backrest upright or only gently sloping backwards. High armrests make it difficult to push on. The seat should be firm but the edge should not be hard. There should be room to tuck the legs under the front part of the seat to make standing easier. The covering material is also important: too rough and it restricts movement, too smooth and the patient may slip.

The armrests should be padded and the side supports solid to pre-

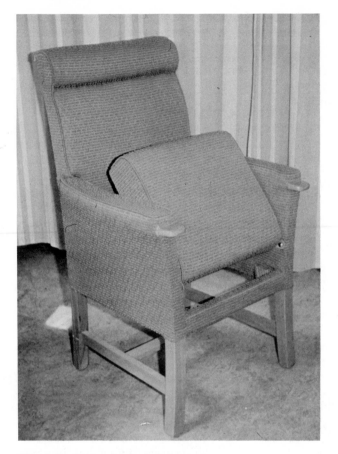

Fig. 4.3   Spring-loaded seat

vent books or knitting falling on to the floor. A wide seat allows easier frequent change of position. If the patient has discomfort within the first ten minutes of sitting down he or she will be very uncomfortable within twenty minutes [71].

Community management

Whatever the success of an inpatient rehabilitation programme, the major problem remains maintaining optimal levels of care over the longer term. It is one thing to carry out full range-of-movement exercises while being supervised in hospital; it is altogether different trying to carry this on away from the 'therapeutic environment'.

There is evidence that home management is more effective than attending a multiprofessional outpatient clinic [72], and great interest has been shown in the role of health visitors in the longer term management of the arthritic patient [73–75].

Patients and their relatives often seek advice on coping at home. The following guide lines can be offered:

- Avoid fatigue. This includes obtaining a good sleep at night.
- Diet should be well controlled. Many rheumatoid patients are anorexic, while others become obese owing to a combination of lack of activity and a tendency to excessive eating from boredom. Both conditions will make the functional ability worse.
- Regular activity is required to maintain the optimal level of muscle power and range of movement of the joints. The chief carer should be taught how to assist, supervise and encourage the patient in a daily exercise programme.
- The patient and relatives should be taught the principles of good posture to be maintained at all times.
- Attention should be paid to the bowels. Inactivity and analgesics often combine to produce constipation. This will require the usual management of constipation in the elderly.
- Arrange furniture to make it easier to move around.
- Plan the day carefully. For instance, carry out upstairs chores before coming down in the morning to avoid frequent and unnecessary climbing of stairs.
- A lightweight duvet assists bed making and causes less pressure on the feet and legs.
- In general it is best to use the largest joint and the strongest muscles which can carry out a particular activity (e.g. use the arm rather than the fingers for carrying). Also, the load should be distributed over two joints (e.g. either the whole arm or both hands).
- Avoid exhaustion.
- Avoid keeping the joints in one position for a long period of time.

References

1. Paolino, J.S. (1971) Rheumatic diseases of the aged: diagnosis and management. *Journal of the American Geriatrics Society*, **19**: 240–51.
2. Gibson, T. and Grahame, R. (1973) Acute arthritis in the elderly. *Age and Ageing* **2**: 3–13.
3. Heimer, R., Levin, F.M. and Rudd, E. (1963) Globulins resembling rheumatoid factor in serum of the aged. *American Journal of Medicine* **35**: 175–81.
4. Meenan, R.F., Yelin, E.H., Nevitt, M. *et al.* (1981) The impact of chronic disease: a sociomedical profile of rheumatoid arthritis. *Arthritis and Rheumatism* **25**: 544–9.
5. Moesmann, G. (1968) Subacute rheumatoid arthritis in old age. *Acta Rheumatica Scandinavica* **14**: 14–23.
6. Ehrlich, G.E., Katz, E.A. and Cohen, S.H. (1970) Rheumatoid arthritis in the aged. *Geriatrics* **25**: 103–13.

7. Cecil, R.L. and Kammerer, W.A. (1951) Rheumatoid arthritis in the aged. *American Journal of Medicine* **10**: 439–45.
8. Adler, E. (1966) Rheumatoid arthritis in old age. *Israel Journal of Medical Science* **2**: 607–13.
9. Moesmann, G. (1968) Clinical features in subacute rheumatoid arthritis in old age. *Acta Rheumatica Scandinavica* **14**: 285–97.
10. Lush, B. (1952) Ulnar deviation of the fingers. *Annals of Rheumatic Disease* **11**: 219–21.
11. Vainio, K. and Ako, M. (1953) Ulnar deviation of the fingers. *Annals of Rheumatic Disease* **12**: 122–4.
12. Brewerton, D.A. (1957) Hand deformities in rheumatoid arthritis. *Annals of Rheumatic Disease* **16**: 183–97.
13. Wigzell, F.W. (1976) Ulnar deviation of the fingers as a clinical sign in the elderly. *Age and Ageing* **5**: 132–40.
14. Hakstain, R.W. and Tubiana, R. (1967) Ulnar deviation of the fingers. *Journal of Bone and Joint Surgery* **49A**: 299–316.
15. Wigzell, F.W. (1982) Further observations on ulnar deviation of the fingers in the elderly. *Journal of Clinical Experimental Gerontology* **4**: 97–108.
16. Karten, I., Lee, M. and McEwen, C. (1973) Rheumatoid arthritis: five year study of rehabilitation. *Archives of Physical Medicine and Rehabilitation* **54**: 120–8.
17. Duthie, J.J.R., Brown, P.E., Knox, J.D.E. and Thompson, M. (1957) Course and prognosis in rheumatoid arthritis. *Annals of Rheumatic Disease* **16**: 411–24.
18. Duthie, J.J.R., Brown, P.E., Truelove, L.H. *et al*. (1964) Course and prognosis in rheumatoid arthritis: a further report. *Annals of Rheumatic Disease* **23**: 193–204.
19. Conarty, J.P. and Nickel, V.L. (1971) Functional incapacitation in rheumatoid arthritis, a rehabilitation challenge. A correlative study of function before and after hospital treatment. *Journal of Bone and Joint Surgery* **53A**: 624–37.
20. Barraclough, D., Alderman, W.W. and Popert, A.J. (1976) Rehabilitation of nonwalkers in rheumatoid arthritis. *Rheumatology and Rehabilitation* **15**: 287.
21. Hawkes, J., Care, G., Dixon, J.S. *et al*. (1985) Comparison of three physiotherapy regimes for hands with rheumatoid arthritis. *British Medical Journal* **291**: 1016.
22. Lawrence, J.S., Bremner, J.M. and Bier, F. (1966) Osteoarthrosis: prevalence in the population and relationship between symptoms and X-ray changes. *Annals of Rheumatic Disease* **25**: 1–24.
23. Gordon, T. (1966) Osteoarthrosis in US adults. In: *Population Studies of the Rheumatic Disease*, Proceedings of the Third International Symposium, New York, pp. 391–7. Excepta Medica Foundation.
24. Kellgren, J.H. and Lawrence, J.S. (1957) Radiological assessment of osteoarthrosis. *Annals of Rheumatic Disease* **16**: 494–501.
25. Caird, F.I., Webb, J. and Lee, P. (1973) Osteoarthrosis of the hands in the elderly. *Age and Ageing* **2**: 150–6.
26. Stecher, R.M. (1955) Heberden's nodes: a clinical description of osteoarthritis of the finger joints. *Annals of Rheumatoid Disease* **14**: 1–10.
27. Labi, M.L.C. and Rathey, U.K. (1982) Hand function in osteoarthritis. *Archives of Physical Medicine and Rehabilitation* **63**: 438–40.
28. Cohen, A.S. (1966) A plea for conservative therapy in rheumatoid arthritis. In: *Controversy in Internal Medicine*, p. 543 (Eds: Inglefinger, F.J., Reiman, A.S. and Finland, M.). W.B. Saunders, Philadelphia.
29. Glick, E.N. (1967) Asymmetrical rheumatoid arthritis after poliomyelitis. *British Medical Journal* **3**: 26–8.
30. Coventry, M.B. (1973) Osteotomy about the knee for degenerative and rheuma-

toid arthritis. *Journal of Bone and Joint Surgery* **55A**: 23–48.
31. Muller, E.A. (1970) Influence of training and of inactivity on muscle strength. *Archives of Physical and Rehabilitation* **51**: 449–62.
32. Nicholas, J.J. and Ziegler, G. (1977) Cylinder splints: their use in the treatment of arthritis of the knee. *Archives of Physical Medicine and Rehabilitation* **58**: 264–267.
33. Harris, R. and Copp, E.P. (1962) Immobilization of the knee joint in rheumatoid arthritis. *Annals of Rheumatic Disease* **21**: 353–9.
34. Partridge, R.E.H. and Duthie, J.J.R. (1963) Controlled trial of the effect of complete immobilization of the joints in rheumatoid arthritis. *Annals of Rheumatic Disease* **22**: 91–9.
35. Gault, S.J. and Spyker, J.M. (1969) Beneficial effect of immobilisation of joints in rheumatoid arthritides: a splint study using sequential analysis. *Arthritis and Rheumatism* **12**: 34–44.
36. Agudelo, C.A., Schumacher, H.R. and Phelps, P. (1972) Effect of exercise on urate crystal induced inflammation in canine joints. *Arthritis and Rheumatism* **15**: 609–16.
37. Feinberg, J. and Brandt, K.D. (1981) Use of resting splints by patients with rheumatoid arthritis. *American Journal of Occupational Therapy* **35**: 173–8.
38. Nicholas, J.J., Gruen, H., Weiner, G. *et al.* (1982) Splinting in rheumatoid arthritis. I: Factors affecting patient compliance. *Archives of Physical Medicine and Rehabilitation* **63**: 92–4.
39. Oakes, T., Ward, J., Gray, R. *et al.* (1970) Family expectations and arthritis patient compliance to a hand resting splint regime. *Journal of Chronic Disease* **22**: 751–4.
40. Scott, J.T. (1960) Morning stiffness in rheumatoid arthritis. *Annals of Rheumatic Disease* **19**: 361–8.
41. Wright, V., Dowson, D. and Longfield, M.D. (1969) Joint stiffness – its characterisation and significance. *Biomedical Engineering* **4**: 4–14.
42. Ehrlich, G.E. and DePiero, A.M. (1971) Stretch gloves: nocturnal use to ameliorate morning stiffness in arthritic hands. *Archives of Physical Medicine and Rehabilitation* **52**: 479–80.
43. Askari, A., Moskowitz, R.W. and Ryan, C. (1974) Stretch gloves: study of objective and subjective effectiveness in arthritis of the hands. *Arthritis and Rheumatism* **17**: 263–65.
44. Culic, D.D., Battaglia, M.C., Wichman, C. and Schmid, F.R. (1979) Efficacy of compression gloves in rheumatoid arthritis. *American Journal of Physical Medicine* **58**: 278–84.
45. Swezey, R.L., Spiegel, T.M., Cretin, S. and Clement, P. (1979) Arthritic hand response to pressure gradient gloves. *Archives of Physical Medicine and Rehabilitation* **60**: 375–7.
46. McKnight, P.T. and Schomburg, F.L. (1982) Air pressure splint effects on hand symptoms of patients with rheumatoid arthritis. *Archives of Physical Medicine and Rehabilitation* **63**: 560–4.
47. Polley, H.F. and Hunder, G.G. (1978) In: *Rheumatological Interviewing and Physical Examination of the Joints*, 2nd Edn. W.B. Saunders, Philadelphia.
48. Pegg, S.M.H., Littler, T.R. and Littler, E.N. (1969) A trial of ice therapy and exercise in chronic arthritis. *Physiotherapy* **55**: 51–6.
49. Mannheimer, C., Lund, S. and Carlsson, C.-A. (1978) The effect of transcutaneous electrical nerve stimulation (TNS) on joint pain in patients with rheumatoid arthritis. *Scandinavian Journal of Rheumatology* **7**: 13–16.
50. Taylor, P., Hallett, M. and Flaherty, L. (1981) Treatment of OA of the knees with TENS. *Pain* **11**: 233–40.

51. Kumar, V.N. and Redford, J.B. (1982) Transcutaneous nerve stimulation in rheumatoid arthritis. *Archives of Physical Medicine and Rehabilitation* **63**: 595–6.
52. Adams, J.E. (1976) Naloxone reversal of analgesia produced by brain stimulation in humans. *Pain* **2**: 161–6.
53. Griffin, J.W. and McClure, M. (1981) Adverse responses to transcutaneous electrical nerve stimulation in a patient with rheumatoid arthritis. *Physical Therapy* **61**: 354–5.
54. Loeser, J.D., Black, R.G. and Christman, A. (1975) Relief of pain by transcutaneous stimulation. *Journal of Neurosurgery* **42**: 308–14.
55. Richardson, R.R., Meyer, P.R. and Raimondi, A.J. (1979) Transabdominal neurostimulation in acute spinal injuries. *Spine* **4**: 47–51.
56. Eriksson, M., Schuller, H. and Sjolund, B. (1978) Hazard from transcutaneous nerve stimulation in patients with pacemakers. *Lancet* **17**: 1319.
57. Nicholas, J.J., Gruen, H., Weiner, G. *et al.* (1982) Splinting in rheumatoid arthritis. II: Evaluation of lightcast II fiberglass polymer splints. *Archives of Physical Medicine and Rehabilitation* **63**: 95–6.
58. Fried, D.M. (1969) Splints for arthritis. In: *Arthritis and Physical Medicine*, Chapter 13 (Ed: Licht, S.). Waverly Press, Baltimore.
59. Smith, E.M., Juvinall, R.C., Corell, E.B. *et al.* (1970) Bracing the unstable knee. *Archives of Physical Medicine and Rehabilitation* **51**: 22.
60. Brattstrom, M. (1973) *Principles of Joint Protection in Chronic Rheumatic Disease*. Wolfe Medical, London.
61. Leach, R.E., Baumgard, S. and Brown, J. (1973) Obesity: its relationship to osteoarthrositis of the knee. *Clinical Orthopaedics* **93**: 271–3.
62. Bennett, R.L. (1965) Orthotic devices to prevent deformities in the hand in rheumatoid arthritis. *Arthritis and Rheumatism* **8**: 1006–18.
63. Convery, F.R., Conarty, J.P. and Nickle, V.L. (1968) Dynamic splinting of the rheumatoid hand. *Orthotics and Prosthetics* **22**: 41–5.
64. Melvin, J.L. (1982) In: *Rheumatic Disease: Occupational Therapy and Rehabilitation*, 2nd Edn. F.A. Davis, Philadelphia.
65. Convery, F.R., Conarty, J.P. and Nickle, V.L. (1971) Flexion deformities of the knee in rheumatoid arthritis. *Clinical Orthopaedics and Related Research* **74**: 90–3.
66. Lehmann, J.F., Masock, A.J., Warren, C.G. and Koblanski, J.N. (1970) Effect of therapeutic temperatures on tendon extensibility. *Archives of Physical Medicine and Rehabilitation* **51**: 481–7.
67. deAndrade, J.R., Grant, C. and Dixon, A. St L. (1965) Joint distension and reflex muscle inhibition in the knee. *Journal of Bone and Joint Surgery* **47A**: 313–22.
68. Vasey, J.R. and Crozier, L.W. (1980) A neuromuscular approach to knee joint problems. *Physiotherapy* **66**: 193–4.
69. Atherton, J., Chatfield, J., Clarke, A.K. and Harrison, R.A. (1980) Chair comfort and the arthritic patient. *British Journal of Occupational Therapy* **43**: 366–7.
70. Munton, J. (1981) Seating for the arthritic. *Reports on Rheumatic Diseases* No. 78. Arthritis and Rheumatism Council.
71. Atherton, J., Chatfield, J., Clarke, A.K. and Harrison, R.A. (1980) *Easy Chairs for the Arthritic*. DHSS Aids Assessment Programme.
72. Katz, S., Vignos, P.J., Moskowitz, R. *et al.* (1968) Comprehensive outpatient care in rheumatoid arthritis. *Journal of the American Medical Association* **206**: 1249–54.

73. Firth, D., Roberts, M., Wright, J.G. *et al.* (1973) The value of health visitors in a rehabilitation unit. *Rheumatology and Rehabilitation* **12**: 143–7.
74. Vignos, P.J., Thompson, H.M., Katz, S. *et al.* (1972) Comprehensive care and psychosocial factors in rehabilitation in chronic rheumatoid arthritis: a controlled study. *Journal of Chronic Disease* **25**: 457–67.
75. Healey, L.A. (1975) An alternative to hospitalisation for acute rheumatoid arthritis. *Medical Times* **103**: 173–8.

5

Spinal conditions

The spine is particularly prone to degenerative changes with increasing age. Trauma is less common as a cause in the elderly, although the amount of trauma required to produce damage is lower than in younger people owing to the higher incidence of metabolic bone disease in the elderly.

The cervical spine

The prevalence of degenerative changes in the cervical spine increases with age [1]. About 80 per cent of people aged 65–74 have radiological evidence of cervical spondylosis [2], though in the majority this is asymptomatic [3,4].

Cervical spondylosis

In cervical spondylosis disc degeneration results in narrowing of the disc space and there are associated bony bars formed by osteophytes. These deformities result in a number of symptoms. For example, *neck pain* may be due to:

- degeneration of the apophyseal joints resulting in limitation of neck movement and reflex muscle spasm;
- cervical disc protrusion producing pressure on the nerve roots, though acute prolapse is more common in younger people;
- osteophyte occlusion of the neural foramina producing nerve compression [3];
- root sleeve fibrosis [5];
- abnormal intervertebral movement produced by ligament laxity [6].

Dizziness or light-headedness may be due to:

- osteophytes from the neurocentral and/or apophyseal joints compressing the vertebral artery as it passes through the foremen on the

transverse process [7–10];
- occlusion of a tortuous vertebral artery owing to shortening of the cervical spine associated with narrowing of the vertebral bodies and intervertebral discs;
- decreased feedback from the receptors in the apophyseal joints [11, 12].

Pyramidal long tract signs may be due to cervical myelopathy.

Cervical myelopathy

As many as one-sixth of patients referred for assessment of gait disturbances have myelographic evidence of compression myelopathy due to cervical spine disease [13]. The compression may be due to factors that decrease the area of the spinal canal, including cervical spondylosis [14]; infolding of the ligamentum flava [15]; calcification of the longitudinal ligament [16, 17]; vertebral subluxation [18, 19]; subaxial subluxation in rheumatoid arthritis [20–24]; or vertebral ankylosing hyperostosis [25, 26].

The clinical features of myelopathy vary widely and usually develop slowly. Weakness, heaviness or clumsiness of the arm is common and may be associated with muscle wasting, though this is rarely severe, at a level dependant on the site of the compression. Upper limb tendon reflexes may be increased or depressed depending on whether the pyramidal tracts or the anterior horn cells have been damaged. Long tract damage presents as a tendency to drag the feet, a sensation of the legs being too heavy with signs of ataxia and/or increased spasticity. There may also be anaesthesia or paraesthesia in the arms or the legs, and vibration and position sense loss may be the predominant feature.

Management of cervical spine disorders

The rehabilitation approach largely depends on the clinical features. For instance, a cervical collar may be helpful for radicular pain but may exacerbate symptoms of dizziness by limiting movement at the apophyseal joints.

In radiculopathy where pain is localized in the absence of other neurological symptoms, simple heat therapy sometimes helps to decrease the muscle spasm and allow gentle neck exercises. This can then be supplemented by the use of a cervical collar. Although, theo-retically, a rigid plastic collar which holds the chin in a cup and extends over the upper part of the chest and back is required to immobilize the neck, it is rare to find an elderly person who will wear this unless symptoms are severe and the relief dramatic. In practice a 'Plastazote' collar is sufficient to give some support, and the heat retention helps to relieve the muscle spasm, providing symptomatic relief.

It must be recognized that a collar is uncomfortable, and so it is reasonable to advise the patient that the important times to wear it are when carrying out household duties or when out walking. It is common to find that the patient has been advised to wear the collar day and night. This is usually counterproductive by decreasing compliance. It is acceptable to suggest that it can be removed during rest periods and in bed.

In severe cases bed rest or even traction may be necessary; but, in general, traction, collars, shortwave diathermy or exercise do not seem to influence the natural history of acute neck pain [27, 28], though they do provide temporary symptomatic relief.

Traction has certain disadvantages and side effects. It has been noted that some obese patients tended to faint during traction [29], and this may have been due to the pressure on the chest from the traction harness. It is also recorded in both normal healthy young people [30] and in patients [31] that ventilatory function can be compromised. Care should be taken with patients who have respiratory problems.

It is not too clear why traction works. Although the disc space does increase on X-ray examination during traction [32, 33], there is no evidence that the pressure within the disc is affected; and it may actually rise [34], probably owing to reflex muscle activity during traction.

Excessive activity of the arms which may increase the compressive forces should be avoided: lifting heavy shopping bags or digging in the garden are examples.

Where there is obvious evidence of myelopathy a surgical opinion should be sought. Acute herniation of an intervertebral cervical disc is uncommon in the elderly, but requires immobilization of the neck to reduce the pressure on the disc. This will mean the patient either lying flat in bed, or sitting with the head supported in a rigid cervical brace or even traction. A slight degree of neck flexion is preferred since the anteroposterior diameter of the spinal canal is decreased in neck extension. In general, surgical intervention will not be required. Indeed, elderly patients do not seem to respond well to surgical intervention, especially laminectomy [35]. Anterior interbody fusion may give better results [35, 36], although there are doubts as to whether even this produces better results than conservative treatment [37].

In the more chronic form of cervical myelopathy, neck support with a well-fitting cervical collar decreases the symptoms and possibly slows down the progress of the disease [38]. About 50 per cent of patients will improve symptomatically without any form of treatment [39].

The dorsal spine

Spondylosis is common but rarely produces pain. When pain does occur it is usually localized and can be produced by percussion or rotating the upper trunk with the hips kept still. Vertebral body collapse is most common in the mid- or low-thoracic regions.

Metastatic or myelomatous deposits are another possibility. Lesions in the dorsolumbar spine result in five characteristic features [40]:

1. *The 'iliac crest point' sign.* Pain and deep tenderness is detected over the iliac crest at a point that corresponds to the cutaneous emergence of the posterior branches of the affected spinal nerves.
2. *Thickening and hypersensitivity of the skin and subcutaneous tissues of the gluteal and iliac crest region.* This may be noted when a fold of the skin and subcutaneous tissues is gently rolled between the thumb and forefinger. The non-affected side can be used for comparison, but it is a difficult sign to elicit in obese patients.
3. *Local signs in the thoracolumbar region.* When pressure is applied vertically and tangentially on the spinous processes in turn, tenderness is detected on reaching the involved segment.
4. *Tenderness of the apophyseal joints.* Tenderness can be elicited by deep palpation over these joints.
5. *Diagnostic block.* Injecting local anaesthetic into the suspected apophyseal joint results in pain relief.

The lumbar spine

As many as 60 per cent of males and 44 per cent of females over the age of 35 years have radiological evidence of lumbar spinal degeneration [2]. In middle age there is a tendency for various combinations of degenerative abnormalities to occur in the annulus and/or nucleus of the intervertebral disc. In the younger person the fluidity of the nucleus pulposus supported by an elastic annular fibrosus allows the vertical forces to be transmitted into horizontal forces without damage being produced. With advancing age collagen precipitates within the nucleus and the annulus loses its elasticity, so that the disc becomes a fibrous mass. Vertical forces are then no longer diffused without producing outward bulging of the disc [41]. Changes in the vertebral bodies result in them losing height and increasing in breadth [42].

These changes eventually result in increased hypermobility of the spine which, with degeneration of the facet joints and the intervertebral disc, lead to further narrowing of the spinal canal. To some extent the decrease in lordosis compensates for the degenerative changes.

Osteoporosis

Osteoporosis increases with advancing age and is especially marked in women, although because women have less bone in middle age the proportional loss of bone is greater in elderly men [43]. Osteoporosis, especially affecting the trabecular bone, is a common cause of compression fractures of the lower thoracic and upper lumbar vertebrae [43], and spontaneous fractures of the sacrum have also been reported [44].

The medical treatment of osteoporosis is still controversial. Nordin [43], with his vast experience, believes that further deterioration can be prevented and the vertebral fracture rate decreased [45] by calcium replacement and treatment with norethistone 5 mg daily if there is evidence of rapid bone absorption in an elderly woman and vitamin D if there is evidence of malabsorption.

Lumbar spinal stenosis

In spinal stenosis the anterior, posterior and lateral dimensions of the spinal canal are narrower than normal, with associated abnormality of the shape of the canal. When the narrowing is severe there is compression of the cauda equina. Although there is a developmental form, most cases in the elderly are associated with osteoarthritis of the spine and are most marked opposite the intervertebral discs and the posterior articular process. In this case the stenosis is often segmental, with normal dimensions between the stenotic areas. Other causes include Paget's disease [46] and spondylolisthesis.

Symptoms vary according to the level and the severity of the stenosis. The most commonly reported feature is intermittent claudication due to cauda equina compression [47–56]. Other symptoms are radiculitis [56], and back or leg pain which may be constant or intermittent. The characteristic pain is one which comes on shortly after walking but which is relieved after a while by rest and is sometimes associated with paraesthesia and occasionally weakness. It is also thought that this might be one of the causes of 'drop attack'. Straight leg raising, though limited, is not as markedly affected as with disc lesions. Sensory abnormalities are variable and there are often abnormal reflexes in the legs.

The rehabilitation programme is similar to that for backache (see below). If the pain is severe or muscle weakness occurs, then a surgical approach should be considered, though even this may not relieve the symptoms entirely.

Back pain

Back pain is so common that 50–80 per cent of people suffer from it at some stage in life [57–61]. The prevalance increases with advancing age in women but is almost constant from the age of 30 in men [62].

According to a prospective study by Biering-Sorensen [63], the associated clinical features of backache for people in their sixties are (figures in per cent) disturbed sleep (males 31, females 40); and pain aggravated by sitting (males 18, females 47), standing (males 19, females 28) or stooping (males 61, females 70). Lying down aggravated the pain in 13 per cent of men and 21 per cent of women but was also one of the commonest relieving factors (men 40, women 51). It is also of note that one-half of the women and one-third of the men found that walking eased the pain. One other aggravating factor, which is not commonly recognized, was the pain on bowel movement (males 12, females 20).

Causes of back pain

The potential causes of back pain include not only disorders of the vertebral column and supporting structures, but also lesions within the spinal canal or thoracic and abdominal cavities. This complicates finding a satisfactory treatment for 'backache'.

Non-specific cases

Most cases of back pain in the elderly fall into a group where there are no specific X-ray or laboratory test findings. About 50 per cent of these patients have symptoms relating to one iliac crest, and the symptoms can be abolished by injecting the posterior iliac crest with a local anaesthetic [64]; this is the 'iliolumbar syndrome'. Similar relief of pain has been produced by injecting facet joints [65].

Sacroiliac pain can be tested for by 'springing' the sacroiliac joints by pressing the iliac crests inwards, or pressing downwards on the superior iliac spines, when the patient is lying supine; or by pressing down on the sacrum when the patient is lying prone. Pain felt in the sacroiliac joints indicates inflammation of the joint. It must be noted that pain and tenderness over the iliac crest on superficial palpation may be due to lesions in the dorsolumbar area [40].

Spondylosis

On examination there is a decrease in the normal lumbar curve and marked limitation of movement in all directions. There may be associated radicular pain, producing sciatica owing to osteophyte compression of the nerve roots. Compression of the nerves produces para-esthesia whereas inflammation results in pain on movement.

Disc herniatation

This produces pain which to some extent is limited by the size of the spinal canal – the smaller the canal the earlier the pain will be produced.

It is not unusual for higher lumbar discs to be involved in the elderly, producing pain in the groin or anterior thigh which may be interpreted as being due to hip involvement. The femoral nerve stretch test, in which pain is felt in the front of the thigh when the knee is flexed with the patient lying prone, helps to differentiate. The pain usually settles with a few days of bed rest. It is rare to require traction. Even in younger patients only about 5 per cent of those treated conservatively eventually required laminectomy [66].

Epidural injection of methyl prednisolone can have dramatic results [67], though the technique may be difficult in the elderly owing to osteoarthritis.

Spondylolisthesis

A corset is usually sufficient to treat the symptoms. Where this fails, surgical spinal fusion may be required.

Muscle or ligament damage

Pain from muscles or ligaments may produce symptoms similar to that of disc prolapse [68]. This can be seen from the experimental injection of hypertonic saline into ligaments, a joint capsule, periosteum or annulus, which results in a deep, ill-defined ache that may be referred to the buttocks, sacroiliac area or legs [65, 68].

Crush fracture of a vertebral body

This is usually due to osteoporosis but may occur secondary to a neoplastic deposit. Osteoporotic collapse is responsible for 45 per cent of the non-malignant causes of backache, occurring most frequently in the lower thoracic vertebrae [69], whereas disc degeneration is the commonest predisposing cause in the lumbar region.

Tumours

A spinal tumour is suggested by pain that is worse on lying down and improved by sitting up, although often the pain is constant and not influenced by movement.

Spinal stenosis

This produces intermittent claudication of cauda equina.

Paget's disease

This usually presents with pain of a deep boring nature.

Other mechanisms have been suggested for backache, such as irritation by acidic materials from degenerating disc [70], intraosseous hypertension or genetic factors.

Diagnostic pointers

There are several pointers which may give some clue as to the cause of the pain.

Onset

The majority of spinal conditions result in pain with a gradual onset. Acute onset after unaccustomed exertion or after trauma suggests a prolapse of an intervertebral disc or a crush fracture of the body of a vertebra.

Site

Crush fractures are most common in the mid or low-thoracic region. Spondylotic pain is most common at the lumbar concavity (L4–S1 region), although it can be quite widely spread from T10 to L5 secondary to disc degeneration [71]. Disc prolapse is most common in the 7th thoracic disc in females and 8th in males [2], though L3/4 disc is also commonly affected.

Pain characteristics

The commonest pain is a constant ache which is generally associated with chronic pathology of a degenerative nature. Stabbing pain is more related to acute conditions like disc prolapse or crush fracture. Deep, boring pain is more characteristic of bone disorders than articular lesions and is suggestive of underlying neoplastic disease or Paget's disease.

Radiation

Radiation of pain usually implies nerve root involvement, the site depending on the level of the lesion.

Effect of movement

Most back pains are made worse by movement and relieved by rest. Pain that is worse at rest suggests either ankylosing spondylitis or malignancy.

Range of movement

Patients with degenerative lesions have marked limitation of flexion and extension movements but lateral movement is less involved. In inflammatory lesions lateral movements tend to be affected early.

Management of back pain

Nearly all descriptions of the management of back pain, and certainly most of the research, has been carried out on young or middle-aged patients. It is not always possible to extrapolate from these studies for the management of the elderly, where work and sexual activities play a much smaller part and the psychological overlay of back pain is less predominant. Many of the recognized techniques such as traction, manipulation and exercises are not acceptable to the frail elderly person.

One of the problems is that the patient is primarily concerned with the symptoms. If the pain is relieved by analgesia many patients seems less interested in preventing further damage by means of unattractive exercises, control of sitting posture and environmental changes.

The vast majority of back pains settle within a few days and do not require medical intervention. For more persistent pain simple analgesia and heat therapy may be all that is required [72]. For very persistent pain admission to hospital is required, especially for those living alone. The simple process of admitting into a caring environment has amazing effects on backache even before analgesics or physiotherapy have been started. Part of this may be due to the psychological relief that something is 'being done', but it may also be due to the decrease in work which has to be done and the firmer hospital beds.

A number of simple approaches can be used. Normally a firm mattress on the bed is sufficient to provide support, but some patients benefit from lying on a bead pillow mattress (see Chapter 3) which allows firmer support to be provided under the lumbar spine.

Lying supine produces the least pressure in the lumbar discs, while there is a slight increase when lying in the lateral position. The pressure is also higher when sitting, especially in a flexed position, than when standing erect [73]. Certainly in younger patients there is evidence from a controlled trial that bed rest is more effective than remaining ambulatory [74]. The position which seems to give optimal relief for many patients is lying flat with only one pillow under the head (to discourage flexion of the spine) and one under the knees (to tilt the pelvis).

The philosophy of a hard mattress need not be adhered to rigorously since some patients cannot tolerate a very firm surface, though most seem to gain some benefit. Although the more rigid support is probably helpful in lesions affecting L5 or S1 by producing a decrease in tension on the nerve roots [75], flexion will produce less stretch on the L2 or L3 roots and therefore a softer bed may be more comfortable.

Since prolonged bed rest has major disadvantages in the elderly, the patient should be allowed up for short periods during the day, and certainly to use the toilet – there is no place for a bedpan for the patient with back pain. Some patients gain comfort from lying on the floor with the hips and knees at right angles supported on a chair.

The role of traction is also debatable. It is difficult to imagine displaced material becoming realigned, though it may help inflammation to settle. However, research evidence does not provide support for the benefit of traction [76, 77].

Standing from a chair can be difficult. If the chair has no arms then the patient may find it easiest to stand with one leg in front, and the other at the side, of the seat and push up with the hands on the seat.

Others benefit, for both lying and sitting, from being splinted in a simple vacuum posture controller (see Chapter 3) which maintains a more reasonable alignment of the lumbar spine.

It is often assumed that weak trunk flexor muscles [73], extensor muscles [78, 79] or both groups of muscles [78, 80] add to the problems of spinal dysfunction, though there is little evidence that strengthening the muscles prevents further pain [81].

Traditionally exercises fall into three groups: strengthening of the paravertebral muscles (extension exercises), 'mobilizing exercises' which are predominantly flexion in nature, and isometric contraction of abdominal muscle to increase the intra-abdominal pressure, thereby splinting the spine.

There are several schools of thought on approaches to the physiotherapy of back pain. Some regard the pain as being due to deviations in the normal posture of the spine and therefore advocate flexion exercises to obtain a 'flat' back [82]. Others believe that the lumbar lordosis prevents disc protrusion and advocate manipulation and mobilization of the joints [83]. Studies of different approaches have been unable to show statistically significant differences between various exercise programmes [84–86], or that physiotherapy is any better than placebo in improving muscle strength or spinal mobility in patients with back pain [87].

Some physiotherapists use heat and other modalities to decrease the muscle spasm and 'tension' in the spinal muscles which they claim is producing the pain. Their view has been supported by the finding that electromyographic activity of the back muscle was higher in back-pain sufferers than in those without back pain while both groups underwent stressful situations [88]. However, in another study back-pain sufferers showed greater paralumbar tension during relaxation training than did those without back pain [89]. This latter study has been challenged on the grounds that the technique of electromyographic recording was likely to produce erroneous results: from their own study Kravitz *et al.* [90] could find no difference in the resting electromyographic recordings between those with and those without back pain. This may be significant when considering the role of relaxation therapy in lower back pain. On the other hand, heat can reduce muscle spasm [91], and this may account for some of the pain relief from ultrasound or other heat modalities.

Other methods of value, in addition to analgesics, are simple exercises, heat treatment and lumbar support in a corset, all of which have some contribution to play with none being superior to the others [92]. Doran and Newill's trial was on middle-age back-pain sufferers. Manipulation sometimes produced quick results but there was no way of identifying in advance those patients who would benefit. Corsets were slower but the long-term effects were equally good. Analgesia on its own was less effective than when combined with physiotherapy.

The role of other modalities is uncertain. A number of studies have suggested that physiotherapy does not influence the clinical course of backache [84, 93, 94]. In younger patients back extension exercises are less effective than those which build up abdominal muscle tone [95], especially when combined with intermittent traction [96], which supports the theory that weak abdominal muscles are an important contributory cause of back pain. Lidstrom and Zachrisson [96] compared 'conventional' treatment (mobilization and strengthening exercises along with heat and massage) with 'alternative' therapy (intermittent pelvic traction and isometric exercises) and found that there was no statistically significant difference between the two forms of treatment.

The effectiveness of modalities such as transcutaneous nerve stimulation [97], acupuncture [98] and heat is still doubtful. Other treatments such as electrotherapy, electromassage, deep manual massage or ethyl-chloride sprays, although commonly used, especially in the United States, do not seem to have been submitted to adequate research analysis.

In general it seems that most forms of therapy are used because at least some patients benefit symptomatically, but there is little evidence that any is more effective than another [77, 92, 99].

Advice about the type of chair is important. No sitting position can produce the degree of lumbar lordosis present in standing [100]. Indeed, sitting is more often an aggravating than a relieving factor in backache [63]. A sitting trunk – thigh angle of 135° is required to produce a near-normal lordosis and this is difficult to achieve in the elderly. The best compromise is to provide a firm support behind the lumbar curve.

Surgical corsets

The role of lumbar support by a surgical corset is uncertain. It is thought that by compensating for the weak abdominal musculature there is an increase in the efficiency of the thoracic and abdominal cavities to support and extend the spine [101]; that is, some of the stresses are transmitted through the abdominal contents rather than through the vertebral column, which seems to be important especially during activity. Theoretically, compression of the abdominal contents helps to splint the lumbar spine by increasing intra-abdominal pressure. The evidence for this is conflicting, with some studies showing that it does [102] and others that it does not [103, 104].

It has been suggested that spinal supports act by decreasing movement of intervertebral joints, raising the intra-abdominal pressure, decreasing the lumbar lordosis, providing psychological support, providing heat and encouraging muscle relaxation [105]. Rigid braces actually seem to increase the movement at the lumbar–sacral segment [106, 107]. Corsets do, however, seem to decrease the pressure within the intervertebral disc by about 30 per cent [108] although only in some exercises such as extension or holding weights, whereas pressure is increased in flexion [104]. They do not immobilize the spine in the lumbar, sacral region (106). Forces from the corsets are concentrated at or near the thoracolumbar junction; in some patients lumbar–sacral flexion was greater with than without the brace. Similar findings have been found for the limitation of rotation at the lumbar–sacral level [109] and for electrical activity of the trunk muscles [105] (and therefore muscle effort), although corsets do not seem to alter the myoelectric activity during walking [105].

Ideally the lumbar support should:

- have metal ribs which support the normal lumbar lordosis;
- be long enough posteriorly to splint from the lower thoracic region to the sacrum;
- have a lower abdomen compression support;
- be fastened tightly;
- he specially designed for the individual patient.

These characteristics make it uncomfortable and difficult to put on for many elderly people. Experience shows that many elderly people gain sufficient relief from a temporary elasticated 'pull-on' corset. It has also been suggested that a broad belt with a lumbar pad or roll can give some degree of comfort by encouraging better maintenance of the lumbar lordosis [104], although this has not been tested on the elderly.

One of the problems with a surgical corset is the physical effort required to fasten it tight enough to be effective. This often proves to be a great stumbling block for elderly people, especially those living alone. There is also the danger that splinting for too long will result in disuse atrophy.

Precautionary note for staff

Management of the elderly disabled often induces backache in the carers [111], including nursing staff and therapists. It is therefore important to ensure that all carers know the appropriate techniques for transferring and lifting disabled people. All staff should be taught the techniques of personal back care, including the use of hoists and the wearing of elasticated supports when involved in moving heavy patients.

Trousers and tunics instead of dresses allow greater freedom of movement.

References

1. Mikklesen, E.M., Duff, I.F. and Dodge, H.J. (1970) Age-specific prevalence of radiographic abnormalities of the joints of hands, wrist and cervical spine of adult residents of Tecumseh. *Journal of Chronic Disease* **23**: 151-9.
2. Lawrence, J.S., De Graffe, R. and Laine, V.A.I. (1963) Degenerative joint disease in random samples and occupational groups. In: *The Epidemiology of Chronic Rheumatism*, Vol.1, p. 98 (Eds: Kellgren. J.H., Jeffrey, M.R. and Ball, J.). Blackwell Scientific Publications, Oxford.
3. Pallis, C.A., Jones, A.M. and Spillane, J.D. (1954) Cervical spondylosis. *Brain* **77**: 274-89.
4. Adams, K.R.H., Yung, M.W., Lye, M. and Whitehouse, G.H. (1986) Are cervical spine radiographs of value in elderly patients with vertebrobasilar insufficiency? *Age and Ageing* **15**: 57-9.
5. Frykholm, R.J. (1947) Deformities of dural pouches and strictures of dural sheaths in cervical region producing nerve-root compression: contribution to

etiology and operative treatment of brachial neuralgia. *Journal of Neurosurgery* **4**: 403–13.

6. Verbiest, H. (1973) The management of cervical spondylosis. *Clinical Neurosurgery* **20**: 262–94.

7. Sheehan, S., Bauber, R.B. and Meyer, J.S. (1960) Vertebral artery compression in cervical spondylosis: arteriographical demonstration during life of vertebral artery insufficiency due to rotation and extension of the neck. *Neurology* **10**: 968–86.

8. Williams, D. and Wilson, T.G. (1962) The diagnosis of major and minor syndromes of basilar insufficiency. *Brain* **85**: 741–74.

9. Kubala, M.J. and Millikan, C.H. (1964) Diagnosis, pathogenesis and treatment of 'drop attacks'. *Archives of Neurology* **11**: 107–13.

10. Kameyama, M. (1965) Vertigo and drop attacks: with special reference to cerebrovascular disorders and atherosclerosis of the vertebrobasilar systems. *Geriatrics* **20**: 892–900.

11. De Jong, P.T.V.M., De Jong, J.M.B.V., Cohen, B. and Jongkees, L.B.W. (1977) Ataxia and nystagmus induced by injection of local anaesthetics in the neck. *Annals of Neurology* **1**: 240–6.

12. Wyke, B.D. (1979) Cervical articular contributions to posture and gait: their relation to senile disequilibrium. *Age and Ageing* **8**: 251–8.

13. Sudarsky, L. and Ronthal, M. (1983) Gait disorders among elderly patients. *Archives of Neurology* **40**: 740–3.

14. Peterson, D.I. and Dayes, L.A. (1977) Myelopathy associated with cervical spondylosis. *Journal of Family Practice* **4**: 233–6.

15. Adornato, B.T. and Glasberg, M.R. (1980) Diseases of the spinal cord. In: *Neurology Science and Practice of Clinical Medicine*, Vol. 5, pp. 392–433 (Ed: Rosenberg, R.N. Grune and Strattin, New York).

16. Murkami, N., Muroga, T. and Sobue, I. (1978) Cervical myelopathy due to ossification of the posterior longitudinal ligament: a clinical study. *Archives of Neurology* **35**: 33–6.

17. Hanai, K., Adachi, H. and Ogasawara, H. (1977) Axial transverse tomography of the cervical spine narrowed by ossification of the posterior longitudinal ligament. *Journal of Bone and Joint Surgery* **59B**: 481–4.

18. Stoops, W.L. and King, R.B. (1962) Neural complications of cervical spondylosis, their response to laminectomy and foramenotomy. *Journal of Neurosurgery* **19**: 986–99.

19. Epstein, J.A., Carras, R., Epstein, B.S. and Levine, L.S. (1970) Myelopathy in cervical spondylosis with vertebral subluxation and hyperlordosis. *Journal of Neurosurgery* **32**: 421–6.

20. Ball, J. and Sharp, J. (1971) Rheumatoid arthritis of the cervical spine. In: *Modern Trends in Rheumatology*, Vol. 2, pp. 117–38. Butterworths, London.

21. Boyle, A.C. (1971) The rheumatoid neck. *Proceedings of the Royal Society of Medicine* **64**: 1161–5.

22. Bland, J.H. (1974) Rheumatoid arthritis of the cervical spine. *Journal of Rheumatology* **1**: 319–41.

23. Cabot, A. and Becker, A. (1978) The cervical spine in rheumatoid arthritis. *Clinical Orthopaedics* **131**: 130–40.

24. Park, W.M., O'Neill, M.O. and McCall, I.V. (1979) The radiology of rheumatoid involvement of the cervical spine. *Skeletal Radiology* **4**: 1–7.

25. Gibson, T. and Schumacher, H.R. (1976) Ankylosing hyperostosis with cervical cord compression. *Rheumatology and Rehabilitation* **15**: 67–70.

26. Epstein, J.A., Epstein, B.S., Levine, L.S. and Carras, R. (1978) Cervical

myeloradiculopathy caused by arthrotic hypertrophy of the posterior facets and laminae. *Journal of Neurosurgery* **49**: 387–92.
27. British Association of Physical Medicine (1966) Pain in the neck and arm: a multicentre trial of the effects of physiotherapy. *British Medical Journal* **1**: 253–8.
28. Goldie, I. and Lanquist, A. (1970) Evaluation of the effects of different forms of physiotherapy in cervical pain. *Scandinavian Journal of Rehabilitation Medicine* **2**: 117–21.
29. Lehmann, J.F. and Brunner, B.S. (1958) A device for application of heavy lumbar traction: its mechanical effects. *Archives of Physical Medicine and Rehabilitation* **39**: 696–700.
30. Quain, M.B. and Tecklin, J.S. (1985) Lumbar traction: its effects on respiration. *Physical Therapy* **65**: 1343–6.
31. Scott, B.O. (1955) A universal traction frame and lumbar harness. *Annals of Physical Medicine* **2**: 258–60.
32. Goldie, I.F. and Reichmann, S. (1977) The biomechanical influence of traction on the cervical spine. *Scandinavian Journal of Rehabilitation Medicine* **9**: 31–4.
33. Gupta, R.C. and Ramarad, S.V. (1978) Epidurography in reduction of lumbar disc prolapse by traction. *Archives of Physical Medicine* **59**: 322–7.
34. Anderson, G.B.J., Schultz, A.B. and Nachemson, A.L. (1983) Intervertebral disc pressure during traction. *Scandinavian Journal of Rehabilitation Medicine* **Suppl.9**: 88–91.
35. Gregorius, F.K., Estrin, T. and Crandall, P.H. (1976) Cervical spondylotic radiculopathy and myelopathy. *Archives of Neurology* **53**: 618–25.
36. Crandall, P.H. and Batzdorf, U. (1966) Cervical spondylotic myelopathy. *Journal of Neurosurgery* **25**: 57–66.
37. Lunsford, L.C., Bissionette, P.A.C. and Zorub, D.S. (1980) Anterior surgery for disc disease. 2: Treatment of cervical spondylotic myelopathy in 32 cases. *Journal of Neurosurgery* **53**: 12–19.
38. Wilkinson, M. (1976) The clinical aspects of myelopathy due to cervical spondylosis. *Acta Neurologica Belgium* **76**: 276–8.
39. Less, F. and Turner, J.W. (1963) Natural history and prognosis of cervical spondylosis. *British Medical Journal* **i**: 1607–10.
40. Maigne, R. (1980) Low back pain of thoracolumbar origin. *Archives of Physical Medicine and Rehabilitation* **61**: 389–95.
41. Kieffer, S.A., Stadlan, E.M., Mohandas, A. *et al.* (1969) Discographic–anatomical correlation of developmental changes with age in the intervertebral disc. *Acta Radiological Diagnosis* **9**: 733–9.
42. Vernon-Roberts, B. and Perie, C.J. (1977) Degenerative changes in the intervertebral discs of the lumbar spine and their sequelae. *Rheumatology and Rehabilitation* **16**: 13–21.
43. Nordin, B.E.C. (1983) Osteoporosis. In: *Bone and Joint Disease in the Elderly* (Ed: Wright, V.). Churchill Livingstone, Edinburgh.
44. Lourie, H. (1982) Spontaneous osteoporotic fracture of the sacrum: an unrecognised syndrome in the elderly. *Journal of the American Medical Assocation* **248**: 715–7.
45. Nordin, B.E.C., Horsman, A., Crilly, R.G. *et al.* (1980) Treatment of spinal osteoporosis in post-menopausal women. *British Medical Journal* **280**: 451–4.
46. Sadar, E.S., Walton, R.J. and Gossman, H.H. (1972) Neurological dysfunction in Paget's disease of the vertebral column. *Journal of Neurosurgery* **37**: 661–5.
47. Blau, J.N. and Logue, V. (1961) Intermittent claudication of the cauda equina. *Lancet* **i**: 1071–86.

48. MacNab, I. (1971) Negative disc exploration. *Journal of Bone and Joint Surgery* **3A**: 891–903.
49. Brish, A., Lerner, M.B. and Braham, J. (1964) Intermittent claudication from compression of the cauda equina by a narrowed spinal canal. *Journal of Neurosurgery* **21**: 207–11.
50. Cooke, T.D.V. and Lehmann, P. (1968) Intermittent claudication of neurogenic origin. *Canadian Journal of Surgery* **11**: 151–9.
51. Evans, J.G. (1964) Neurogenic intermittent claudication. *British Medical Journal* **2**: 985–7.
52. Joffe, R., Appleby, A. and Arjona, V. (1966) Intermittent ischaemia of the cauda equina due to stenosis of the lumbar canal. *Journal of Neurology, Neurosurgery and Psychiatry* **29**: 315–8.
53. Kavanaugh, G.J., Svien, H.J., Holman, C.B. and Johnson, R.M. (1968) 'Pseudoclaudication' syndrome produced by compression of the cauda equina. *Journal of The American Medical Association* **206**: 2477–81.
54. Silver, R.A., Schude, H.L., Stack, J.K., Conn, J. and Bergan, J.J. (1969) Intermittent claudication of neurospinal origin. *Archives of Surgery* **98**: 523–9.
55. Spanos, N.C. and Andrew, J. (1966) Intermittent claudication and lateral lumbar disc protrusions. *Journal of Neurology, Neurosurgery and Psychiatry* **29**: 273–7.
56. Munro, D. (1956) Lumbar and sacral compression radiculitis. *New England Journal of Medicine* **254**: 243–52.
57. Hult, L. (1954) The Munkfors investigation. *Acta Orthopaedica Scandinavica* **Suppl. 16**: 1–76.
58. Nachemson, A. (1971) Low back pain, its etiology and treatment. *Clinical Medicine* **7–8**: 18–24.
59. Chaffin, D.B. and Park, K.S. (1973) A longitudinal study of low back pain as associated with occupational weight-lifting factors. *American Industrial Hygiene Association Journal* **34**: 513–24.
60. White, A.A. and Gordon, S.L. (1982) Synopsis: Workshop on indiopathic low back pain. *Spine* **7**: 141–9.
61. Deyo, R.A. (1983) Conservative treatment for low back pain. *Journal of the American Medical Association* **250**: 1057–62.
62. Biering-Sorensen, F. (1983) A prospective study of low back pain in a general population. I: Occurrence, recurrence and aetiology. *Scandinavian Journal of Rehabilitation Medicine* **15**: 71–9.
63. Biering-Sorensen, F. (1983) A prospective study of low back pain in a general population. II: Location, character, aggravating and relieving factors. *Scandinavian Journal of Rehabilitation Medicine* **15**: 81–8.
64. Hirschberg, G.G., Froetscher, L. and Naeim, F. (1979) Iliolumbar syndrome as a common cause of low back pain: Diagnosis and prognosis. *Archives of Physical Medicine and Rehabilitation* **60**: 415–19.
65. Mooney, V. and Robertson, J. (1976) The facet syndrome. *Clinical Orthopaedics* **115**: 149–56.
66. Johnson, E.W. and Fletcher, F.R. (1981) Lumbosacral radiculopathy: Review of 100 consecutive cases. *Archives of Physical Medicine and Rehabilitation* **62**: 321–3.
67. Dilke, T.F.W., Burry, H.C. and Grahame, R. (1973) Extradural corticosteroid injection in the management of lumbar nerve root compression. *British Medical Journal* **2**: 635.
68. Kellgren, J.H. (1977) The anatomical source of back pain. *Rheumatology and Rehabilitation* **16**: 3–12.

82   *Spinal conditions*

69. Fornasier, V.L. and Czitrom, A.A. (1978) Collapsed vertebrae: a review of 659 autopsies. *Clinical Orthopaedias* **131**: 261–5.
70. Nachemson, A. (1969) Intradisc measurement of pH in patients with lumbar rhizopathies. *Acta Orthopaedica Scandinavica* **40**: 23–42.
71. Lawrence, J.S. (1969) Disc degeneration: its frequency and relationship to symptoms. *Annals of Rheumatic Diseases* **28**: 121–38.
72. Dillane, J.B., Fry, J. and Kalton, G. (1966) Acute back syndrome – a study from general practice. *British Medical Journal* **2**: 82–4.
73. Nachemson, A. (1975) Towards a better understanding of low back pain: a review of the mechanics of the lumbar disc. *Rheumatology and Rehabilitation* **14**: 129–43.
74. Wiesel, S.W. and Rothman, R.H. (1980) Acute low back pain: an objective analysis of conservative therapy. *Spine* **5**: 324–30.
75. Charnley, J. (1951) Orthopaedic signs in the diagnosis of disc protrusion with special reference to straight leg raising. *Lancet* **1**: 186–92.
76. Matthews, J.A. (1968) Dynamic discography: a study of lumbar traction. *Annals of Physical Medicine* **9**: 275–80.
77. Matthews, J.A. and Hickling, J. (1975) Lumbar traction: a double blind controlled study of sciatica. *Rheumatology and Rehabilitation* **14**: 222–5.
78. Nordgren, B., Schele, R. and Lindroth, K. (1980) Evaluation and prediction of back pain during military field service. *Scandinavian Journal of Rehabilitation Medicine* **12**: 1–8.
79. McNeill, T., Warwick, D., Andersson, G. and Shultz, A. (1980) Trunk strengths in attempted flexion, extension and lateral bending in healthy subjects and patients with low-back disorders. *Spine* **5**: 529–38.
80. Alston, W., Carlson, K.E., Feldman, D.J., Grimm, Z. and Gerontinos, E. (1966) A quantitative study of muscle factors in chronic low back syndrome. *Journal of American Geriatrics Society* **14**: 1041–7.
81. Reynolds, P.M.G. (1975) Measurement of spinal mobility: a comparison of three methods. *Rheumatology and Rehabilitation* **14**: 180–5.
82. Cailliet, R. (1971) In: *Low Back Pain Syndrome*, 2nd Edn. F.A. Davis Co., Philadelphia.
83. Cyriax, J. (1975) *Textbook of Orthopaedic Medicine* Vol. 1: *Diagnosis of Soft Tissue Lesions*, 6th Edn. Williams and Wilkins, Baltimore.
84. Glover, J.R., Morris, J.G. and Khosla, T. (1974) Back pain: a randomized clinical trial of rotational manipulation of the trunk. *British Journal of Industrial Medicine* **31**: 59–64.
85. Rohinger, C. (1963) Pilot study on low back pain. *Journal of Canadian Physiotherapy Association* **15**: 16–18.
86. Zylbergold, R.S. and Piper, M.C. (1981) Lumbar disc disease: comparative analysis of physical therapy treatments. *Archives of Physical Medicine and Rehabilitation* **62**: 176–9.
87. Martin, P.R., Rose, M.J., Nicholas, P.J.R. *et al.* (1986) Physiotherapy exercises for low back pain: process and clinical outcome. *International Rehabilitation Medicine* **8**: 34–8.
88. Holmes, T.H. and Wolff, H.G. (1952) Life situations, emotions, and backache. *Psychosomatic Medicine* **14**: 18–33.
89. Grabel, J.A. (1973) Electromyographic study of low back muscle tension in subjects with and without chronic low back pain. *Dissertation Abstracts International* **34B**: 2929-B.
90. Kravitz, E., Moore, M.E. and Glaros, A. (1981) Paralumbar muscle activity in chronic low back pain. *Archives of Physical Medicine and Rehabilitation* **62**: 172–6.

91. Fountain, F.P., Gersten, J.W. and Sengir, O. (1960) Decrease in muscle spasm produced by ultrasound, hot packs and infra-red radiation. *Archives of Physical Medicine* **41**: 293-8.
92. Doran, D.M.I. and Newill, D.T. (1975) Manipulation in the treatment of low back pain: a multi-centre study. *British Medical Journal* **2**: 161-4.
93. White, A.W.M. (1969) Low back pain in men receiving workmen's compensation. *Canadian Medical Association Journal* **95**: 50-6.
94. Kane, R.L., Olsen, D., Leymaster, C., Woolley, F.R. and Fischer, F.D. (1974) Manipulating the patient: a comparison of the effectiveness of physician and chiropractor care. *Lancet*: **1**: 1333-6.
95. Kendall, P.H. and Jenkins, J.M. (1968) Exercises for backache: a double blind controlled trial. *Physiotherapy* **53**: 154-7.
96. Lidstrom, A. and Zachrisson, M. (1970) Physical therapy on low back pain and sciatica. *Scandinavian Journal of Rehabilitation Medicine* **2**: 37-42.
97. Thorsteinsson, G., Stonnington, H.H., Stillwell, G.K. and Elveback, L.R. (1977) Transcutaneous electrical stimulation: a double blind trial of efficiency in pain. *Archives of Physical Medicine and Rehabilitation* **58**: 8-13.
98. Edelist, G., Gross, A.E. and Langer, F. (1976) Treatment of low back pain with acupuncture. *Canadian Anaesthetics Society Journal* **23**: 303-7.
99. Sims-Williams, H., Jayson, M.I.V., Young, S.M. *et al.* (1978) Controlled trial of mobilisation and manipulation for patients with low back pain in general practice. *British Medical Journal* **2**: 1333-40.
100. Keegan, J.J. (1953) Alterations of the lumbar curve related to posture and seating. *Journal of Bone and Joint Surgery* **35A**: 589-603.
101. Morris, J.M. (1974) Low back bracing. *Clinical Orthopaedics* **102**: 126-32.
102. Morris, J.M., Lucas, D.B. and Bresler, B. (1961) Role of the trunk in stability of the spine. *Journal of Bone and Joint Surgery* **43A**: 327-51.
103 Grew, N.D. and Deane, G. (1978) Lumbar spinal orthoses. *Oxford Orthopaedic Engineering Centre Annual Report*, 23-9.
104. Nachemson, A., Shultz, A. and Anderson, G. (1983) Mechanical effectiveness studies of lumbar spine orthoses. *Scandinavian Journal of Rehabilitation Medicine* **Suppl. 9**: 139-48.
105. Waters, R.L. and Morris, J.M. (1970) Effect of spinal supports on the electrical activity of muscles of the trunk. *Journal of Bone and Joint Surgery* **52-A**: 51-60.
106. Norton, P.L. and Brown, T. (1957) The immobilizing efficiency of back braces: Their effect on the posture and motion of the lumbosacral spine. *Journal of Bone and Joint Surgery* **39-A**: 111-39.
107. Lumsden, R.M. and Morris, J.M. (1968) An *in vivo* study of axial rotation and immobilization of the lumbar sacral joint. *Journal of Bone and Joint Surgery* **50-A**: 1591-1602.
108. Nachemson, A. and Morris, J.M. (1964) Lumbar discometry: lumbar intradisc pressure measurement *in vivo*. *Lancet* **i**: 1140-2.
109. Lumsden, R.M. and Morris, J.M. (1968) An *in vivo* study of axial rotation and immobilization at the lumbosacral joint. *Journal of Bone and Joint Surgery* **50-A**: 1591-1602.
110. Carabelli, R.A. (1986) Waistbelt lumbar sacral support. *Physical Therapy* **66**: 231-2.
111. Rawlins, S. (1983) How physios can prevent back pain in hospitals. *Remedial Therapist*, 3 June: 4.

6

Fracture of the neck of the femur

General features

Although fracture of the neck of the femur is usually regarded as an orthopaedic problem, in reality it is a surgical interlude in a medical problem: the patient has disorders which result in a fall which, in turn, results in a fracture. This may not always be the case, since there is some evidence that a few fractures occur spontaneously and produce falls [1-4]. In view of the large medical and social component it is appropriate that patients with fracture of the femur receive care from a surgeon and a physician.

As with most degenerative disorders the incidence of fracture of the hip increases with age, the rate after the age of 60 doubling every five years for women and seven years for men [5]. The incidence rates from four studies [1, 6-8] are shown in Table 6.1. In common with other studies [9-11], they show that the incidence in females is two to three times that in males, although there is a tendency for these to converge in very advanced age [6, 7]. This pattern is not universal, with a predominance of males with fracture of the femur occurring in Singapore [12] and Hong Kong [13].

For some reason the incidence of fracture of the femur seems to be rising [14], with a rate of increase of 6 per cent a year between 1970 and 1977 and 10 per cent thereafter. For women over 75 the incidence per thousand rose from 8 a year in 1971 to 16 a year in 1981. Other studies have been unable to confirm this trend [7, 15]. These figures must be taken into account when considering the demographic trend of further increases in the very old population over the next decade or so, since they are relevant to the organization of orthopaedic services. In Britain, for example, patients with fracture of the proximal femur occupy about half of the available orthopaedic beds [16, 17].

One finding that is difficult to explain is the predominance of left-sided fractures [13, 18]. Alffram [1] reported this laterality in 55 per cent of 1024 intracapsular fractures and 54 per cent of all hip fractures. Evans [19] pointed out that this was only true for men under 60,

Table 6.1 Incidence of fractures of the femoral neck by age and sex per 10 000 population

Age range	Alffram (1964) [1] M	F	Donaldson et al. (1979) [6] M	F	Evans (1979) [7] M	F	Kreutzfeldt (1984) [8] M	F
30–39	2	6	15	5				
40–44	8	5						
45–49	22	15	21	33				
50–54	51	23						
55–59	80	45						
60–64	150	67	70	170	100	160	90	170
65–69	280	104			160	360	260	590
70–74	491	257			250	660		
75–79	830	372	270	176	480	1190		
80–84	1577	565			1530	1980	840	1980
85–89			1120	1670				
90–94					2610	2470		
95+			*	5530				

and especially for those where the fracture was due to a road traffic accident; he suggested that the difference may be due to the dynamics of automobile accidents. The laterality could also be due to stronger bones developing from the predominant use of the right leg. Below the age of 60 years, experimentally, there is no difference between the two sides in the femoral neck resistance to compression force [20], though after this age one side is weaker (they did not say which). Virtama [21] has shown in active individuals (though not in the elderly with osteoporosis) that ash weights in bones are higher in the right than the left limbs.

The incidence of second fractures is about 7–10 per cent [22–24]. In a study of 500 patients admitted with fracture of the femoral neck, 10.6 per cent had had a second fracture, of which 38 per cent had occurred within one year of the original fracture [24]. It is also of note that 74 per cent of patients with recurrent fractures had originally sustained an intracapsular fracture, 58 per cent an intracapsular fracture on both occasions and 25 per cent extracapsular fractures on both occasions.

Classification

At the simplest level fracture of the femoral neck can be either intracapsular or extracapsular. Extracapsular fractures nearly always unite if there is correct surgical fixation. Intracapsular fractures are more vulnerable to avascular necrosis because of the disruption of the blood supply to the femoral head.

There is some confusion as to which is the more common site for the fracture. Some studies have reported that trochanteric fractures are more common than intracapsular fractures [25–27], with the frequency increasing with advancing age. However, others have found that cervical fractures are more common [28, 29], though patients with trochanteric fractures were significantly older than those with cervical fractures [25], had a longer length of stay in hospital and were less likely to return home.

Halpin and Nelson [30] classified patients into the following three groups according to the goals that are set:

1. For the bedridden group, pain relief and ease of nursing are the primary goals of treatment.
2. For semi-active patients who are not able to comply with the postoperative treatment regimes that require restricted weight bearing, the goal is to resume preoperative walking as soon as possible to prevent further deterioration.
3. With fully active, mentally alert patients with prolonged life expectations, the goal is to obtain union of the fracture without avascular necrosis to provide a pain-free hip.

Influencing factors

Osteoporosis

The rapid rise in the incidence of fractures with advancing age suggests that there is some weakening of the bone structure which makes it more likely to break under stress. There is increased prevalence of osteoporosis in elderly patients with fracture of the upper femur [31–33], and it has been suggested that there is a 'fracture threshold' for bone mass below which fracture risk increases [34]. However, Exton-Smith [35] found that, although the mean metacarpal/cortical bone ratios were lower in patients with fracture of the femur, there was a very wide scatter of values and many were in the high percentile range, suggesting that there is unlikely to be a single critical level for the fracture.

What is probably more important is the relationship of the bone mass to the forces it has to withstand. Thus, whether the bone fractures will depend on the weight of the patient and the type of fall or knock.

Osteomalacia

There is a very strong association between fractures and osteomalacia [36, 37]. About 40 per cent of men and 20–30 per cent of women with fracture of the femoral neck have osteomalacia on bone biopsy [32]. Even when the classical features of osteomalacia are absent, some studies have found an association between low vitamin D levels and a fractured femur [38, 39], although others have not [41, 42]. Some of the association may be related to the amount of sunshine since there is a positive correlation between latitude and hip fracture [43] (Jerusalem and Johannesburg are notable exceptions). However, there are likely to be many other variables which have an influence on these figures.

A relationship of osteomalacia to the site of the fracture is possible since patients with trochanteric fractures have significantly lower levels of 25-hydroxy vitamin D [44] and higher levels of metabolic bone disease [45] than do patients with cervical fractures. This may account for the seasonal variation of subcapital fractures, which have a peak in winter, whereas the intertrochanteric fractures occur at a constant rate throughout the year [37].

Injury

The commonest association with fracture of the femur is a fall, though the degree of trauma varies. Muckle [4] found that only 38 per cent of subcapital and 42 per cent of trochanter fractures occurred following a definite incident such as a fall from steps, a wall or a platform. In the other cases the leg suddenly 'gave way' while walking or turning. In Sheldon's study of falls, 12 per cent of patients sustained a fracture of the femur [46]. Both fracture of the femur and falls are common in old age but only a small proportion of falls result in a fracture. Brocklehurst *et al.* [22] found that, although a history of falls was obtained more often in the fractured femur group than in controls, this only reached statistically significant levels for those over the age of 85 years, of whom 70 per cent of the fracture group and 46 per cent of the controls had experienced falls in the previous year. Similarly, Baker [48] was unable to demonstrate a greater prevalence of falls in patients with fracture of the femur than in community controls.

Whatever the statistical relationship between the fracture group and controls, there is no doubt that some form of fall is strongly associated with fracture of the femur. In a study of 450 women with fracture of the femur, 71 per cent occurred within or near to the patient's home and a further 4 per cent were residents in old persons' homes [2]. The commonest falls (46 per cent) were due to trips, stumbles, slips or overbalancing; 16 per cent were due to drop attacks; 13 per cent to accidents associated with chairs or beds; and only 8 per cent to giddiness.

The high association with institutional care [2, 48, 49] suggests that general frailty plays a major role for both the fall and the tendency to fracture.

Associated diseases and disorders

Most studies have found a large number of concurrent medical problems associated with fracture of the femur [2, 50–53], with only one-third of patients with fracture of the femur having no definable medical problem prior to the fracture [54].

Commonly associated diseases and disorders reported are: chronic brain failure [24, 28, 53], diabetes mellitus [26, 52, 53], Parkinson's disease [24, 26, 53], heart disease [53, 54], rheumatoid arthritis [1], lung disease [53] and stroke [1, 24, 54, 55]. It is of note that in hemiplegia the fracture is nearly always on the hemiplegic side [1]. This is probably not surprising since other neurological disorders producing disuse of a limb are associated with osteoporosis in the affected limb [55–57].

The influence of drug therapy in fracture of the femur is uncertain. Although taking medication is common this is probably in keeping with the general prescribing patterns for the elderly [29]. It has been suggested that the drugs themselves may have a direct association with the fracture. For instance, Muckle [4] observed that 70 per cent of patients with fracture of the femoral neck due to minor injury were on long-term medication (such as hormones, anticonvulsants and diuretics, which could affect bone density) compared with only 22 per cent of those with significant injury (e.g. falling from steps).

In general, the physical state [24] and mobility [8] is much poorer in patients with fracture of the femur than in age–sex matched controls, especially for those over the age of 75. It is obvious that those who fall are usually those with a combination of underlying bone disease and medical conditions resulting in an increased tendency to fall. This emphasizes the importance of the geriatricians involvement in management of patients with fractures of the femur.

Outcome

The advent of an aggressive surgical approach to fracture of the femur has led to a reduction of both the mortality [58–61] and morbidity [60, 61] following the injury.

Mortality

Mortality is reported to be quite high, especially in men [19], following fracture of the femur, with about 40 per cent dying within six months of the injury [19, 58] and 50 per cent by the end of the first year [26, 62]; though other studies report only about half of these levels [29, 53, 63, 64]. A high mortality is particularly likely in patients admitted from institutional care, while hospital mortality correlates well with the pre-fracture dependency levels [63, 65] and other medical conditions [8].

Morbidity

The aim of the rehabilitation programme is to return the patient to his or her pre-fracture ability. Barnes [65] examined 70 elderly patients referred for rehabilitation and found that 40 per cent returned to their pre-fracture level; but there did not appear to be an association between the level of recovery and the sex of the patient, the surgical technique, the side of fracture, the motivation or orientation of the patient, or the presence or absence of postoperative leg pain. The only two features which showed a significant association with ability to reach the pre-fracture ambulation status were a previous leg fracture and the number of physiotherapy sessions received. Similar ambulation levels have been found in other studies [58, 61], with a greater proportion of younger patients showing complete recovery [1, 26, 61].

Early surgery has been shown to improve the functional status following a fractured femur, with 70 per cent of the operated group, but only 54 per cent of the conservatively treated group, reaching normal activity [67]. Most recovery occurs in the first six months, although it can continue for up to two years [27]. Once recovery is achieved it is usually maintained [27]. This, however, is age-related, with 72 per cent of those under 70 years, 45 per cent of those 70–79 years and only 26 per cent of those 80 years and over having a sustained return of activities of daily living function [27].

Postoperative complications

Pressure sores

Pressure sores are theoretically preventable. However, since many patients have been lying on a hard surface for a long time prior to admission to hospital, sores can develop before nursing attention is received. The elderly are particularly vulnerable, about one-quarter developing pressure sores – and half of these are deep [53]. Most pressure sores following hip operations occur in women over 70 years of age, and the majority start soon after admission, particularly on the day of operation [68].

The introduction of surgical internal fixation of the fracture has helped to reduce the frequency of pressure sores [67] by about 50 per cent. There is also evidence (69–71) that a single dose of ACTH pre-operatively can help to decrease the incidence of pressure sores following fracture of the femur [69–71].

Deep-vein thrombosis

Deep-vein thrombosis is difficult to detect without special investigation. Campbell [53] reported only 4 per cent of patients requiring anti-coagulant therapy for deep-vein thrombosis in the calf. A similar figure was found by Pimpinelli and Cerulli [67] in their surgically treated group; but they did not report any from their conservatively treated patients, suggesting that thrombophlebitis is a complication of surgery rather than being due to the fracture itself.

Incontinence of urine or faeces

Urinary incontinence is very common around the time of fracture of the femur. About 50 per cent of elderly patients are treated for urinary retention or incontinence either pre- or postoperatively, though this resolves within three days in about 60 per cent of cases [53]. About 40 per cent of patients become faecally incontinent owing to impaction of faeces or confusion [53]. All elderly patients admitted to hospital should be presumed to have constipation until proved otherwise.

Avascular necrosis and non-union

The purpose of internal fixation is to position the fracture parts so that the bone heals in good alignment. Non-union has been reported occurring in 7 per cent of fractures with perfect alignment, but this rises to 34 per cent when the alignment angle is less than 150° or greater than 185° [72]. The rate of non-union also closely parallels the severity of the osteoporosis [73]. In general the non-union rates for intracapsular fractures is 5–15 per cent [74–78], with later segmental collapse of 7–10 per cent [75, 79, 80].

Avascular necrosis of intracapsular fractures increases from about 12 per cent for undisplaced fractures to about 27 per cent for those that are displaced [74]. Others have found no avasular necrosis when there was good fixation [81]. However, even when the only evidence of poor reduction is an anterior angulation of less than 30°, about one-fifth develop avascular necrosis [82, 83]. Good surgical reduction is essential if avascular necrosis is to be avoided [54, 83], although it occurs even when fractures are adequately reduced.

A very large study found that a delay of up to one week before operation had no significant effect on the incidence of non-union or late segmental collapse [84]. However, Manninger *et al.* [85] found that early fracture reduction and fixation reduced the incidence and severity of avascular necrosis when compared with those whose operation was delayed. This may be because the blood supply to the head of the femur is not necessarily ruptured but may be compressed by the displaced fractured tissue [86, 87], thereby producing reversible ischaemia. In addition, newer operative techniques, such as the sliding screw plate [88], have improved the union rate and decreased the incidence of avascular necrosis.

Shortening of the leg

About one-third of patients develop shortening of the affected leg [66]. Three-quarters of these patients do not reach pre-fracture ambulatory levels, compared with 52 per cent of those without shortening (though this did not reach statistically significant levels).

Hip pain

Some localized pain is common following the operation. Part of this is due to tissue trauma; but if it persists the patient should be investigated for infection, bending of the plate or slipping of the prosthesis. Barnes [66] found that 54 per cent of patients had pain sufficient to interfere with walking during the rehabilitation programme, and 61 per cent of these did not reach pre-fracture ambulatory status. Pain is more likely to be present in non-operated patients [67], but even in those with internal fixation 23 per cent developed pain on weight bearing and 4 per cent had continuous pain.

Limping

Many patients limp after the operation. In many cases this is natural cautiousness about putting weight on the 'broken' leg, although this is often reinforced by the rehabilitation team who try to encourage partial weight bearing. About two-thirds of the patients who limp do so because of pain although there is often some evidence of weakness of the gluteal muscles [67].

Local infection

About 6-8 per cent of surgically treated patients developed signs of local infection following the operation [67, 89]. Much of this depends on the site of the fracture and the duration of the surgery [29]. Local infection in the orthopaedic patient is always of concern because of the danger of infecting the bone. The essential treatment is as for infection at any site – good drainage and antibiotics.

Repeat surgery

Slipping of the prosthesis or avascular necrosis results in a second operation in a small proportion of patients, varing from 2 per cent [53] to 14 per cent [28], especially for cervical fractures (21 per cent) [28].

Functional outcome

Functional recovery should be good following a rehabilitation programme. Ceder *et al.* [28] found that preoperatively most of their patients had been able to manage basic activities but only 70 per cent had been carrying out more demanding activities such as cooking, kitchen work, housework or shopping. However, most of those who had carried out these functions regained them. Only a few patients were walking out of doors at the time of discharge, but most eventually did so.

The commonest cause of poor functional outcome is the mental state of the patient [90, 91]. Those most likely to reach a good level of independence are younger male patients, with a good pre-fracture medical condition, good mental state and high initial activities of daily living score [91]. Since none of these can be influenced by medical treatment, special management techniques will be required.

Even after discharge from hospital only about one-third walk unaided, one-eighth use a quadraped and half requiring a walking stick [92]. However, it has to be recognized that one-third of all patients admitted with a fracture of the femur had been using a walking aid prior to the fracture.

Organization

Length of stay

The average hospital stay following fracture of the femur is about three to four weeks [6, 28, 61, 74], which increases with age in both sexes up to the ninth decade, after which it begins to fall [7], presumably owing to the high mortality in the very old. However, median length of stay does not show a direct correlation with age, suggesting that the rising mean length of stay with age is determined by a small group requiring long-stay care [7]. Patients with trochanteric fractures tend to have a prolonged length of stay [29, 44]. Length of stay has markedly decreased since the advent of surgical fixation of the fracture [67].

Geriatric–orthopaedic units

A number of combined geriatric–orthopaedic (GO) units have been described [53, 64, 90, 93, 94]. The advantages of the GO units are, according to Campbell in a prospective study [53]:

1. The geriatrician has particular experience of the medical problems and post operative complications in the elderly.
2. The patient benefits from the rehabilitation and nursing skills of the geriatric unit.
3. There is a close association between the geriatric unit and the social agencies which may be required by the patient after discharge.

Probably one of the major differences between an orthopaedic ward and a GO unit is the nursing approach. On the GO unit patients are more likely to be encouraged to dress in their indoor clothes, and there is an educational attitude of the rehabilitation environment.

Devas [93] states that 'there is no place in a geriatric orthopaedic unit for the bedridden patient'. This emphasizes the specialist role of the unit in selecting those patients who will most benefit from the combined approach of the orthopaedic surgeon and the geriatric rehabilitation team. Some units regard themselves as specialized in the same way as an intensive care unit; that is, when the patient no longer requires or will benefit from the specialized skills, then alternative accommodation must be found by the original transferring ward. This is necessary if the specialist skills are to be used effectively.

The patients most likely to benefit from a GO unit are those with fracture following a minor fall indicating a general frailty and deteriorating condition [94]. Those who have had a true accident and were previously fit usually do not require admission to the GO unit and can be discharged directly from the orthopaedic ward within a week or two of the operation.

The close relationship between orthopaedic and geriatric units can extend to the provision of a full medical assessment of the patient by the geriatrician *before* the operation. The patient then gains the benefit of both medical and surgical skills and therefore starts off with optimal opportunities for full and good recovery. Castleden [95] has argued that the geriatrician's role on the orthopaedic ward is to provide medical advice to the orthopaedic team rather than being responsible for the rehabilitation and long-stay management.

The effectiveness of the GO unit is difficult to determine. Boyd *et al.* [64] compared turnover of patients in the year before, and the year after, the introduction of a GO unit. They found that the average length of stay fell from 66 to 48 days with a saving of 27 per cent of bed-days and an increase in the proportion of patients returning home.

An alternative approach adopted by Sikorski *et al.* [96] is to treat the fracture surgically as soon as possible and return the patient home as soon as treatment of a highly sophisticated nature is no longer required. However, patients are excluded from the scheme if there are medical or surgical problems which in themselves require admission to hospital; if the fracture is so unstable that early weight bearing cannot be allowed; if the patient lives more than 15 miles from the hospital; if they live alone, are mentally or physically incompetent or unreliable or have an inadequate home environment; or where the patient or the family refuse to allow discharge. Most of those living at home with support are able to return there, but only 27 per cent of those living alone manage to be rapidly discharged. All those in residential institutional care return there. This approach, therefore, has its limitations for a large proportion of elderly people with fracture of the femur.

Social outcome

Figures vary for the number of patients who can be discharged, from 30–38 per cent [53, 63] through 54–59 per cent [90, 97] to 87 per cent [8] for those previously living at home. About one-half of patients continue to deteriorate socially over the first two years following the fracture, especially those transferred to institutional care [98]. The sex of the patient does not seem to influence the timing of the discharge from hospital, but the older the patient the less were the chances of returning home [28]. Almost all in the 50–64 age group returned home and all were at home by the end of the first year; fewer of those 65–79 years returned home, but they remained at home during the first year; whereas the discharge rate for those over 80 years was very much lower and only about two-thirds of these were still at home after four months. Patients were more likely to return home if they had previously been living with someone than if they lived alone [28].

As many as 25 per cent of those patients discharged home become dependent [62]. This has important implications for social services, with a large amount of community support being required by about two-thirds of the patients discharged [53]. However, many patients had previously been dependent on social services [28].

Prognostic indicators

Cluster analysis suggests that there are two main types of variables associated with prediction of discharge [99]. The first group are background variables such as age, general medical condition, type of fracture, sex and living with someone. The second type are the functional variables such as pre-fracture ability to visit someone and to shop, ability to walk and to manage activities of daily living at two weeks following surgery.

Poor prognostic signs are a previous history of dependency at home [28, 62], previous poor health [28, 61, 91, 100], inability to walk at two weeks following surgery [28, 91] and living alone [28, 62, 97]. Although advancing age is a poor prognostic sign [61, 62, 91, 100], it is less important than concurrent disease [28], although this is also associated with advancing age. Neurological disease, especially dementia, is a particularly poor prognostic sign for discharge from hospital [28, 61, 76].

Many of the prognostic features are less specific and the physiotherapist's assessment of balance, stamina, weight bearing, motivation and mental state is probably a more accurate assessment than the specific rating systems [101].

Rehabilitation

The value of rehabilitation

There is very little research information available about the value of rehabilitation in the management of patients with fracture of the femur. In an uncontrolled trial, the only two factors that were associated with the patient reaching prefracture ambulatory status were the absence of a previous fracture and the amount of physical therapy received [66]. However, a number of factors, such as the potential for recovery, could have influenced the provision of physiotherapy. In addition, some patients left the rehabilitation programme before their full potential had been reached.

In another uncontrolled trial, patients receiving an intensive rehabilitation programme were compared with a nonrehabilitated group matched for age, sex, socioeconomic status and prior disability [102]. The non-rehabilitated group gained poorer levels of walking compared with pre-fracture status and more of them had marked deficits in activities of daily living function compared with the rehabilitated group. The authors do not state why those in the non-rehabilitated group did not receive the rehabilitation programme, and this complicates interpretation of the findings.

Operatively unfit patients

The generally accepted policy is to operate on patients with fracture of the femur to immobilize the fracture and mobilize the patient. However, there are occasions when the patient remains unfit for surgery. This usually results in management by traction for several weeks with the risk of all the complications of bed rest.

One approach of providing immediate weight bearing without operation is the light weight hip spica [103]. This provides a three-point fixation of the fracture and supports the injured limb with a weight-bearing lateral beam. The splint is inflated and the spica adjusted to the shape of the patient's trunk and thigh by tightening adjustable lacings. The spica then tightly encloses the leg, thigh and pelvis and the patient can be stood up, allowing full weight bearing. This approach is usually painfree provided the spica has been correctly adjusted. Care has to be taken to avoid the limb 'rolling out' at the fracture site, causing external rotation.

Non-displaced fractures

The decision on whether to treat conservatively or not is more difficult for non-displaced fractures. This is more likely to occur in younger patients, although a few elderly people present with fractures obviously having walked on the leg for several days or even weeks. Several authors have reported the results of conservative non-weight-bearing mobilization [54, 104–107]. Disimpaction occured in 6–16 per cent, which then required operation. Avascular necrosis occurred in 8–20 per cent of conservatively treated patients, a figure similar to that for patients treated by internal fixation. Conservative treatment is probably only indicated for patients who present with an impacted femoral neck fracture several weeks after their injury and are walking without pain [107].

Displaced fractures

The conservative approach for displaced fractures requires prolonged bed rest with either positioning using a hip spica or traction to maintain abduction and internal rotation. This, however, has major disadvantages in the elderly with thrombophlebitis, hypostatic pneumonia, urinary tract infections, constipation, pressure sores and disuse atrophy. There is no doubt that immobilization results in accelerated bone loss [108], and bed exercises, as opposed to weight bearing, do not reverse this trend [109]. There can be very few indications for such damaging non-treatment.

Demented patients

The foregoing comments are not particularly helpful when considering the very demented and previously immobile patient. Even though De Palma [110] suggested that the poorer the general condition of the patient, the more urgent the early surgical intervention, even Devas [111] – who is renowned for his enthusiasm for surgical treatment of elderly persons with fracture of the femur – points out the very poor prognosis in patients where the fracture is just one further feature of impending dissolution. Lyon and Nevins [112], in an uncontrolled trial of patients with severe organic mental syndromes, compared those receiving surgical treatment for fracture of the femur with conservative management and concluded that non-operative management was a reasonable alternative provided that good nursing care was available.

For severely demented immobile patients who are not fit for operation, there is no contraindication to sitting in a chair since the degree of fracture displacement is irrelevant. Control of the pain is then the most important goal.

Time to operation

There is no firm agreement as to the optimal time to operation. Some surgeons argue that there is no reason to operate on the patient immediately since time should be allowed for the patient to be made as medically fit for surgery as possible. Others feel that deterioration occurs so rapidly following the trauma of the fracture that early, if not immediate, operation is important.

As far as healing of the bone is concerned, the time to operation does not seem to make too much difference [65, 113], although this view has been disputed [85].

Early *versus* late weight bearing

Non-weight bearing, often for many months, has been regarded as essential to allow healing. Banks [54] thought that even five months after operation might be too soon to bear weight and that there should be radiological evidence of union before weight bearing was allowed. It has been suggested that early compression results in necrosis of the femoral head [114], but weight bearing at about two weeks following the operation has not been shown to increase the complication rate [83, 115–120]. Indeed, necrosis of the head has been found to be higher in the late weight-bearing group [113], and compression of the fracture seems to have a beneficial effect on the union of cancellous bone [121].

Theoretically, internal fixation should allow immediate weight bearing, although there has been an understandable fear of allowing the patient to do so. Ainsworth [120] described his 10-year experience of immediate weight bearing and found no increase in mortality or morbidity. He states that immediate weight bearing is justified only if there is adequate reduction in both planes, the immobilizing nail is inserted in the correct line of weight bearing, and the nail telescopes to allow for impaction on weight bearing.

In practice it is extremely difficult to control the amount of weight bearing in an elderly person, owing to their lack of understanding of what is meant by 'partial weight bearing' and a natural hesitancy to put weight on the 'broken' leg even when encouraged to do so. Several approaches have been used to help the patient to be aware of the amount of weight being put through the affected side. One uses a pressure detecting device fitted into the shoe which sets of a buzzer when a predetermined pressure level is reached. Another approach is to include a weight measuring device into the walking stick which then assesses when 30–50 per cent of the weight is being taken through the stick [122]: when the predetermined level is exceeded, a feedback mechanism alerts the patient.

Physiotherapy

The main aim of physiotherapy is to maintain a good range of joint movement and muscle power. Early mobilization aims to prevent deep-vein thrombosis and the other complications of bed rest, especially disuse muscle atrophy and balance disturbances.

General muscle weakness is not uncommon in the elderly. Farrow [123], describing his personal experience following an intertrochanteric fracture, pointed out the importance of the triceps which are required to stabilize the balance and are used for mobilization on crutches; on climbing stairs they have to lift the whole weight on the body, and on descending stairs they are required to check the descent. Farrow also pointed out that the shortening of the psoas muscle due to the avulsion at its lower attachment causes difficulty in many tasks. For instance, when leaning forwards in the sitting position the psoas is about the same length as when fully contracted. Any attempt at further contraction only succeeds in raising the foot a few inches from the floor, causing great difficulty when attempting to put on shoes or stockings.

Taking the above factors into account, the basic pattern of management is as follows. Within 24 hours of the operation the physiotherapist starts passive movement of the affected limb to maintain the range of movement and to encourage proprioceptive awareness. On the second day the patient can normally be allowed to sit out of bed since the load on the nail is similar whether the patient is nursed in bed or on a chair [124]. Within two or three days the patient can take assisted exercises and start weight bearing. Although partial weight bearing is often attempted in theory, in practice this is much more difficult to achieve. Either the patient will not put any weight on the affected limb or is unable to understand the concept of 'partial weight bearing'. Since the compression pressure seems to improve the rate of bone formation, there seems little point in attempting to be too strict about this with the patient.

Normally walking starts between parallel bars but can usually progress rapidly to the use of a walking frame. The standard frame encourages a stop – start gait and offers greater opportunity to avoid weight bearing. For this reason a wheeled frame is preferable since it encourages a reciprocal gait pattern. As confidence is gained through the improvement in walking and balance, the patient may progress on to a stick or no aid at all. Since most elderly people who require a geriatric rehabilitation approach are frail, most will continue to require a walking aid even if this is only the furniture within the home.

Where the patient is reluctant to take weight through the affected side in the absence of complications, the flexible standing frame (see Chapter 3) can be useful in providing security and gradually increasing the amount of weight taken through each leg.

Much of the rehabilitation programme for the frail person with fracture of the femur is increasing confidence, increasing muscle strength, improving balance and, where necessary, controlling pain.

References

1. Alffram, Per-A. (1964) An epidemiological study of cervical and trochanteric fractures of the femur in an urban population. *Acta Orthopaedica Scandinavica* **Suppl.65**: 47–64.
2. Clark, A.N.G. (1968) Factors in fracture of the female femur: a clinical study of the environmental, physical, medical and preventative aspects of this injury. *Gerontologia Clinica* **10**: 257–60.
3. Reeves, B. (1977) What comes first, the fracture or the fall? *Journal of Bone and Joint Surgery* **59B**: 375.
4. Muckle, D.S. (1979) Iatrogenic factors in femoral neck fractures. *Injury* **8**: 98–101.
5. Knowelden, J., Buhr, A.J. and Dunbar, O. (1964) Incidence of fractures in persons over 35 years of age. *British Journal of Preventative and Social Medicine* **18**: 130–41.
6. Donaldson, L.J., Stoyle, T.F. and Clarke, M. (1979) Fractured neck of femur in Leicestershire. *Public Health London* **93**: 285–9.
7. Evans, J.G. (1979) Fractured proximal femur in Newcastle upon Tyne. *Age and Ageing* **8**: 16–24.

8. Kreutzfeldt, J., Haim, M. and Bach, E. (1984) Hip fracture among the elderly in a mixed urban and rural population. *Age and Ageing*. **13**: 111–19.
9. Levine, S., Makin, M., Menczel, J. *et al.* (1970) Incidence of fractures of the proximal end of the femur in Jerusalem. *Journal of Bone and Joint Surgery* **52A**: 1193–202.
10. Alhava, E.M. and Puittenen, J. (1973) Fractures of the upper end of the femure as an index of senile osteoporosis in Finland. *Annals of Clinical Research* **5**: 398–403.
11. Wallace, W.A. (1983) The increasing incidence of fractures of the proximal femur: an orthopaedic epidemic. *Lancet* **i**: 1413–4.
12. Wong, P.C.N. (1966) Fracture epidemiology in a mixed South East Asian community (Singapore). *Clinical Orthopaedics and Related Research* **45**: 55–61.
13. Chalmers, J. and Ho, K.C. (1970) Geographical variations in senile osteoporosis. The association with physical activity. *Journal of Bone and Joint Surgery* **52B**: 667–75.
14. Lewis, A.F. (1981) Fracture of neck of the femur: changing incidence. *British Medical Journal* **283**: 1217, 1220.
15. Nilsson, B.E. and Obrant, K.J. (1978) Secular tendencies of the incidence of fracture of the upper end of the femur. *Acta Orthopaedica Scandinavica* **49**: 389–91.
16. Department of Health and Social Security (1981) *Orthopaedic Services: Waiting Time for Out-patient Appointment and In-patient Treatment.* HMSO, London.
17. Evans, J.G., Prudham, D. and Wanless, I. (1979) A prospective study of fractured proximal femur: incidence and outcome. *Public Health London* **93**: 235–41.
18. Jensenius, H. (1956) Osteosynthesis of medial fractures of the femoral neck. *Acta Chirgura Scandinavica* **111**: 322–32.
19. Evans, J.G. (1982) Epidemiology of proximal femoral fractures. In: *Recent Advances in Geriatric Medicine*, Vol. 2, pp. 201–14 (Ed: Isaacs, B). Churchill Livingstone, Edinburgh.
20. Hirsch, C. and Brodetti, A. (1956) The weight bearing capacity of structural elements in femoral neck. *Acta Orthopaedica Scandinavica* **26**: 15–23.
21. Virtama, P. (1960) Variations in the ash contents of bones of the extremities. *Annales Medicinae Experimentalis et Biologiae Fenniae* **38**: 127–32.
22. Brocklehurst, J.C., Exton-Smith, A.N., Lempert-Barber, S.M. *et al.* (1978) Fracture of the femur in old age. *Age and Ageing* **7**: 7–15.
23. Gallagher, M.D., Melton, L.J., Riggs, B.L. *et al.* (1980) Epidemiology of fractures of the proximal femur in Rochester, Minnesota. *Clinical Orthopaedics and Related Research* **150**: 163–71.
24. Boston, D.A. (1982) Bilateral fractures of the femoral neck. *Injury* **14**: 207–10.
25. Katz, S., Ford, A.B., Heiple, K.G. and Newill, V.A. (1964) Studies of illness in the aged: recovery after fracture of the hip. *Journal of Gerontology* **19**: 285–93.
26. Beals, R. (1972) Survival following hip fractures: Long term follow up of 607 patients. *Journal of Chronic Disease* **25**: 235–44.
27. Crane, J.G. and Kerneck, C.B. (1983) Mortality associated with hip fractures in a single geriatric hospital and residential health facility: a ten year review. *Journal of the American Geriatrics Society* **31**: 472–5.
28. Ceder, L., Thorngren, K-G. and Wallden, B. (1980) Prognostic indicators and early home rehabilitation in elderly patients with hip fractures. *Clinical Orthopaedics and Related Research* **152**: 173–84.
29. Beringer, T.R.O., McSherry, D.M.G. and Taggart, H. McA. (1984) A microcomputer based audit of fracture of the proximal femur in the elderly. *Age and Ageing* **13**: 344–8.

30. Halpin, P.J. and Nelson, C.L. (1980) A system of classification of femoral neck fractures with special reference to choice of treatment. *Clinical Orthopaedics and Related Research* **152**: 44–8.
31. Stevens, J., Freeman, P.A., Nordin, B.E.C. *et al.* (1962) The incidence of osteoporosis in patients with femoral neck fractures. *Journal of Bone and Joint Surgery* **44B**: 520–7.
32. Aaron, J.E., Gallagher, J.C., Anderson, J. *et al.* (1974) Frequency of osteomalacia and osteoporosis in fractures of the proximal femur. *Lancet* **i**: 229–33.
33. Pogrund, H., Makin, M., Robin, G. *et al.* (1977) Osteoporosis in patients with fractured femoral neck in Jerusalem. *Clinical Orthopaedics and Related Research* **124**: 165–72.
34. Newton-John, H.F. and Morgan, D.B. (1968) Osteoporosis: disease or senescence? *Lancet* **i**: 232–3.
35. Exton-Smith, A.N. (1976) The management of osteoporosis. *Proceedings of the Royal Society of Medicine* **69**: 931–4.
36. Galagher, J.C., Aaron, J., Nicholson, M. *et al.* (1972) The role of osteoporosis and osteomalacia in fractures of the femoral neck. *Journal of Bone and Joint Surgery* **54B**: 192.
37. O'Driscoll, M. (1973) Subcapital fracture types and osteomalacia and vitamin D deficiency. *Journal of Bone and Joint Surgery* **55B**: 882.
38. Faccini, J.M., Exton-Smith, A.N. and Boyde, A. (1976) Disorders of bone and fracture of the femoral neck. *Lancet* **i**: 1089–92.
39. Brown, I.R.F., Bokowska, A. and Millard, P.H. (1976) Vitamin D status of patients with femoral neck fractures. *Age and Ageing* **5**: 127–31.
40. Baker, M.R., McDonnell, H., Peacock, M. and Nordin, B.E.C. (1979) Plasma 25-hydroxy vitamin D concentrations in patients with fractures of the femoral neck. *British Medical Journal* **1**: 589.
41. Lund, B., Sorensen, O.H. and Christensen, A.B. (1975) 25 (OH) D3 and fractures of the proximal femur. *Lancet* **2**: 300–2.
42. Weisman, Y., Salama, R., Harell, A. and Edelstein, S. (1978) Serum 24, 25-dihydroxy vitamin D and 25-hydroxy vitamin D concentrations in femoral neck fracture. *British Medical Journal* **2**: 1196–7.
43. Lewinnek, G.E., Kelsey, J., White, A.A. and Kreiger, M.P.H. (1980) The significance of a comparative analysis of the epidemiology of hip fractures. *Clinical Orthopaedics and Related Research* **152**: 35–43.
44. Lawton, J.O., Baker, M.R. and Dickson, R.A. (1983) Femoral neck fractures – two populations. *Lancet* **ii**: 70–2.
45. Wicks, M., Garrett, R., Vernon-Roberts, B. and Fazzalari, N. (1982) Absence of metabolic bone disease in the proximal femur in patients with fracture of the femoral neck. *Journal of Bone and Joint Surgery* **64B**: 319–22.
46. Sheldon, J.H. (1960) On the natural history of falls in old age. *British Medical Journal* **2**: 1685–90.
47. Baker, M.R. (1980) *The Epidemiology and Aetiology of Femoral Neck Fracture.* MD thesis, University of Newcastle upon Tyne.
48. Leitch, I.H., Knowelden, J. and Seddon, H. (1964) Incidence of fractures, particularly neck of the femur, in patients in mental hospitals. *British Journal of Preventive and Social Medicine* **18**: 142–5.
49. Bennett, A.E., Deane, M., Elliott, A. and Holland, W.W. (1968) Care of old people in residential homes. *British Journal of Preventive and Social Medicine* **222**: 193–8.
50. Sweet, M.B.M., Mendelow, A., Kotler, M.N. *et al.* (1967) Fractured neck of femur. Associated morbidity and mortality. *South African Journal of Surgery* **5**: 57–64.

51. Riska, E.B. (1970) Factors affecting the primary mortality in the treatment of hip fractures. *Injury* **2**: 107–15.
52. Andersen, B. and Ostberg, J. (1972) Long-term prognosis in geriatric surgery: 2–17 year follow up of 7922 patients. *Journal of the American Geriatrics Society* **20**: 255–28.
53. Campbell, A.J. (1976) Femoral neck fractures in elderly women: a prospective study. *Age and Ageing* **5**: 102–9.
54. Banks, H.H. (1962) Factors influencing the result in fractures of the femoral neck. *Journal of Bone and Joint Surgery* **44A**: 931–64.
55. Abramson, A.S. (1948) Bone disturbances in injuries of the spinal cord and cauda equina. *Journal of Bone and Joint Surgery* **30A**: 982–7.
56. Whedon, G.D. (1952) Calcium loss in paralytic poliomyelitis and its quantitive relationship to the development of demonstrable osteoporosis. *Journal of Clinical Investigation* **31**: 672–3.
57. Gillespie, J.A. (1954) The nature of bone changes associated with nerve injuries and disuse. *Journal of Bone and Joint Surgery* **36B**: 464–73.
58. Niemann, K.M.W. and Mankin, H.J. (1968) Fractures about the hip in an institutionalised population. *Journal of Bone and Joint Surgery* **50A**: 1327–40.
59. Naden, D. and Denbesten, L. (1969) Fractures of the neck of femur in the aged: review of 224 consecutive cases. *Journal of the American Geriatrics Society* **17**: 198–204.
60. Braatz, J.H. and Pino, A.E. (1972) Therapy and rehabilitation for psychogeriatric patients with hip fracture. *Geriatrics* **27**: 101–6.
61. Miller, C.W. (1978) Survival and ambulation following hip fractures. *Journal of Bone and Joint Surgery* **60A**: 930–4.
62. Thomas, T.G. and Stevens, R.S. (1974) Social effects of fractures of the neck of femur. *British Medical Journal* **3**: 456–8.
63. Jensen, J.S., Tondevold, E. and Sorensen, P.H. (1979) Social rehabilitation following hip fractures. *Acta Orthopaedica Scandinavica* **50**: 777–85.
64. Boyd, R.V., Comptom, E., Hawthorne, J. and Kemm, J.R. (1982) Orthogeriatric rehabilitation ward in Nottingham: a preliminary report. *British Medical Journal* **285**: 937–8.
65. Barnes, B., Brown, J.T., Garden, R.S. *et al.* (1976) Subcapital fractures of the femur: a prospective review. *Journal of Bone and Joint Surgery* **58B**: 2–24.
66. Barnes, B. (1984) Ambulation outcome after hip fracture. *Physical Therapy* **64**: 317–21.
67. Pimpinelli, G. and Cerulli, G. (1979) Survival and quality of recovery of patients with pertrochanteric fractures of the femur. *Italian Journal of Orthopaedics and Traumatology* **5**: 111–26.
68. Versluysen, M. (1985) Pressure sores in elderly patients: the epidemiology related to hip operations. *Journal of Bone and Joint Surgery* **67B**: 10–13.
69. Barton, A.A. and Barton, M. (1968) The inhibition of decubitus ulceration with ACTH. *Journal of Pathology and Bacteriology* **96**: 345–51.
70. Barton, A.A. and Barton, M. (1969) ACTH and decubitus ulceration: an experimental study. *British Journal of Pharmacology* **36**: 219–24.
71. Barton, A.A. and Barton, M. (1981) Drug based inhibition of pressure sores. *Care, Science and Practice* **1**: 14–16.
72. Garden, R.S. (1964) Low angle fixation in fractures of the femoral neck. *Journal of Bone and Joint Surgery* **46B**: 630–47.
73. Barnes, R. (1970) Femoral neck fracture. *Proceedings of the Royal Society of Medicine* **63**: 1119–20.
74. Fielding, J.W., Wilson, S.A. and Ratzan, S. (1974) A continuing end result study of displaced intracapsular fractures of the neck of the femur treated with

Pugh nail. *Journal of Bone and Joint Surgery* **56A**: 1464–72.

75. Arnold, W.D., Lyden, J.P. and Minkoff, J. (1974) Treatment of intracapsular fractures of the femoral neck – with special reference to percutaneous Knowles pinning. *Journal of Bone and Joint Surgery* **56A**: 254–62.
76. Baker, G.I. and Barrick, E.F. (1978) Deyerle treatment for femoral neck fractures. *Journal of Bone and Joint Surgery* **60A**: 269–71.
77. Chapman, M.W., Stehr, J.H., Eberle, C.F. *et al.* (1975) Treatment of intracapsular hip fracture by the Deyerle method: a comparative review of one hundred and nineteen cases. *Journal of Bone and Joint Surgery* **57A**: 735–44.
78. Johnson, J.T.H. and Crothers, O. (1975) Nailing versus prosthesis for femoral neck fractures: a critical review of long term results in 239 consecutive private patients. *Journal of Bone and Joint Surgery* **57A**: 686–95.
79. Metz, C.W., Sellars, T.D., Feagin, J.A. and Levine, M.I. (1970) The displaced intracapsular fracture of the neck of the femur. *Journal of Bone and Joint Surgery* **52A**: 113–27.
80. Meyers, M.H., Harvey, J.P. and Moore, T.H. (1973) Treatment of displaced subcapital and transcervical fracture of the neck of the femur by muscle pedicle bone graft and internal fixation. *Journal of Bone and Joint Surgery* **55A**: 257–74.
81. Garden, R.S. (1974) Reduction and fixation of subcapital fractures of the femur. *Orthopaedic Clinics of North America* **5**: 683–712.
82. Arnold, C.C. and Lemberg, R.K. (1977) Fracture of the femoral neck. *Clinical Orthopaedics and Related Research* **129**: 217–22.
83. Brown, J. and Abrami, G. (1964) Transcervical femoral fracture. *Journal of Bone and Joint Surgery* **46B**: 648–63.
84. Barnes, R., Brown, J.T., Garden, R.S. and Nicoll, E.A. (1976) Subcapital fractures of the femur: a prospective review. *Journal of Bone and Joint Surgery* **58B**: 2–24.
85. Manninger, J., Kazar, G., Fekete, E. *et al.* (1985) Avoidance of avascular necrosis of the femoral head following fracture of the femoral neck, by early reduction and internal fixation. *Injury* **16**: 437–48.
86. Rowe, C.R. and Lowell, J.D. (1961) Prognosis of fracture of the acetabulum. *Journal of Bone and Joint Surgery* **43A**: 30–59.
87. Soto-Hall, P. and Johnson, L.H. (1964) Variations in the intra-articular pressure of the hip joint in injury and disease. *Journal of Bone and Joint Surgery* **46A**: 509–16.
88. Nordkild, P., Sonne-Holm, S. and Jensen, J.S. (1985) Femoral neck fracture: sliding screw plate versus sliding nail plate – a randomised trial. *Injury* **16**: 449–54.
89. Murray, D.G. (1964) Wound infection after surgery for fractured hip. *Journal of the American Medical Association* **190**: 505–8.
90. Clark, A.N.G. and Wainwright, D. (1986) Management of fractured neck of femur in the elderly female. *Gerontologia Clinica* **8**: 321–6.
91. Carroll, D.G. (1969) Prediction of performance of patients with hip fracture. *Maryland State Medical Journal* January: 69–74.
92. Ceder, L., Eklund, L., Inerot, S. *et al.* (1979) Rehabilitation after hip fracture in the elderly. *Acta Orthopaedical Scandinavica* **50**: 681–8.
93. Devas, M.B. (1974) Geriatric orthopaedics. *British Medical Journal* **1**: 190–2.
94. Devas, M.B. (1976) Geriatric orthopaedics. *Annals of the Royal College of Surgeons of England* **58**: 16–21.
95. Castleden, C.M. (1977) Who is responsible for the elderly patients on orthopaedic wards? *Geriatrics*, **July**: 65–8.
96. Sikorski, J.M., Davis, N.J. and Senior, J. (1985) The rapid transit system for

patients with fracture of proximal femur. *British Medical Journal* **290**: 439–43.

97. Ceder, L., Lindberg, L, and Odberg, E. (1979) Differentiated care of hip fracture in the elderly. Mean hospital days and results of rehabilitation. *Acta Orthopaedica Scandinavica* **51**: 157–61.

98. Jensen, J.S. and Bagger, J. (1982) Long term social prognosis after hip fractures. *Acta Orthopaedica Scandinavica* **53**: 97–101.

99. Ceder, L., Svensson, Thorngren K-G. (1980) Statistical prediction of rehabilitation in elderly patients with hip fractures. *Clinical Orthopaedics and Related Research* **152**: 185–90.

100. Katz, S., Heiple, K.G., Downs, T.D. *et al.* (1967) Long term course of 147 patients with fracture of the hip. *Surgery Gynaecology and Obstetrics* **124**: 1219–30.

101. Cobey, J.C., Cobey, J.H., Conant, L. *et al.* (1976) Indicators of recovery from fractures of the hip. *Clinical Orthopaedics and Related Research* **117**: 258–62.

102. Katz, S., Jackson, B.S., Jaffe, M.W. *et al.* (1962) Multidisciplinary studies of illness in aged persons. VI: Comparison study of rehabilitated and nonrehabilitated patients with fracture of the hip. *Journal of Chronic Disease* **15**: 979–84.

103. Patrick, J.H. (1981) Intertrochanteric hip fracture treated by immediate mobilisation in a splint. *Lancet* **i**: 301–3.

104. Flatmark, A.L. and Lone, T. (1962) The prognosis of abduction fractures of the neck of the femur. *Journal of Bone and Joint Surgery* **44B**: 324–7.

105. Crawford, H.B. (1969) Impacted femoral neck fractures. *Clinical Orthopaedics and Related Research* **66**: 99–106.

106. Hillboe, T.W., Staple, T.W., Lansche, E.W. and Reynolds, F.C. (1970) The non-operative treatment of impacted fractures of the femoral neck. *Southern Medical Journal* **63**: 1103–6.

107. Bentley, G. (1980) Treatment of nondisplaced fractures of the femoral neck. *Clinical Orthopaedics and Related Research* **152**: 93–101.

108. Issekutz, B., Blizzard, J.J., Birkhead, N.C. *et al.* (1966) Effect of prolonged bed rest on urinary calcium output. *Journal of Applied Physiology* **21**: 1013–20.

109. Hantman, D.A., Vogel, J.M., Donaldson, C.L. *et al.* (1973) Attempts to prevent disuse osteoporosis by treatment with calcitonin, longitudinal compression and supplementary calcium and phosphorus. *Journal of Clinical Endocrinology and Metabolism* **36**: 845–58.

110. DePalma, A.F. (1970) Fractures of the upper end of femur. In: *The Management of Fractures and Dislocations*, pp. 1236–1325 (Ed: DePalma, A.F.). W.B. Saunders, Philadelphia.

111. Devas, M. (1976) Orthopaedics, In: *Cowdry's Care of the Geriatric Patient*, 5th Edn., pp. 258–74 (Ed: Steinberg, S.I.). C.V. Mosby Co., St Louis.

112. Lyon, L.J. and Nevins, M.A. (1977) Nontreatment of hip fractures in senile patients. *Journal of the American Medical Association* **238**: 1175–6.

113. Graham, J. (1968) Early or delayed weight bearing after internal fixation of transcervical fracture of the femur. *Journal of Bone and Joint Surgery* **50B**: 166–71.

114. Rokkanen, P. and Slatis, P. (1967) Effect of compression on the healing of subcapital osteotomies of the femoral neck and the avascularized femoral head. *Acta Orthopaedica Scandinavica* **38**: 163–73.

115. Bonnin, J.G. and Cashman, B. (1963) Early weight bearing in low angle nailing of the femoral neck. *British Journal of Surgery* **50**: 640–8.

116. Abrami, G. and Stevens, J. (1964) Early weight bearing after internal fixation of transcervical fracture of the femur. *Journal of Bone and Joint Surgery* **46B**: 204–5.

117. Hullinger, C.W. (1967) Intracapsular fractures of the neck of the femur. *International Surgery* **47**: 166–71.
118. Gibson, J.M.C. (1964) Early weight bearing in fractures of the femoral neck. *Journal of the Royal College of Surgeons, Edinburgh* **9**: 213–14.
119. Haggqvist, S-O (1969) Results of early weight-bearing in cases of operated subcapital neck fractures. *Acta Orthopaedica Scandinavica* **40**: 684–5.
120. Ainsworth, T.H. (1971) Immediate full weight bearing in the treatment of hip fractures. *Journal of Trauma* **11**: 1031–40.
121. Charnley, J. and Baker, S.L. (1952) Compression arthrodesis of the knee: a clinical and histological study. *Journal of Bone and Joint Surgery* **34B**: 187–99.
122. Engel, J., Amir, A., Messer, E. and Caspi, I. (1983) Walking cane designed to assist partial weight bearing. *Archives of Physical Medicine and Rehabilitation* **64**: 386–8.
123. Farrow, R. (1977) Rehabilitation of intertrochanteric fractures at home: an insight. *Practitioner* **219**: 246–50.
124. Frankel, V.H., Burstein, A.H., Brown, R.H. and Lygre, L. (1971) Biolemetry from the upper end of the femur. *Journal of Bone and Joint Surgery* **53A**: 1023.

7

Peripheral vascular disease

General features

Peripheral vascular disease is almost impossible to detect in its early stages since it starts in childhood and progresses at a variable rate throughout the remainder of life. Even where an artery is lined with atheromata it may remain patent and perfusion pressure may not fall until the lumen in decreased to one-third of its diameter.

When considering peripheral vascular disease it is important to distinguish between muscle and skin blood flow. At rest the muscle requires only a small blood flow, which increases by a factor of about ten on walking; skin, on the other hand, is viable with a very small blood flow. The site of the circulatory disturbance influences the symptoms produced: disease of larger blood vessels results in intermittent claudication, and disease of distal small vessels in skin changes.

Intermittent claudication

By definition intermittent claudication does not occur at rest but results from muscle ischaemia during activity. The cause of the pain is uncertain but it is assumed to be due to a build-up of the products of muscle metabolism within muscles. Pain is classically felt in the calf (72 per cent), although it may occur in the sole of the foot (18 per cent) or the buttocks (8 per cent) [1]. It usually starts after a relatively standard distance, which will be shortened by hurrying or on inclines.

Epidemiology

Little epidemiological information is available about peripheral vascular disease. One of the difficulties is that the elderly seem to present late for medical or surgical treatment, possibly because limited activity results in the disease progressing before symptoms are produced. In a population study of people aged 62 years and over, 10 per

106

Table 7.1 Prevalence of peripheral vascular disease in the elderly (Hale *et al.* [4])

	Claudication	Cold hands/feet
Men		
65–69	7.3	20.7
70–74	11.9	20.6
75–79	17.3	23.3
80–84	21.2	27.8
>84	20.3	35.9
Women		
65–69	11.0	26.6
70–74	11.7	23.8
75–79	11.9	29.6
80–84	17.7	34.0
>84	12.7	46.3

cent of men and 3 per cent of women had evidence of intermittent claudication based on clinical history and an examination of the foot pulses [2]. A study of a younger population (45–69 years), using a history of pain on walking which was relieved by rest and with a fall in ankle blood pressure after exercise, found a prevalence of 2.2 per cent of men and 1.2 per cent of females in this age range [3]. In another large community study of symptoms in the elderly, intermittent claudication was present in 18 per cent of females and 21 per cent of males in the 80–84 age group (Table 7.1), with symptoms of cold feet being present in a much higher proportion.

In the Framingham longitudinal study the annual incidence of intermittent claudication was about one-quarter that of coronary heart disease at the age of 45–54 and about one-fifth that in the 55–64 age group [4]. The prevalence increased with age, though this was not as marked as for coronary artery disease.

Intermittent claudication is commoner in men than in women, though this varies widely between the various studies, from 62 per cent [5] to 92 per cent [6] being male.

A number of factors are strongly associated with intermittent claudication. A history of smoking is nearly always present [3, 7, 8]. The risk increases by a factor of fifteen in men and seven in women [3] and is proportional to the number of cigarettes smoked. Although pipe and cigar smokers have a lower prevalence of intermittent claudication, they have a higher risk than non-smokers [3].

Other factors associated with intermittent claudication are hypertension, hyperglycaemia [3], hyperfibrinogen and hyperuricaemia [33, 9, 10]. The role of blood lipids is less clear [11, 12].

The natural progression of intermittent claudication is variable. In the elderly there may be little change over a 5-year period, with 78–90 per cent showing no deterioration or improving [13, 14]; about 7 per cent will eventually require amputation [13, 15] and nearly of all these will also have diabetes mellitus.

Intermittent claudication is associated with a high 5-year mortality rate, usually due to cardio- or cerebrovascular disease [16], and is especially high when there is concomitant ischaemic heart disease or diabetes mellitus. The relative mortality is, however, higher for younger than for older patients [17]. The 5-year survival for those 35–44 years of age is about 90 per cent, and this progressively falls with advancing age to about 40 per cent for those 75 years and over [15]. In effect, the life expectancy is equivalent to a person about 10 years older [18].

Assessment

There are many methods of assessing peripheral vascular disease. However, invasive methods like angiography, muscle pH and pO_2, the use of electromagnetic flow meters and isotope clearance techniques are impractical in general geriatric practice, as is the non-invasive technique of impedence plethysmography [19].

Doppler measurement of the systolic blood pressure at the ankle [20–22] is simpler and has the advantage that it can be carried out in general departments. When the ankle pressure is less than 75 per cent that of the brachial blood pressure [23], there is a drop in the ankle pressure on exercise [24]; or when there is a difference between the two ankles of 20 per cent [25] then there is significant arterial insufficiency. Measurement of the systolic ankle pressures using Doppler techniques is not easy in the elderly, owing to arteries being difficult to locate or being incompressible through calcification [26]. In addition the arterial pressure gradient may not be affected until only 20–30 per cent of the lumen is patent [27], while symptoms may occur at levels of much less occlusion. The pressures can only be measured at rest, but this can be overcome to some extent by the use of transcutaneous oxygen tension monitoring [26, 28, 29]. Although this requires expensive specialist equipment, the technique is more easily available in vascular departments.

For rehabilitation purposes a functional approach is more practicable. This involves measuring the time to the initial onset of pain and the maximum walking tolerance (i.e. the distance at which the patient has to stop because the pain in no longer tolerable). These parameters are considered to be more reliable and reproducible, especially on a treadmill, than the patients' own opinion of walking distances [30], although Gerdle *et al.* [31] found a close correlation between the laboratory measurement of work carried out and the patients' own estimation of walking distance.

Management of intermittent claudication

General comments

The general approach is to advise the patient on protective techniques. The feet should be kept warm and dry, although local heat should be avoided because it increases the metabolic rate. Woollen socks are generally preferable to nylon or man-made fibre stockings. Regular chiropody is important to prevent excessive growth of the nails and to prevent callosities, especially in the diabetic who often has a combination of a peripheral neuropathy and arteriopathy. Tight stockings, garters or elastic bands should not be worn. Sitting with the legs crossed should be avoided, but compliance is often difficult to achieve. Shoes should fit well and have no pressure areas. Some recommend a soft insole to prevent the development of callosities, especially where there is a foot deformity.

Smoking

It is essential that patients stop smoking. Even elderly, long-standing smokers can do so. Avoiding other drugs that are likely to affect the peripheral vascular tree, especially beta-blockers, has obvious implications for the prescribing clinician. Management of conditions that are likely to affect the oxygenation of the blood, especially anaemia, lung disease and congestive heart failure, also makes common sense.

Drug therapy

Drug therapy is generally thought to have little or no effect on the outcome [32–34], and the long-term results of surgery are poor [35–38]. Although vasodilators can increase the blood flow to muscle at rest, there is no evidence that they are effective on exercise [39]. The pain of intermittent claudication is probably due to the build-up of metabolites in the tissues, and this may account for some of the symptomatic relief of pain from naftidrofuryl oxalate. This is worth trying since the effect seems to be more marked in the elderly [40, 41].

Passive exercises

Traditionally Buerger's exercises have been taught to improve the circulation, using the effect of gravity to improve the blood flow and elevation of the leg to improve venous drainage. The technique involves the patient lying on the bed with the leg elevated until there is blanching; the leg is then hung over the side of the bed until it is flushed; it is then placed horizontal until a normal colour returns. This is carried out several times three of four times a day. There is very little evidence that the technique is effective, and at least one study did not show any significant improvement in the blood flow to the ischaemic limb [42]. Nevertheless, when sitting there is a rise in the blood pressure at the ankle [43] and perfusion in the ischaemic leg [44] which is greater than the levels associated with rest pain and non-healing of skin ulcers. This certainly fits in with the experience that many patients find relief by hanging the affected leg out of bed. Although a rise in the orthostatic blood pressure in the leg is usually associated with an increase in vasoconstriction, this is probably less likely to occur in the ischaemic limb owing to the build-up of ischaemic metabolites [45] or in diabetes mellitus [46].

Active exercises

Progressively increasing exercises of the lower limbs is thought to increase the development of the collateral circulation [47, 48] with associated symptomatic improvement [47–56]. These exercises do not have to be specific. For instance, in one controlled trial unsupervised daily walking improved the walking ability of patients in the treatment group even though there was no statistically significant increase in the maximum blood flow to the muscles [47]. Similar findings have been demonstrated using a bicycle ergometer [50].

Studies of the effect of exercise using venous-occlusion strain-plethysmography have not shown an improvement in blood flow [55–57], suggesting that symptomatic recovery is not due to improvement in the collateral circulation and may indicate a metabolic effect or adaptation to exercise. There is, however, conflicting evidence from other studies where an increase in blood flow was found following an exercise programme [48, 49, 51, 58].

Some of the effect of exercise is probably related to metabolic changes in ischaemic muscle similar to those seen in normal muscle after exercise, especially an increase in succinic oxidase [59, 60]. There is evidence that the metabolic abnormalities can be improved after an exercise programme without there being significant change in the blood flow [53–55].

A number of suggestions have been put forward for the symptomatic improvement, including improved glycolytic and oxidative metabolism, improved utilization of oxygen [50], redistribution of blood flow within the leg, increased pain tolerance or improved walking technique [61].

The patients most likely to benefit from an exercise programme are those without symptomatic coronary artery insufficiency and those without rest pain [62]. It is generally thought that the more proximal the arterial stenosis the poorer the response to exercise, although not all studies have been unable to confirm this [62, 63]. The patients least likely to complete an exercise programme are those with cardiac disease, rapid progression of the disease, intercurrent disease or social reasons [55].

For exercise to be effective it must be continued in the long term since ceasing a training programme results in a decrease in walking tolerance [58]. Techniques basically fall into two groups, supervised and unsupervised. Supervised exercises are effective [63] and to a greater level than home treatment [30]. The encouragement stimulates the patient to continue activities at a higher level than he or she would otherwise perform and offers the opportunity for monitoring basic parameters, such as blood pressure, as well as the organization of a planned programme. It does, however, have the disadvantages of the patient having to travel to the hospital and assessment in an artificial environment.

Most exercise programmes require the use of an exercise bicycle, pedalator [64] or treadmill [65–67], which is usually electrically driven at a set speed, with or without a slight incline. The pedalator provides reciprocal dorsal and plantar flexion of the ankles on hinged foot-boards set against resistance. It has the advantage that it can also be used whilst the patient is sitting or lying, it is therefore suitable for patients with breathlessess or balance problems and has less effect on the cardiovascular system than does the treadmill [64].

Bicycle exercises are not as effective as a treadmill in improving walking ability [68], suggesting that some form of walking exercise is preferred. Walking has the advantage that it can be carried out unsupervised, the patient being told to increase the walking distance gradually using a technique of walking as quickly as possible until the pain is difficult to tolerate, resting until it settles and then repeating the exercise. Elderly patients are often limited as much by breathlessness or arthritis as by intermittent claudication, and encouraging them to walk at their optimal pace is the best that can be achieved.

The programme described by Dahllöff *et al.* [30], excluding those where the ischaemic symptoms were present at rest or with gangrene and those in heart failure, was as follows: walking (5 minutes); jogging (3 minutes); dynamic exercises of the legs in the erect position (3 minutes); stretching exercises (7 minutes); relaxation movements for the calf and feet (5 minutes); the programme ending with further jogging (4 minutes), then walking (3 minutes) assisted by musical accompaniment. These times are likely to require modification for the elderly.

There is evidence that electrical stimulation of normal calf muscles in animals [69, 70] and man [71-74] increases the blood flow to the muscles. There is less evidence that it has any direct effect in the presence of vascular disease.

Patients occasionally ask for advice on exercises they can carry out at home. Although the best exercise seems to be to go out for a daily walk of progressively increasing distance, this is not always feasible owing to weather conditions, the type of local environment (steep hills or uneven ground) or social difficulties. A number of exercises can be carried out at home [75]:

- *Lying*: Flex, extend and rotate the ankle. Elevate the extended leg for three or four seconds, repeating by alternating the legs 10 times. Flex and extend the knee.
- *Sitting*: Stand up and sit down several times, preferably without using the arms if possible.
- *Standing*: Holding on to a support (e.g. the back of a chair), stand on the toes and then bend slowly down into a crouching position, or as far as possible. Repeat this several times.

Intermittent pneumatic compression

The value of intermittent pneumatic compression in peripheral vascular disease is discussed in Chapter 3.

Other modalities

Heat has been used in the past to increase the vasodilatation of the tissues. Since the affected arteries are already maximally dilated within the limits of the arteriosclerosis, heating the affected limb possibly causes vasodilatation of more normal vessels resulting in blood being diverted away from the ischaemic area. There is, however, an argument for using heat at other parts of the body, such as over the abdomen, to produce reflex vasodilation, although there is no evidence that this is effective in peripheral vascular disease.

Cutaneous ischaemia

The foregoing discussion has concentrated on the more dramatic form of peripheral vascular disease (i.e. pain). However, earlier symptoms may relate more to cutaneous than to muscle ischaemia. These vary from simple cold feet to gangrene, often associated with numbness of the feet, especially when walking. As the vascular disease deteriorates then ulcers which are slow to heal appear related to minor areas of trauma. They are most common on the tips of the toes or over the head of the fifth metatarsal and may be the result of careless nail-paring.

Management largely depends on protection and care of the ischaemic foot. In general this means protecting the foot against trauma, avoiding and treating infection, and maintaining an exercise programme to improve the circulation.

Foot protection requires the patient to wear appropriate well-fitting shoes which have no local areas of compression, the wearing of warm wollen socks and the provision of regular competent chiropody. These are especially important when there is an associated diabetic neuropathy.

Skin changes may be associated with rest pain, especially when a constant pain occurs while lying down. The rest pain may be due to a combination of a decreased blood flow due to the horizontal position and increased metabolic rate due to the warmth of the bed. For this reason patients seek comfort by sitting up and placing the foot on the floor. The pain will be made worse if the patient develops dependent oedema by spending too much time sitting up.

When gangrene does occur a number of measures can be taken. The traditional management of bed rest is counterproductive, resulting in a decreased blood flow to the leg and producing disuse muscle atrophy and decreasing the venous return.

Unfortunately many elderly patients with peripheral vascular disease are unfit for general anaesthesia and reconstructive surgery. However, there are reports of good results from phenol lumbar sympathectomy in elderly patients [76–78] This has the advantage of being simple with very few complications.

Muscle cramps

Muscle cramps – sudden, painful muscle contractions, usually at rest and lasting for several minutes – are associated with peripheral vascular disease although they may be precipitated by water and electrolyte disturbances, hypotension and drugs such as nifedipine [79] or beta-adrenergic stimulants.

Most patients find their own approach to dealing with the cramps. These include massaging the muscle, using heat from a hot water bottle, or ice packs. It is difficult to know whether these have any real effect since the condition is usually self-limiting and the activity required to obtain the appropriate remedy may also influence the outcome. Some patients find using elasticated stockings helps to prevent attacks when they are frequent. The acute attack can be shortened by stretching the offending muscle, though this increases the pain in the short term. Symptomatic relief can be obtained by getting out of bed and putting weight through the affected foot, thereby stretching the calf muscles.

References

1. Gillespie, J.A. and Douglas, D.M. (1961) *Obliterative Vascular Disease of the Lower Limb*. Livingstone, Edinburgh.
2. Milne, J.S. and Williamson, J. (1972) Intermittent claudication and peripheral pulses in older people. *Age and Ageing* 1: 146-51.
3. Hughson, W.G., Mann, J.I. and Garrod, A. (1978) Intermittent claudication: prevalence of risk factors. *British Medical Journal* 1: 1379-81.
4. Hale, W.E., Perkins, L.L., May, F.E. *et al.* (1986) Symptom prevalence in the elderly: an evaluation of age, sex, disease and medication use. *Journal of American Geriatrics Society* 34: 333-40.
5. Kannel, W.B., Skinner, J.J., Schwartz, M.J. and Shurtleff, D. (1970) Intermittent claudication: incidence in the Framingham study. *Circulation* 41: 875-83.
6. Widmer, L.K., Greensher, A. and Kannel, W.B. (1964) Occlusion of peripheral arteries: a study of 6400 working subjects. *Circulation* 30: 836-52.
7. Juergens, J.L., Barker, N.W. and Hines, E.A. (1960) Arteriosclerosis obliterans: review of 520 cases with special reference to pathogenic and prognostic factors. *Circulation* 21: 188-95.
8. Janzon, L. (1975) Risk factors in peripheral arterial disease. *Acta Chirurgica Scandinavica* 141: 596-9.
9. Dormandy, J.A., Hoare, E., Colley, J. *et al.* (1973) Prognostic significance of rheological and biochemical findings in patients with intermittent claudication. *British Medical Journal* 4: 581-3.
10. Medalie, J.H., Papier, C.M., Goldbourt, U. and Herman, J.B. (1975) Major factors in the development of diabetes mellitus in 1000 men. *Archives of International Medicine* 135: 811-17.
11. Greenhalgh, R.M., Lewis, B., Rosengarten, D.S. *et al.* (1971) Serum lipids and lipoproteins in peripheral vascular disease. *Lancet* 2: 947-50.
12. Skrede, S. and Kvarstein, B. (1975) Hyperlipidaemia on peripheral atherosclerotic arterial disease. *Acta Chirurgica Scandinavica* 141: 333-40.
13. McAllister, F.F. (1976) The fate of patients with intermittent claudication managed nonoperatively. *American Journal of Surgery* 132: 593-5.
14. Kakkar, V. (1979) Peripheral vascular disease. *Medicine* 22: 1118-24.
15. Boyd, A.M. (1962) Natural course of arteriosclerosis of the lower extremities. *Proceedings of the Royal Society of Medicine* 55: 591-3.
16. Hughson, W.G., Mann, J.I. and Tibbs, D.J. (1978) Intermittent claudication: factors determining outcome. *British Medical Journal* 1: 1377-9.
17. Källerö, K.S. (1981) Mortality and morbidity in patients with intermittent claudication as defined by venous occlusion plethysmography: a ten-year follow-up study. *Journal of Chronic Disease* 34: 455-62.
18. Bloor, K. (1961) Natural history of arteriosclerosis of the lower extremities. *Annals of the Royal College of Surgeons of England* 28: 36-52.
19. Fajgelj, A., Haeger, K., Lindell, S.E. and Olsson, N.M. (1967) Arteriography, plethysmography and walking distance in artrial obliteration of the legs. *Vascular Disease* 4: 280-9.

20. Yao, J.S.T. and Takaki, S. (1978) Technique of measuring lower limb arterial pressures. In: *Clinical Surgery*: Vol. 14: *Vascular Surgery and Reticulo-Endothelial System*, p. 62 (Ed: Bernstain, E.F.). C.V. Mosby Co., St Louis.

21. Nicolaides, A.N. (1978) The value of noninvasive tests in the investigation of lower limb ischaemia. *Annals of the Royal College of Surgeons* 60: 249–52.

22. Lepantalo, M., Lindfors, O. and Pekkola, P. (1983) The ankle/arm blood pressure ratio as a screening test for arterial insufficiency of the lower limb. *Annals Chirurgiae et Gynaecologiae* 72: 57–61.

23. Lennihan, R. and Mackereth, M.A. (1973) Ankle pressures in arterial occlusive disease involving the legs. *Surgical Clinics of North America* 53: 657–66.

24. Strandness, D.E. (1970) Exercise testing in the evaluation of patients undergoing direct arterial surgery. *Journal of Cardiovascular Surgery* 11: 192–6.

25. Froneck, A., Johansen, K.H., Dilley, R.B. and Bernstein, E.F. (1973) Noninvasive physiologic tests in the diagnosis and characterization of peripheral arterial occlusive disease. *American Journal of Surgery* 126: 205–14.

26. Holdich, T.A.H., Reddy, P.J., Walker, R.T. and Dormandy, J.A. (1986) Transcutaneous oxygen tension during exercise in patients with claudication. *British Medical Journal* 292: 1625–8.

27. Fiddian, R.V., Byar, D. and Edwards, E.A. (1964) Factors affecting blood flow through a stenosed vessel. *Archives of Surgery* 88: 83–90.

28. Byrne, P., Provan, J.L. and Ameli, F.M. (1984) The use of transcutaneous oxygen tension measurements in diagnosis of peripheral vascular insufficiency. *Annals of Surgery* 200: 159–65.

29. Takagi-Smith, M., Bryne, P., Ameli, F.M. *et al.* (1984) The measurement of transcutaneous oxygen tension ($PtcO_2$) and its application in the vascular laboratory. *Bruit* 8: 213–16.

30. Dahllöf, A.G., Holm, J. and Schersten, T. (1983) Exercise training of patients with intermittent claudication. *Scandinavian Journal of Rehabilitation* Suppl. 9: 20–26.

31. Gerdle, B., Hedberg, B., Angquist, K.-A. and Fugl-Meyer, A. (1986) Isometric strength and endurance in peripheral arterial insufficency with intermittent claudication. *Scandinavian Journal of Rehabilitation Medicine* 18: 9–15.

32. Coffman, J.D. and Mannick, J.A. (1972) Failure of vasodilator drugs in arteriosclerosis obliterans. *Annals of Internal Medicine* 76: 35–9.

33. Gundersen, J. (1972) Segmental measurements of systolic blood pressure in the extremities including the thumb and the great toe. *Acta Chirurgica Scandinavica (Supplement)* 426: 1–90.

34. Mashiah, A., Patel, P., Schraibman, I. and Charlesworth, D. (1978) Drug therapy in intermittent claudication: an objective assessment of the effects of three drugs on patients with intermittent claudication. *British Journal of Surgery* 65: 342–5.

35. Martin, P. (1973) Surgery for atherosclerosis below the inguinal ligament: the value of profundoplasty. *Progress in Surgery (Basel)* 12: 128–49.

36. Denck, H. (1975) Reocclusion rate after arterial reconstructive surgery. *Journal of Cardiovascular Surgery* 16: 352.

37. Terpstra, J.L. and Thomeer, H. (1975) Causes of rethrombosis following arterial reconstructions below the renal arteries. *Journal of Cardiovascular Surgery* 16: 392–400.

38. Hammarsten, J., Holm, J. and Schersten, T. (1976) Peripheral arterial insufficiency: experiences from 299 operated limbs. *Journal of Cardiovascular Surgery* 17: 503–8.

39. Zetterquist, S. (1968) Muscle and skin clearance of antipyrene from exercising

ischaemic legs before and after vasodilating trials. *Acta Medica Scandinavica* **183**: 487–96.
40. Waters, K.J., Craxford, A.D. and Chamberlain, J. (1980) The effect of naftidrofuryl (Praxilene) on intermittent claudication. *British Journal of Surgery* **67**: 249–351.
41. Clyne, C.A., Galland, R.B., Fox, M.J. *et al.* (1980) A controlled trial of naftidrofuryl (Praxilene) in the treatment of intermittent claudication. *British Journal of Surgery* **67**: 347–8.
42. Wisham, L.H., Abramson, A.S. and Ebel, A. (1953) Value of exercise in peripheral arterial disease. *Journal of American Medical Association* **153**: 10–12.
43. Coni, N.K. (1983) Posture and the arterial pressure of the ischaemic foot. *Age and Ageing* **12**: 151–4.
44. Eickhoff, J.H. (1980) Forefoot vasoconstrictor response to increased venous pressure in normal subjects and in arteriosclerotic patients. *Acta Chirurgica Scandinavica* **146 (Suppl. 502)**: 7–14.
45. Lewis, D.H. and Mellander, S. (1962) Comparative effects of sympathetic control and tissue metabolites on resistance and capacitance vessels and capillary filtration in skeletal muscle. *Acta Physiologica Scandinavica* **56**: 162–7.
46. Raymar, G., Hassan, A. and Tooke, J.E. (1986) Blood flow in the skin of the foot related to posture in diabetes mellitus. *British Medical Journal* **292**: 87–90.
47. Larsen, O.A. and Lassen, N.A. (1966) Effect of daily muscular exercise in patients with intermittent claudication. *Lancet* **2**: 1093–6.
48. Sanne, H. and Sivertsson, R. (1968) The effect of exercise on the development of collateral circulation after experimental occlusion of the femoral artery of the cat. *Acta Physiologica Scandinavica* **73**: 257–63.
49. Alpert, J.S., Larsen, O.A. and Lassen, N.A. (1969) Exercise and intermittent claudication: blood flow in the calf muscle during walking studied by the Xenon-133 clearance method. *Circulation* **39**: 353–9.
50. Zetterquist, S. (1970) Effect of daily training on the nutritive blood flow in exercising ischaemic legs. *Scandinavian Journal of Clinical Laboratory Investigation* **25**: 101–11.
51. Ericsson, B., Haeger, K. and Lindell, S.E. (1970) Effect of physical training on intermittent claudication. *Angiology* **21**: 188–92.
52. Blumchen, G., Landry, F., Kiefer, H. and Schlosser, V. (1970) Haemodynamic responses of claudicating extremities: evaluation of a long range exercise program. *Cardiology* **55**: 114–27.
53. Dahllöf, A.G., Bjorntorp, P., Holm, J. and Schesten, T. (1974) Metabolic activity of skeletal muscle in patients with peripheral arterial insufficiency: effects of physical training. *European Journal of Clinical Investigation* **4**: 9–15.
54. Sorlie, D. and Myhre, K. (1978) Effects of physical training in intermittent claudication. *Scandinavian Journal of Clinical Laboratory Investigation* **38**: 217–22.
55. Ekroth, R., Dahllöf, A.G., Gunderall, B. *et al.* (1978) Physical training of patients with intermittent claudication: indications, methods and results. *Surgery* **84**: 640–3.
56. Skinner, J.S. and Strandness, D.E. (1967) Exercise and intermittent claudication. II: Effect of physical training. *Circulation* **36**: 23–9.
57. Dahllöf, A.G., Holm, J., Schersten, T. and Sivertssen, R. (1976) Peripheral arterial insufficiency: effect of physical training on walking tolerance, calf blood flow and blood flow resistance. *Scandinavian Journal of Rehabilitation Medicine* **8**: 19–26.
58. Lepäntalo, M., Sundberg, S. and Gordin, A. (1984) The effect of physical training and flunarizine on walking capacity in intermittent claudication. *Scandinavian Journal of Rehabilitation Medicine* **16**: 159–62.

59. Schersten, T., Holm, J. and Bjorntorp, P. (1971) Metabolic adaptation in muscle tissue in patients with arterial insufficiency. *European Journal of Clinical Investigation* **1**: 390.
60. Holm, J., Bjorntorp, P. and Schersten, T. (1972) Metabolism activity in human skeletal muscle: effect of peripheral arterial insufficiency. *European Journal of Clinical Investigation* **2**: 321–5.
61. Schoop, W. (1973) Mechanism of beneficial action of daily walking training of patients with intermittent claudication. *Scandinavian Journal of Clinical and Laboratory Investigation* **128 (Suppl.)**: 197–200.
62. Jonason, T., Jonzon, B. Ringqvist, I. and Öman-Rydberg, A. (1979) Effect of physical training on different categories of patients with intermittent claudication. *Acta Medica Scandinavica* **206**: 253–8.
63. Clifford, P.C., Davies, P.W., Hayne, J.A. and Baird, R.N. (1980) Intermittent claudication: is a supervised class worth while? *British Medical Journal* **1**: 1503–4.
64. Lee, K.H., Gutierrez, I. and Smiehorowski, T. (1980) Pedalator assessment of occlusive arterial disease of the lower extremies. *Archives of Physical Medicine and Rehabilitation* **61**: 265–9.
65. Yao, S.T. (1970) Haemodynamic studies in peripheral arterial disease. *British Journal of Surgery* **57**: 761–6.
66. Raines, J.K., Darling, C., Buth, J. *et al.* (1976) Vascular laboratory criteria for management of peripheral vascular disease in the lower extremities. *Surgery* **79**: 21–9.
67. Strandness, D.E. and Bell, J.W. (1964) Evaluation of haemodynamic response of claudicating extremity to exercise. *Surgery Gynaecology and Obstetrics* **119**: 1237–42.
68. Kitamora, K., Miyamura, M. and Matsui, H. (1976) Blood flow of the lower limb in maximal treadmill and bicycle exercise. *Journal of the Physiological Society of Japan* **38**: 457–9.
69. Wakim, K.G. (1953) Influence of frequency of muscle stimulation on circulation in the stimulated extremity. *Archives of Physical Medicine* **34**: 291–5.
70. Randall, B.F., Imig, C.J. and Hines, H.M. (1953) Effect of electrical stimulation upon blood flow and temperatures in skeletal muscle. *American Journal of Physical Medicine* **32**: 22–6.
71. Currier, D.P., Petrilli, C.R. and Threlkeld, A.J. (1986) Effect of graded electrical stimulation on blood flow to healthy muscle. *Physical Therapy* **66**: 937–43.
72. Folkow, B, and Halicka, H.D. (1968) A comparison between 'red' and 'white' muscle with respect to blood supply, capillary surface area and oxygen uptake during rest and exercise. *Microvascular Research* **1**: 1–4.
73. Petrofsky, J.S., Phillips, C.A., Sawka, M.N. *et al.* (1981) Blood flow and metabolism during isometric contractions in cat skeletal muscle. *Journal of Applied Physiology* **50**: 493–502.
74. Hecker, B., Carron, H. and Schwartz, D.P. (1985) Pulsed galvanic stimulation: effects of current frequency and polarity on blood flow in healthy subjects. *Archives of Physical Medicine and Rehabilitation* **66**: 369–71.
75. Hayne, J.A. (1980) The effect of exercise with early claudication. *Physiotherapy* **66**: 260–1.
76. Mashiah, A., Soroker, D., Pasik, S. and Mashiah, T. (1982) Salvage of an ischaemic limb by phenol sympathectomy. *Age and Ageing* **11**: 127–9.
77. Walker, P.M. and Johnston, K.W. (1980) Predicting the success of sympathectomy: a prospective study using discriminant function and multiple regression analysis. *Surgery* **87**: 216–21.

78. Reid, W., Watt, J.K. and Gray, T.G. (1970) Phenol injection of the sympathetic chain. *British Journal of Surgery* **57**: 45–50.
79. Keidar, S., Binenboim, C. and Palant, A. (1982) Muscle cramps during treatment with nifedipine. *British Medical Journal* **285**: 1241–2.

8

Lower-limb amputation

Introduction

In the United Kingdom there are about 1.6 lower-limb amputees per 1000 of the population [1], 80 per cent being over the age of 60 years and with a male:female ratio of 9:1 [2]. Over three-quarters of amputations are carried out because of vascular disease [3-4], although in the elderly this rises to over 90 per cent [2].

Diabetes mellitus is present in up to 50 per cent of patients with amputation for vascular disease. This is important since it affects pre-operative preparation as well as post operative management, the level of amputation (primarily small vessel disease), wound healing and the long-term management.

Preoperative preparation

Preoperative psychological preparation is important [5]. Parkes and Napier [6] have suggested that this should include:

- an adequate explanation of why the operation is necessary;
- an explanation, in simple terms, of what the operation entails;
- a prediction of how the patient can expect to feel after the operation, including a description of the phantom reactions and stump pain (not all workers agree about the latter);
- instructions on what to do about pain (e.g. relaxation exercises);
- reassurance that the pain will pass;
- introduction to, and explanation of, the limb fitting service;
- realistic information regarding the probable effect of the operation on his or her future activities.

An opportunity for the patient to talk with someone who has successfully adapted to an amputation can be helpful at this stage. This peer support can be more convincing than the professional approach, although it needs to be used in conjuction with, and not instead of, the rehabilitation team's support. It must be recognized that peer support is based on personal experience and assumptions which may not be clinically relevant or true. Experience of having had an amputation does not automatically improve the tact of an individual, nor does it necessarily produce an understanding of the needs of the patient.

Since the elderly are likely to have a number of other medical problems the geriatrician should be involved at an early stage. It is helpful if there can be a preoperative team discussion involving the surgeon, physician, therapists, nurses, prosthetist and social worker, along with the patient and the family to ensure that the correct preparations are being made and that the appropriate goals are being set.

A number of preventive measures can be carried out at the preoperative stage. These include:

1. *Prevention of contractures.* Correct bed positioning and exercises are relevant here.
2. *Prevention of pressure sores.* Extra care must be taken of the least-affected leg, which is very vulnerable.
3. *Muscle exercises.* A successful adaptation to a prosthesis will depend on the strength of the patient, especially the arms and the good leg. It is also good psychology to start the exercises at this stage.
4. *Training in walking techniques.* Since the patient will need to use some form of walking aid, this technique can be taught in the preoperative stages, as can the technique of balancing on one leg. Some units have used a strap-on prosthesis on which the patient kneels to give the experience of weight bearing on an artificial limb [7].

Early postoperative care

Prevention of postoperative complications

This includes the normal activities to prevent chest infections, deep-vein thrombosis and pressure sores. Special attention will also need to be paid to the intact leg.

Prevention of contractures

Contractures seriously hamper the rehabilitation programme. They are due to a number of factors, including long-term bed rest (preoperative or postoperative), poor positioning and altered muscle action following surgery. The following positioning of the patient helps to prevent contractures:

1. A pillow should *not* be placed under the knee, nor should the leg be

elevated with the hip and knee flexed. Raising the foot of the bed is a more effective way of treating oedema.

2. When lying on the back the pelvis should be kept level and the legs not abducted; nor should the affected leg be abducted. The patient should be discouraged from hanging the stump over the edge of the bed.

3. Prone lying is effective in discouraging flexion of the hips or knees, provided that the patient does not slip into the side-lying position which particularly encourages flexion of the hips and knees.

4. For side-lying the patient should lie on the non-affected side with the hip slightly flexed. The affected leg should then be supported in a neutral position on a pillow.

5. When sitting the stump should be supported in extension. Sitting with the leg dependent encourages the development of oedema and contractures.

6. A padded resting splint can help to keep the leg extended.

Promotion of wound healing

Wound healing depends on good nutrition, control of diabetes, treatment of anaemia, management of infection and the control of oedema. Stump elevation is required to control oedema, though it is important that the knee is not flexed for prolonged periods since this encourages the development of contractures.

The use of pressure bandaging to control the oedema and 'shape' the stump is debatable. It may do harm, especially if it produces a tourniquet effect thereby increasing the oedema. Pressures of more than 10 mmHg under elastic bandaging can produce venous occlusion [8]. This is relevant since elasticated bandages exerts varying pressure – in one study [9] ranging from 23 to 72 mmHg. Tissues are also particularly susceptible to low constant pressures even for a relatively short time [10].

Dressings

There are a number of possibilities for providing dressing to the stump. *Soft dressings* consisting of gauze pads and bandage secured in place by an elasticated bandage are often used until the wound is healed [2, 11]. They are, however, not without their problems since they do not control the oedema and can actually make it worse.

Semirigid dressings include paste dressings and the inflatable splint. Paste dressings are applied at the time of operation and take several hours to set into a semirigid support. They have the advantage that they are put on before the oedema has developed and provide good protection and prevent oedema development [2, 12–15]. Since the paste bandage has to remain in place for several days, observation of the wound is difficult. It does, however, provide an opportunity for early mobilization in a temporary prosthesis.

The air splint provides a more flexible support while providing easier access to the wound for nursing care [2, 4, 16, 17]. It does have the disadvantage that there is no control of the amount of pressure exerted: it is blown up orally and pressures as high as 35 mmHg can be achieved [8, 16], which may be detrimental to wound healing and venous blood flow.

The concept of the static air splint has further been advanced by pneumatic intermittent compression (see Chapter 3). There is little research evidence for the timing or pressures required, though suggested levels are 40 seconds of compression with 20 seconds of deflation [18], or 20 seconds compression with 60 seconds deflation. It is very difficult to maintain the compression sleeve on a short stump.

Rigid dressings usually consist of plaster of Paris applied at the time of operation [2, 4] and are left in place for about two weeks. Wound healing does seem to be improved by this technique [19].

Rigid braces prevent frequent observation of the wound – some would say this is an advantage! There is, however, the danger that local pressure areas can result in local necrosis. If the fitting is poor or the cast becomes loose, then oedema will not be prevented and damage may occur. Other disadvantages include the need for constant availability of specialized personnel to deal with problems as they arise.

Controlled-environment treatment is a more advanced approach, utilizing a clear PVC bag which, though tightly sealed, allows circulation of air under pressure. It allows constant observation of the wound while providing compression [2, 20, 21]. This system is not yet readily available to geriatric rehabilitation units.

There have been very few studies to indicate the most appropriate dressing. In one study which compared a standard soft dressing with a rigid plaster dressing (with or without early weight bearing), healing was quickest (4 weeks) for the rigid dressing, compared with six weeks for the soft dressing and eight weeks for the rigid dressing with weight bearing [19]. However, only 59 per cent of those treated with soft dressings were able to successfully use a temporary prosthesis, compared with 65 per cent of those with a rigid dressing and 75 per cent of those with a rigid dressing and early weight bearing.

Shaping of the stump

Oedema in the stump makes it difficult to fit a temporary prosthesis. The tendency is, therefore, to attempt to 'shape' the stump using elas-

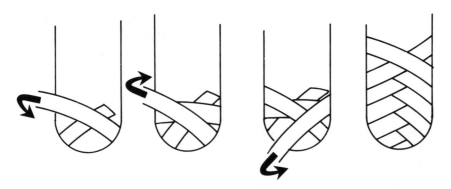

Fig. 8.1 Bandaging the stump of an amputee

ticated bandage or shrinker socks [2]. Unfortunately, when applied over the soft dressing they can produce local areas of pressure and oedema.

To be effective there should be little if any padding under the elasticated bandaging, which should be long enough to provide adequate coverage and wide enough to decrease the areas of local pressure. In general there should be firm tension at the level of the stump which decreases proximally, and the bandage should not overlap by more than two-thirds of its width. Ideally the bandage should be fastened above the proximal joint to prevent it slipping. If slippage is a problem then a cotton sock can be placed over the bandage and attached to a belt at the waist.

There has been some debate as to the most effective way of putting on the bandage. A spiral wrap produces local areas of constriction; and so a figure-of-eight wrap which produces forces diagonally across the leg is more satisfactory (Fig. 8.1), being twice as effective in reducing oedema as the spiral wrap [22]. The figure-of-eight wrap does take longer to apply and requires a longer length of bandage; but these are minor considerations since it is more stable and stays on longer.

Shrinker socks provide elasticated support in the shape of a stump stocking which is fastened to the waist belt for support and used as a secondary dressing [17]. They do not require great expertise in fitting, although as the limb alters socks of different sizes are required. They have also been shown to be more effective in reducing oedema than elastic bandaging [23].

Improvement and maintenance of muscle strength

The amputee depends on the good muscle strength in the arms and the intact leg. Since there has usually been a period of inactivity prior to the operation, muscle strength activities are required pre- and post-operatively. Muscle strength in the residual part of the limb is essential for activity and to maintain muscle bulk for ease of fitting, and comfort of wearing, a prosthesis [24].

Encouragement of mobility and balance

Elderly patients spending too long in bed rapidly develop balance disturbances and loss of muscle power. Active bed exercises include isometric contractions for the gluteals and quadriceps muscles, range-of-movement activities and straight-leg raising. The use of a 'trapeze bar' hanging above the bed assists in care of the pressure areas, transferring activities and for building up arm strength. Transferring techniques are taught within the first two to three days post operatively.

Standing training begins in parallel bars. Weight is taken through both legs using a temporary prosthesis and the weight transferred from one leg to the other and then from heels to toes. Once competent in these activities the amputee can start to take a few steps in the parallel bars, and then later on a frame.

Younger amputees can usually mobilize on crutches, but this is less appropriate for the elderly owing to balance disturbances. For this reason elderly patients usually progress on to a lightweight frame after a period of walk training in the parallel bars. The disadvantage of the frame is that it encourages the patient to hop on the sound leg, with the danger of toppling backwards [25]. This should not be a problem if a temporary prosthesis is used.

Amputation decreases the amount of proprioceptive feedback and increases dependency on vision [26, 27]. It is therefore important to ensure that the treatment environment is well lit and that the patient wears the appropriate spectacles.

Abnormal gait patterns often develop and only a few elderly people achieve the ideal walking patterns of the young traumatic amputee. Nevertheless, good techniques should be taught, and some patients benefit from seeing their difficulties demonstrated on video tape [28].

Transferring techniques

There are several techniques for transferring from a wheelchair to a bed or commode:

- *Side transfer*. The wheelchair is placed parallel to the bed, the arm of the wheelchair removed and the patient slides on to the bed.
- *Diagonal transfer*. The wheelchair is placed diagonally with the

intact leg next to the bed. By standing up and pivoting on the good leg, transfer takes place.

- *Forward transfer.* This can be used for the bilateral amputee. The chair is placed at right-angles to the bed and the patient moves forwards into a sitting position on the bed and then pivots round. This requires good arm strength and most elderly people prefer the side transfer.

Early rehabilitation

Encouragement to stand and walk before the technique has been 'forgotten' is an important part of the rehabilitation programme. It is a useful way of preventing complications such as weakness, balance disturbances and depression, and is an effective way of deciding whether the patient is suitable for a permanent prosthesis [29]. It produces an improvement in the morale of the patient, and a decrease in post-operative mortality and morbidity [30], including primary wound healing [31] and shortening of length of stay in hospital [31]. It also seems to result in a greater number of patients discharged walking on a prosthesis [19, 32, 33].

The major concern about early mobilization is the effect that it has on wound healing. The available evidence is that it does not deter, and may indeed stimulate, wound healing [19]. However, the study did show that the peak time for healing of the tissues was twice as long for a rigid dressing with early weight bearing than for a rigid dressing alone.

Temporary prostheses

There have been a large number of early temporary prosthetic devices. The earlier devices incorporated a footpiece into the plaster of Paris rigid cast applied at the time of surgery. This was rather heavy and had all the disadvantages described above for rigid dressings. There are also problems in obtaining a satisfactory fitting for patients with decreased sensation, persistent pain or skin grafts. Tissue shearing stresses and increased forces have been overcome to some extent by enclosing the stump in Plastazote (a thermoplastic material) as part of the plaster of Paris cast [34].

One way of providing the early mobilization without these disadvantages is by the use of lightweight temporary prostheses. A number of these have been described. Callen [35] has described the use of Hexcelite, a thermoplastic material, which, after being softened in hot water, is wrapped around the stump providing indentations over the patellar tendon to provide a weight-bearing point. It is then left to

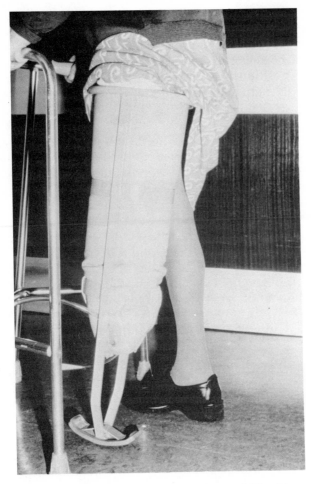

Fig. 8.2   Pneumatic post-amputation mobility aid

cool and harden. A shank, foot and suspension strap is then riveted on to the newly formed socket and the prosthesis is ready for use. Another simple device was described by Devas [36]: this was a foam-lined polyethylene socket which was attached to a foot piece or rocker by two side pieces.

An alternative approach is the use of a pneumatic prosthesis [4, 16, 17, 37–39] (Fig. 8.2). The pneumatic splint consists of a double sleeve which can be inflated. It is first placed around the stump and then in either a fibreglass shell or a metal cage; the bag is inflated to provide a rigid support to the leg. It has several advantages [38, 39]: it is easy to fit and remove, allows easy access for wound inspection, allows early weight bearing and mobilization with minimal discomfort, reduces postoperative pain and swelling, prevents depression, maintains equal pressure avoiding distal oedema, is self-suspending and lightweight, and decreases the risk of knee-flexion contracture. The author has used this technique for one demented amputee who kept falling over because she tried to stand and walk, being unaware that the leg was absent: she responded well to an air splint prosthesis.

It might be expected that this approach can only be used with a unilateral amputation, but there have been reports of bilateral amputees benefiting [40].

The disadvantages of the air splint are that it is bulky and hot for the patient to wear, if punctured loses its effectiveness rapidly, and is difficult to suspend on an above-knee amputee [39].

Prosthetics

The success rate of fitting an artificial limb depends largely on the level of the amputation. Preservation of the knee joint has a marked effect on outcome – a greater proportion of below-knee amputees becoming independent [41].

Stump socks

Prosthetic design and fitting requires specialized skills and will not be considered here. There are, however, a number of points that are important on the general ward.

Patients sometimes complain that the prosthesis does not fit. This is often due to the stump sock rather than to the limb itself [42]. Stump socks are made in a variety of lengths and widths. Usually the sock is made of a wool and cotton combination, although nylon or cotton undersocks are available for those who are sensitive to wool. Although the sock may have been appropriately prescribed at the time of fitting, subsequent shrinkage or increase in oedema may make it unsuitable at a later stage. A sock that is too small will feel tight and will tend to slip into the socket, leaving the rim unprotected. A sock that is too large will prevent a comfortable fitting and have a number of folds which increase local pressure. If the sock continually slips into the socket, a fastening can be attached to fit over the side support of the socket [42].

Patients should be instructed on careful washing of the sock. Socks washed in water that is too hot, or in a detergent that is too concentrated, will shrink and harden. Similar effects are produced if soaking is for too long or if the washing water is hard. Patients should be advised to wash the sock regularly by hand in a dilute detergent and rinse several times in warm water and dry on a flat surface.

Socket discomfort

Some patients will complain of discomfort of the stump within the socket. In an above-knee amputation the aim is to transfer the weight to the ischial tuberosity. This is complicated in the elderly owing to tissue atrophy which makes ischial bearing uncomfortable. In this case the socket may have to be modified to transfer the weight to the gluteal compartment. Most of the earlier problems of tissue breakdown and oedema development can now be overcome by the use of quadrilateral-shaped contact sockets. It must be recognized that there are continuous changes in the size of the stump. Nearly all patients put on weight after amputation [43], and this has to be balanced against the shrinkage. Even mature stumps fluctuate in volume [43].

For the below-knee amputee the aim of the socket is to provide stability as well as load bearing. Although most stumps, even in a patellar bearing prosthesis, take some of the load, there are certain areas – such as the head of the fibula, crest and cut end of the tibia and the area over the hamstring tendons – which tolerate pressure less well than others. If the prosthetist has not designed the socket adequately or there has been a change in the shape of the stump which puts pressure on these areas, then the patient will not tolerate the prosthesis and will require refitting.

Although the socket is designed effectively for walking, it has to be recognized that many elderly amputees spend most of their time sitting down, and therefore a compromise has to be made to make the socket comfortable for this position. This involves ensuring that the posterior wall is not too thick, since this tends to result in compression neuropathy. The anterior brim may also need to be modified to prevent excessive pressure on the femoral neurovascular bundle or the anterior superior iliac spine [44].

Pain in the popliteal fossa may be caused by the posterior part of the socket being too long, or not being flared sufficiently, to avoid compression and abrasions during walking.

Keeping the socket in place also creates problems for the elderly. Although the general trend is to use suction suspension, this is more difficult in the elderly owing to the exertion required to put on the prosthesis and the difficulty in bending forwards [44]. For this reason a pelvic band suspension may be more appropriate, although this needs careful padding and can be uncomfortable, especially when sitting.

Wheelchairs

One of the problems with wheelchairs for the amputee, especially when bilateral, is that the weight distribution tends to tip them over backwards. There have been several approaches to coping with this.

A number of anti-tipping devices have been designed to attach to the back of the chair [45, 46], but these limit manipulating a wheelchair on curbs or around furniture. Repositioning the drive wheels further back gives the chair a longer wheelbase but makes it difficult to manipulate, especially in small spaces [46–48].

Sitting the patient further forward in the chair by placing an insert on the backrest is another possibility [49], but this makes it more difficult to reach the wheels.

Lastly, weights may be added to the foot plate or front frame [45, 50]. Ideally the weights should be as low and as far forward as possible. Although the foot plate is ideal for this, it is not usually required for the bilateral amputee since it creates extra length to be manipulated. However, if the weight is placed on the front frame then the weights need to be about 25 per cent heavier than if on the foot plate [49].

Bilateral amputation

About one-sixth of amputees will have the other leg amputated [51–53]. Bilateral amputation obviously affects the chance of prosthesis success – the greatest loss of independence occurring with bilateral above-knee amputation [54]. Much depends on patient selection and the enthusiasm of the rehabilitation team. The success rate for bilateral above-knee amputees wearing full-length articulated prostheses varies tremendously (from 0 to 71 per cent [55, 56]), as it does for those wearing short pylons (from 10 to 84 per cent [52, 56–58]).

The bilateral, especially above-knee, amputee is more easily rehabilitated on two short rocker pylons [51, 52, 57, 59], often known as 'stubbies'. Their advantages are that the centre of force is nearer the ground, thereby improving balance; there is no requirement for a prosthetic knee joint, thereby giving greater control; and there is possibly less strain on the cardiovascular system [52]. Cosmesis is, however, lost at the expense of safety and energy preservation. They can also be useful in training for longer articulated limbs in suitable patients [59].

One problem with the short rocker pylons is the difficulty in putting them on and taking them off [60]. This can be overcome by putting them on whilst in bed, or a simple foot stool can be made which holds the prostheses while providing the necessary resistance when placing the stumps into the sockets [60].

Stump problems

Pain

When nerves are cut they form neuromata which are sensitive for a period after surgery. These symptoms tend to settle down after a while and often respond to simple analgesia. If the neuroma becomes compressed by the artificial limb then the pain is likely to be more prolonged and may require injecting with a local anaesthetic or even surgical exploration.

Phantom limb

It is almost inevitable that in the early stages the patient feels some sensations interpreted as coming from the amputated part [61, 62]. This is painful in about 35 per cent of cases, of which 14–28 per cent are severe [59, 63]. In one study of 6300 amputees, more than 90 per cent were currently experiencing some phantom limb pain regardless of the time since the amputation [64]. The true incidence of phantom symptoms is unknown, with figures varying by as much as from 0.4 to 50 per cent of amputees [65, 66], largely depending on whether the symptoms are asked about or whether the patient complains spontaneously. It seems that although it is a common sensation only a few will suffer incapacitation and long-standing phantom pain [67].

The cause of the phantom phenomenon is unknown. There are three main theories (65):

1. the *peripheral theory*, in which sensations from the cut nerve endings are interpreted by the brain as coming from the original part served;
2. the *central theory*, in which the phantoms are a conscious process independent of the peripheral sensations;
3. the *mixed theory*, in which self-perpetuating circuits are set up by the disturbed stimulation coming from the periphery which are ineffectively controlled by conscious inhibition.

The mixed theory is probably the most likely. The symptoms and the severity vary so widely between individuals to suggest that much depends on the level of cortical awareness rather than just the degree of peripheral stimulation. This implies that factors other than the physical trauma may be associated, such as previous experience and personality as well as cultural factors [61, 66, 68]. Parkes [66] found that persisting pain in the phantom limb was significantly correlated with a rigid and/or compulsively self-reliant personality, there being many people at home, illness of over one year's duration prior to the amputation, persisting illness with threat to life after amputation, pain in the stump during the first month after the operation, and stump complications persisting at 13 months. It also seems to be more common in people who have experienced pain in the limb prior to amputation and for the quality of the pain to be analogous to the previous pain [69].

Phantom sensation is usually short-lived with a progressive decrease in the perceived size of the amputated sector. There is no doubt that often some patients do feel bizarre sensations, such as the foot sticking out at the side. Unfortunately many patients are 'trained' to expect the phantom limb by well-meaning staff and friends. This should be discouraged rather than reinforced.

Management of phantom pain

The management of phantom pain is extremely difficult. In the first instance analgesics are used. If the pain remains severe then surgical intervention may be required, though this is rarely helpful [70, 71]. Many surgical approaches have been used, including nerve blocks [72, 73], neurectomy [74], sympathectomy for burning type pains [75-77], cordotomy [74, 78, 79], dorsal column stimulation [80-82], thalamic surgery [83-85] and cerebellar section [74]. However, the symptoms are rarely severe enough for these procedures to be considered in geriatric practice.

In the rehabilitation setting a number of techniques have been tried with variable success. These have included electrical stimulation [79, 86-89], percussing the stump end [90, 91], ultrasound [92-94] and acupuncture [69, 95, 96]. One interesting and successful approach [89, 97-99] has been to apply transcutaneous electrical nerve stimulation to the contralateral leg at a site equivalent to the area of pain in the phantom. Similar success has been described [100] from injecting local anaesthetic regularly for two weeks into the equivalent site of the phantom pain on the contralateral leg.

A number of psychological approaches have been used, including hypnotherapy [101], psychotherapy [65, 102-104], behaviour modification [105] and emphasis on attempting to move the phantom. Relaxation therapy has generally been demonstrated to help at least some of the symptoms [106-109].

A large number of drugs have been tried, including carbamazepine [110], chlorpromazine [76, 111], lysergic acid diethylamide [112] and propranolol [113].

The fact that there are so many proposed treatments suggests that none is really effective. The difficulty with most of these studies is that they are reports on a small number of individual cases without controls and rarely follow a single case design type of study. For each of the proposed treatments there are other studies finding that they are ineffective.

It is important to differentiate between a painful phantom and local pain since the management is different. Local pain obviously requires local measures. The phantom pain often settles when the prosthesis is being worn. It is certainly worse at times of stress – thus the need to avoid emphasizing the possibility of the phantom limb.

Complications following amputation

Contractures

As indicated in the foregoing, prevention of contracture development is an important part of early postoperative management. Should a contracture develop it is not only difficult to treat but also limits the ability to provide a suitable prosthesis.

There are several possible approaches to the treatment of knee contracture. Heating the tendon by ultrasound whilst providing stretch using weights (see Chapter 2) can be tried. Pneumatic intermittent compression can be tried, but this is less satisfactory on an amputated leg since it is difficult to develop sufficient torque through the shortened leg.

Another possibility is serial splinting in a plaster of Paris cast. In this technique the knee is extended as much as possible and placed in the cast. After several days a new cast can be applied, the tendon having been stretched further.

A modification of the last approach has been described using a splint consisting of two metal bars positioned along the lateral and medial midlines of the lower extremity and held in place by cylindrical casts above and below the knee, leaving the knee joint exposed [114]. The metal bars are hinged but have a locking device. It is therefore possible to maintain constant tension throughout the day and night but allow active forms of rehabilitation to take place.

Skin changes

Some patients develop blisters, hyperkeratoses, infected hair follicles or a cyanosed and pigmented stump owing to venous congestion. All of these are related to pressure from an ill-fitting socket and require appropriate remodelling.

Psychiatric consequences

Amputation is psychologically traumatic, and it has been estimated that as many as 50 per cent of the amputees need some psychological intervention [115, 116].

There are four elements to psychiatric problems associated with amputation [6]:

- the loss event itself and the individual's reaction to it, i.e. the extent of the amputation and how the patient perceives it;
- deprivation in terms of the long-term effects of the amputation: much of this will depend on the previous activity levels of the patient;
- the effect on the family;
- stigma in terms of how the patient is seen by other people and how he is influenced by other's perception of him.

In addition there is the whole concept of grief over the loss of part of the self [6]. The immediate reaction is that of numbness and a strong tendency to deny the effective reality of the loss [117], followed by pain and distress of varying degrees. This numbness tends to wear off in a few hours to be replaced by pining for aspects of the world which are lost and no longer accessible [117]. This is associated with crying, anxiety and depression. The patient concentrates on, and mourns for, what has been lost.

Adjustment should start *before* surgery, and the professional's role is to ensure that the patient understands the process and that there are no unnecessary anxieties due to misinformation. This will have a great deal of influence on his adaptation to the prosthesis. The patient who is told that he will be given a new leg which will be as good as a normal one is likely to be very disappointed and reject the new prosthesis.

There is a need for help with psychosocial transitions: the need to give up one view of his world and himself in it and to replace it with another view. Kessler [118] has pointed out that:

the emotion most persons feel when told that they must lose a limb has been well compared with the emotion of grief at the death of a loved one. A part of the body is to be irrevocably lost; the victim is 'incomplete', he is no longer a 'whole man'.

Although we tend to think of all amputees as being male, as in fact the majority are, there are differences in the psychological approaches of the two sexes. For instance, 78 per cent of females but only 27 per cent of men had a clear visual memory of the lost limb [117]. It was suggested that this may reflect the importance of physical appearance to females.

Much of the description of psychological and psychiatric reactions to amputations concerns the younger age group. There is some evidence (117, 119) that elderly amputees have less depression and fewer psychological symptoms than younger patients [117, 119]; about half regard the amputation as a minor to moderate upset [120]. However, over the longer term the elderly seem to have greater difficulty coping and this seems to lead to a higher level of reactive depression [117, 121, 122]. As many as 13 per cent of amputees become depressed, 11 per cent have feelings of social isolation and 10 per cent have sensations of helplessness [123]. The helpers should not be forgotten since they too, are markedly affected [123], with 20 per cent having anxiety and depression, 10 per cent feeling socially isolated and 5–7 per cent having extra work or feeling an intrusion into their own life style (with a similar number suffering from a reversal of roles).

The contralateral leg

It is essential to protect the contralateral leg which is at a very high risk of also requiring amputation [51] – as high as 60 per cent in the first five years following amputation. For this reason all the protective techniques used in peripheral vascular disease need to be taken.

In addition there is an increased tendency to develop backache and pain in the contralateral knee owing to the additional load.

Environmental and social factors

Most environmental factors require a common sense approach; for example, avoidance of slippery floors, rugs and obstacles. A patient should be taught how to crawl to a chair to assist standing in case he does fall. Falling and rising techniques are particularly important to the bilateral amputee who may be unable to rise, or even turn over, the prosthesis actually getting in the way.

Stairs may be impossible to negotiate for the elderly amputee, so the usual consideration of bringing the bed downstairs is important. There will need to be adequate room for the wheelchair; and chairs and beds will need to be of the correct height – this is particularly important for the bilateral amputee where lower chairs will be required.

There are a number of reports of the marked psychosocial consequences of amputation [117, 120, 123–128]. Both patient and family suffer a high level of social isolation [123, 128] and often have unmet needs for information about financial help and social activity [123]. One of the difficulties is that patients often react to need by denial. It is, therefore, not surprising that the professional services do not respond. Since many patients do not understand what services are available and do not know who to contact, it is important that the social worker and rehabilitation team take a more active role in counselling.

Prognosis

Mortality

The outcome of amputation in the elderly is poor. In one study one-third of the amputees died before discharge from hospital, with an 80 per cent mortality in those over 80 years of age [129]. Interestingly, none of the deaths occurred in the below-knee amputees. Only one of the 13 diabetics died, previous myocardial infarction did not influence the prognosis, but a previous cerebrovascular accident was associated with a high mortality rate.

Morbidity

To a large extent the amount of mobility obtained will depend on the general fitness of the patient prior to the amputation and the level of the amputation. The latter has an important effect on the energy expenditure required to walk. Even in below-knee amputees a short stump results in a greater energy expenditure than a long stump [130], and this will have obvious implications in the presence of disorders of the cardiovascular, respiratory or haematological systems. Increase in energy expenditure is about 10 per cent for a long below-knee amputation, rising to 40 per cent for a short below-knee amputation, to 65 per cent for an above-knee amputation [130, 131].

Energy expenditure

High energy cost is probably one of the main reasons why only about half as many above- as below-knee amputees gain walking [132]. Much of this variation depends on the conditions under which the tests are carried out, especially the speed of walking expected. In practice the amount of energy expended in terms of millilitres per minute per kilogram is not increased – the amputees walk at the same power cost as normals but at a slower rate [133].

There is very little information about energy expenditure in bilateral amputees, with figures varying from an increase of 41 per cent over normals for bilateral below-knee amputees [130] to 280 per cent for bilateral above-knee amputees [134]. These were studies on younger amputees and the effect on the elderly is unknown.

The non-amputated leg

Another important factor is the vascular state of the 'good' leg. This tends to be poorer in patients who require an above-knee amputation, and there is a stronger correlation on the rehabilitation outcome of the state of the non-amputated leg than the vascular state of the stump [136]. Susak *et. al.* concluded that the amputation removes the most severely affected portion of the leg, and so the 'sound' leg becomes the restricting factor.

Mobility

Few amputees return to a normal lifestyle and as age increases functional independence decreases [41]. Somewhere between 30 and 45 per cent of patients over 55 with an above-knee amputation can walk with a prosthesis [41, 137]. Even of those who are walking on a prosthesis at the time of discharge, about 25–60 per cent revert to a wheelchair life [51, 132, 138–142], though later studies have tended to show 70–80 per cent of above-knee amputees still using the prosthesis one to eight years after the amputation [143–145]. The wide variation probably relates to the change over the last few decades in the selection for the type of surgery and for prosthetic fittings, and the use of temporary prostheses both for assessing and for early training. There has also been a marked change in the style of vascular surgery, with an increase in revascularization procedures. This has resulted in a decrease in the total number of patients coming to amputation, a greater number of below-knee amputations, but a subsequent rise in the age of patients having amputations [146]. Patients with a below-knee amputation are more likely to be fitted with, and continue to use, a prosthesis than are above-knee amputees [142], with only 50 per cent of above-knee amputees and 33 per cent of bilateral amputees fitted with prostheses becoming full-time users [145].

Age itself does not seem to be the important factor in successful use of the prosthesis [147]; other factors such as mental deterioration, congestive heart failure, severe angina pectoris, advanced chronic obstructive airways disease, ulceration or infection of the remaining leg, contractures of the stump [142] or general ill-health [147] are more highly correlated.

A wheelchair existence should not be regarded as a failure since many elderly amputees can still have a good quality of life in a chair. For instance, Clarke-Williams [148] found that, although only 54 per cent of bilateral amputees achieved walking with a prosthesis, as many as 70 per cent gained a genuine improvement in the quality of life by being trained to use a wheelchair correctly. Users often feel safer than trying to balance on weak limbs, especially in the presence of heart or lung disease. It must be recognized, however, that wheelchair mobilization is also costly in terms of energy expenditure, with increases in oxygen consumption and heart rate [131, 149–152]. There is also a decrease in the maximum capacity to drive a wheelchair with advancing age [153]. These factors may then also limit activity to elderly patients, especially those with cardiorespiratory disorders.

References

1. LeBlanc, M. (1973) Patient population and other estimates of prosthetics and orthotics in the USA. *Orthotics and Prosthetics* **27**: 38–42.
2. Kay, H.W. and Newman, J.D. (1975) Relative incidence of new amputations. Statistical comparison of 6000 new amputations. *Orthotics and Prosthetics* **29**: 3–16.
3. Glattly, H.W. (1967) The geriatric amputee and the Medicine Act. *Southern Medical Journal* **60**: 774–6.
4. Kerstein, M.B., Zimmer, H., Dugdale, F.E. and Lesner, E. (1974) Amputation of the lower extremely: a study of 194 cases. *Archives of Physical Medicine and Rehabilitation* **55**: 454–9.
5. Egbert, L., Battit, G.E., Welch, C.E. and Bartlett, M.K. (1964) Reduction of postoperative pain by encouragement and instruction of patients: a study of doctor patient rapport. *New England Journal of Medicine* **270**: 825–7.
6. Parkes, C.M. and Napier, M.M. (1970) Psychiatric sequelae of amputation. *British Journal of Hospital Medicine* **20**: 610–14.
7. Vitali, M. and Redhead, R.G. (1967) The modern concept of the general management of amputee rehabilitation including immediate post operative fitting. *Annals of the Royal College of Surgeons of England* **40**: 251–60.
8. Husni, E.A., Ximenes, J.O.C. and Hamilton, F.G. (1968) Pressure bandaging of the lower extremity: use and abuse. *Journal of the American Medical Association* **206**: 2715–18.
9. Isherwood, P.A., Robertston, J.C. and Rossi, A. (1975) Pressure measurements beneath below knee amputation stump bandages: elastic bandaging, the Puddifoot dressing and pneumatic bandaging techniques compared. *British Journal of Surgery* **62**: 982–6.
10. Kosiak, M. (1961) Etiology of decubitus ulcer. *Archives of Physical Medicine and Rehabilitation* **42**: 982–6.
11. Baker, W.H., Barnes, R.W. and Shurr, D.G. (1977) The healing of below-knee amputations: a comparison of soft and plaster dressings. *American Journal of Surgery* **133**: 716–18.
12. Ghiulamila, R.I. (1972) Semirigid dressing for postoperative fitting of below-knee prosthesis. *Archives of Physical Medicine and Rehabilitation* **53**: 186–90.
13. LaForest, N.T. and Regon, L.W. (1973) The physical therapy program after an immediate semirigid dressing and temporary below-knee prosthesis. *Physical Therapy* **53**: 497–501.
14. Fish, S.L. (1976) Semirigid dressing for stump shrinkage. *Physical Therapy* **56**: 1376.
15. Menzies, H. and Newnham, J. (1978) Semirigid dressings: the best for lower extremity amputees. *Physiotherapy (Canada)* **30**: 225–7.
16. Little, J.M., Gosling, L. and Weeks, A. (1972) Experience with a pneumatic lower-limb prosthesis. *Medical Journal of Australia* **1**: 1300–2.
17. Sher, M.H. (1974) The air splint: an alternative to the immediate postoperative prosthesis. *Archives of Surgery* **108**: 746–7.
18. Redford, J.B. (1973) Experiences in the use of pneumatic stump shrinker. *Prosthetics and Orthotics* **12**: 10–15.

19. Mooney, V., Harvey, J.P., McBride, E. and Snelson, R. (1971) Comparison of postoperative stump management: plaster vs soft dressings. *Journal of Bone and Joint Surgery* **53A**: 241–9.
20. Kegel, B. (1976) Controlled environmental treatment (CET) for patients with below knee amputations. *Physical Therapy* **56**: 1366–71.
21. Burgess, E.M. (1978) Wound healing after amputation: effect of controlled environment treatment. A preliminary study. *Journal of Bone and Joint Surgery* **60A**: 245–6.
22. Whitmore, J.J., Burt, M.M., Fowler, R.S. *et al.* (1972) Bandaging the lower extremity to control swelling: Figure-8 versus spiral technique. *Archives of Physical Medicine and Rehabilitation* **53**: 487–90.
23. Manella, K.J. (1981) Comparing the effectiveness of elastic bandages and shrinker socks for lower extremity amputees. *Physical Therapy* **61**: 334–7.
24. Kegel, B., Burgess, E.M., Starr, T.W. and Daly, W.K. (1981) Effects of isometric muscle training on residual limb volume, strength, and gait of below-knee amputees. *Physical Therapy* **61**: 1419–26.
25. Humm, W. (1977) *Rehabilitation of the Lower Limb Amputee*, 3rd Edn. Bailière Tindall, London.
26. Dornan, J., Fernie, G.R. and Holliday, P.J. (1978) Visual input: its importance in the control of postural sway. *Archives of Physical Medicine and Rehabilitation* **59**: 586–91.
27. Fernie, G.R. and Holliday, P.J. (1978) Postural sway in amputees and normal subjects. *Journal of Bone and Joint Surgery* **60A**: 895–8.
28. Netz, P., Wersen, K. and Wetterberg, M. (1982) Video-tape to improve lower limb amputee training. *International Journal of Rehabilitation Research* **5**: 238–9.
29. Sullivan, R.A. and Tucker, J. (1974) Amputee management using a fitted temporary prosthesis: a preliminary report. *Archives of Physical Medicine and Rehabilitation* **55**: 409–12.
30. Hutton, I.M. and Rothnie, N.G. (1977) The early mobilization of the elderly amputee. *British Journal of Surgery* **64**: 267–70.
31. Alvine, F.G. (1980) Amputation surgery – the immediate fit prosthesis. *South Dakota Journal of Medicine* **33**: 7–11.
32. Golbranson, F.L., Ashbelle, C. and Strand, D. (1967) Immediate post surgical fitting and early ambulation: a new concept in amputee rehabilitation. *Clinical Orthopaedics* **56**: 119–31.
33. Burgess, E.M. and Romano, R.L. (1968) The management of lower extremity amputees using immediate post surgical prosthesis. *Clinical Orthopaedics* **57**: 137–46.
34. McPoil, T.G., Bergtholdt, H.T. and Hunt, G.C. (1980) Modifications of temporary below-knee sockets for amputees with absent or diminished sensation. *Physical Therapy* **60**: 437–8.
35. Callen, S. (1981) Hexcelite temporary prostheses for lower-limb amputees. *Physiotherapy* **67**: 138–9.
36. Devas, M.B. (1971) Early walking of geriatric amputees. *British Medical Journal* **1**: 394–6.
37. Little, J.M. (1971) Pneumatic weight-bearing prosthesis for below knee amputees. *Lancet* **1**: 271–3.
38. Bonner, F.J. and Green, R.F. (1982) Pneumatic Airleg prosthesis: report of 200 cases. *Archives of Physical Medicine and Rehabilitation* **63**: 383–5.
39. Rausch, R.W. and Khalili, A.A. (1985) Air splint in preprosthetic rehabilitation of lower extremity amputated limbs: a clinical report. *Physical Therapy* **65**: 912–14.

40. White, S.A. (1979) Treatment of a bi-lateral amputee using pneumatic post-amputation mobility aids. *Physiotherapy* **65**: 15.
41. Kegel, B., Carpenter, M.L. and Burgess, E.M. (1978) Functional capabilities of lower extremity amputees. *Archives of Physical Medicine and Rehabilitation* **59**: 109-20.
42. Hamilton, A. (1978) Sock care for amputees. *Physiotherapy* **64**: 267-8.
43. Fernie, G.R. and Holliday, P.J. (1983) Volume fluctuations in the residual limbs of lower limb amputees. *Archives of Physical Medicine and Rehabilitation* **63**: 162-5.
44. McCollough, M.C., Sarmiento, A., Williams, E.M. and Sinclair, W.F. (1968) Some considerations in management of the above-knee geriatric amputee. *Artificial Limbs* **12**: 28-35.
45. Hinrichsen, L.C., Nordstrom, C. and Law, D.F. (1984) Device to assist training in balancing on rear wheels of wheelchair. *Physical Therapy* **64**: 672-3.
46. Kamenetz, H. (1969) *Wheelchair Book: Mobility for the Disabled*. Thomas, Springfield.
47. Hamilton, A., Williams, E. and Nichols, P.J.R. (1974) Elderly lower limb amputee. *Update* **9**: 1641-50.
48. Loane, T.D. and Kirby, R.L. (1985) Static rear stability of conventional and lightweight variable-axle-position wheelchairs. *Archives of Physical Medicine and Rehabilitation* **66**: 174-6.
49. Hamilton, E.A., Strange, T. and Luker, C. (1976) Modification of standard 8BL chair for use with double amputees. *Rheumatology and Rehabilitation* **15**: 24-5.
50. Loane, T.D. and Kirby, R.L. (1986) Low anterior counterweights to improve static rear stability of occupied wheelchairs. *Archives of Physical Medicine and Rehabilitation* **67**: 263-6.
51. Mazet, R. (1967) The geriatric amputee. *Artificial Limbs* **11**: 33-61.
52. McKenzie, D.S. (1953) Elderly amputees. *British Medical Journal* **1**: 153-6.
53. Hansson, J. (1964) Leg amputees: a clinical follow up study. *Acta Orthopaedica Scandinavica* **69** (Suppl.): 1-104.
54. Hunter, G.A. and Holliday, P. (1978) Major amputation following vascular reconstructive procedures (including sympathectomy). *Canadian Journal of Surgery* **21**: 456-8.
55. Watkins, A.L. and Liao, S.J. (1958) Rehabilitation of persons with bilateral amputation of lower extremities. *Journal of the American Medical Association* **166**: 1584-6.
56. Sakuma, J., Hinterbuchner, C., Green, R.F. and Silber, M. (1974) Rehabilitation of geriatric patients having bilateral extremity amputations. *Archives of Physical Medicine and Rehabilitation* **55**: 101-11.
57. Lowenthal, M., Posniak, A.O. and Tobis, J.S. (1958) Rehabilitation of elderly above-knee amputees. *Archives of Physical Medicine* **39**: 290-5.
58. Bertelson, A. and Ronn, G. (1960) Prosthetics in geriatrics. *Prosthetics International*, 125-9.
59. Wainapel, S.F., March, H. and Steve, L. (1985) Stubby prostheses: an alternative to conventional prosthetic devices. *Archives of Physical Medicine and Rehabilitation* **66**: 264-6.
60. Figueroa, C., Rivera, D. and Wainapel, S.F. (1980) Table to facilitate donning stubby prostheses by bilateral above-knee amputees. *Physical Therapy* **60**: 909-11.
61. Feinstein, B., Luce, J.C. and Langdon, J.N.K. (1954) The influence of phantom limbs. In: *Human Limbs and their Substitutes*, pp. 79-138 (Eds: Klopsteg, P.E. and Wilson, P.D.). McGraw-Hill, New York.

62. Brown, W.A. (1968) Post-amputation phantom limb pain. *Disorders of the Nervous System* **29**: 301–6.
63. Melzak, R. (1971) Phantom limb pain: implications for treatment of pathologic pain. *Anesthesiology* **35**: 509–19.
64. Sherman, R.A. and Tippens, J.K. (1982) Suggested guidelines for treatment of phantom limb pain. *Orthopaedics* **5**: 1595–1600.
65. Kolb, L. (1954) *The Painful Phantom: Psychology, Physiology and Treatment.* Charles C. Thomas, Illinois.
66. Parkes, C.M. (1973) Factors determining the persistence of phantom pain in the amputee. *Journal of Psychosomatic Research* **17**: 97–108.
67. Soloren, K.A. (1962) The phantom phenomena in Finnish war veterans. *Acta Orthopaedica Scandinavica* **3** (Suppl.): 119–25.
68. Bonica, J.J. (1977) Neurophysiologic and pathologic aspects of acute and chronic pain. *Archives of Surgery* **112**: 750–61.
69. Monga, T.N. and Jaksic, T. (1981) Acupuncture in phantom limb pain. *Archives of Physical Medicine* **62**: 229–31.
70. Morgenstern, F. (1970) Surgical treatment of phantom limb pain. In: *Modern Trends in Psychosomatic Medicine* (Ed: Hill, O.W.). Butterworth, London.
71. Crue, B. (1975) *Pain Research and Treatment.* Academic Press, New York.
72. Tatlow, W. and Oulton, J. (1955) Phantom limbs: with observations on brachial plexus blocks. *Canadian Medical Association Journal* **73**: 170–7.
73. Levy, B.A. (1977) Diagnostic, prognostic and therapeutic nerve blocks. *Archives of Surgery* **112**: 870–9.
74. Loeser, J.D. (1977) Neurosurgical control of chronic pain. *Archives of Surgery* **112**: 880–3.
75. Appenzeller, O. and Bicknell, T. (1968) Effects of nervous system lesions of phantom experience in amputees. *Neurology* **19**: 141–6.
76. Parkes, C.M. (1975) Disease of the CNS: relief of pain: headache, facial neuralgia, migraine and phantom limb. *British Medical Journal* **4**: 90–2.
77. Smith, R. and MacLeod, I.B. (1970) Wounds, healing and wound infection. In: *A Companion to Medical Studies*, Vol. 3, Chapter 2, p. 17 (Eds: Passmore, R. and Robson, J.S.). Blackwell Scientific Publications, Oxford.
78. Raskind, R. (1969) Analytical review of open cordotomy. *International Surgery* **51**: 197–222.
79. Shealy, N. (1974) Transcutaneous electrical stimulation for control of pain. *Clinical Neurosurgery* **21**: 269–77.
80. Miles, J., Hayward, M., Mumford, J. *et al.* (1974) Pain relief by implanted electrical stimulators. *Lancet* **1**: 777–9.
81. Krainick, J., Thoden, U. and Reichert, T. (1975) Spinal cord stimulation in post amputation pain. *Surgical Neurology* **4**: 167–70.
82. Nielson, K., Adams, J. and Hosobuchi, Y. (1975) Phantom limb pain: treated with dorsal column stimulation. *Journal of Neurosurgery* **42**: 301–7.
83. Cooper, I. (1965) Clinical and physiologic implications of the thalamic surgery for disorders of sensory communication. *Journal of Neurological Science* **2**: 493–519.
84. Sugita, K., Mustuga, N., Takoaka, Y. and Doe, T. (1972) Results of sterotaxic thalamotomy for pain. *Confinia Neurologica* **34**: 265–74.
85. Jamieson, K. (1965) Thalamotomy for phantom pain. *Medical Journal of Australia* **1**: 678–9.
86. Long, D.M. (1977) Electrical stimulation for the control of pain. *Archives of Surgery* **112**: 884–8.
87. Indeck, W. and Printy, A. (1975) Skin application of electrical impulses for

relief of pain in chronic orthopaedic conditions. *Minneapolis Medicine* **58**: 305–9.

88. Györy, A.N. and Caine, D.C. (1977) Electric pain control (EPC) of painful forearm amputation stump. *Medical Journal of Australia* **2**: 156–8.
89. Carabelli, R.A. and Kellerman, W.C. (1985) Phantom limb pain: relief by application of TENS to contralateral extremity. *Archives of Physical Medicine and Rehabilitation* **66**: 466–7.
90. Russell, W. (1947) Painful amputation stumps and phantom limb treated by repeated percussion to stump neuroma. *British Medical Journal* **1**: 2024–6.
91. Maroon, J. and Jannetta, P. (1973) following peripheral nerve injuries. *Current Problems in Surgery*, February: 25–8.
92. Kobak, D. (1954) Some physiologic considerations of the therapeutic action of ultrasonics. *American Journal of Physical Medicine* **33**: 21–30.
93. Rubin, D. and Kuitert, J. (1955) Use of ultrasonic vibration in the treatment of pain arising from phantom limbs, scars and neuromas. *Archives of Physical Medicine and Rehabilitation* **36**: 445–52.
94. Anderson, M. (1958) Four cases of phantom limb treated with ultrasound. *Physical Therapy Review* **38**: 419–20.
95. Leung, C. and Spoerel, W. (1974) Effect of auricular acupuncture on pain. *American Journal of Chinese Medicine* **2**: 247–60.
96. Murphy, T.M. and Bonica, J.J. (1977) Acupuncture analgesia and anaesthesia. *Archives of Surgery* **112**: 896–902.
97. Hiedl, P., Struppler, A. and Gessler, M. (1979) TNS evoked long loop effects. *Applied Neurophysiology* **42**: 153–9.
98. Loeser, J.D., Black, R.G. and Christman, A. (1975) Relief of pain by transcutaneous stimulation. *Journal of Neurosurgery* **42**: 308–14.
99. Gessler, M., Struppler, A. and Ottinger, B. (1981) Treatment of phantom pain by transcutaneous stimulation (TNS) of the stump, the limb contralateral to the stump and other extremities. In: *Phantom and Phantom Stump Pain* (Eds: Siegfried, J. and Zimmerman, M.). Springer-Verlag, New York.
100. Gross, D. (1981) Contralateral local anaesthesia for the treatment of postamputation pain. In: *Phantom and Phantom Stump Pain* (Eds: Siegfried, J. and Zimmerman, M.). Springer-Verlag, New York.
101. Solomon, G.F. and Schmidt, M. (1978) A burning issue. *Archives of Surgery* **113**: 185–6.
102. Frazier, S. (1966) Psychiatric aspects of causalgia, the phantom limb and phantom pain. *Diseases of the Nervous System* **27**: 441–50.
103. Blood, A. (1956) Psychotherapy of phantom limb pain in two patients. *Psychiatry Quarterly* **30**: 114–22.
104. Weiss, A. (1956) The phantom limb. *Annals of Internal Medicine* **44**: 668–77.
105. Fordyce, W., Fenton, R. and DeLateur, B. (1975) Case histories and shorter communications. In: *Pain: Clinical and Experimental Perspectives* (Ed: Weisenberg, M.). C.V. Mosby, St Louis.
106. Melzack, R. (1965) Pain mechanisms, a new theory. *Science* **150**: 971–9.
107. McKechnie, R. (1975) Relief from phantom limb pain by relaxation exercises. *Journal of Behaviour Therapy and Experimental Psychiatry* **6**: 262–3.
108. Sherman, R. (1976) Case reports of treatment of phantom limb pain with combination of electromyographic biofeedback and verbal relaxation techniques. *Biofeedback and Self Regulation* **1**: 353.
109. Sherman, R., Gall, N. and Gormly, J. (1979) Treatment of phantom limb pain with muscular relaxation training to disrupt the pain–anxiety–tension cycle. *Pain* **6**: 47–55.

110. Elliot, F., Little, A. and Milbrant, W. (1976) Carbamazepine for phantom limb phenomena. *New England Journal of Medicine* **295**: 678.
111. Miles, J. (1956) Psychosis with phantom limb pain treated with chlorpromazine. *American Journal of Psychiatry* **112**: 1027-8.
112. Fanciullacci, M., Del Benge, E., Franchi, G. and Sicuteri, F. (1977) Phantom limb pain: sub-hallucinogenic treatment with LSD 25. *Headache* **17**: 118-19.
113. Oille, W. (1970) Beta adrenergic blockade and phantom limb. *Annals of Internal Medicine* **73**: 1044-5.
114. Amstutz, M.W. (1981) Unique treatment approach for a patient with a below-the-knee amputation. *Physical Therapy* **61**: 37-9.
115. Randall, G.C., Ewalt, J.R. and Blair, H. (1945) Psychiatric reaction to amputation. *Journal of the American Medical Association* **128**: 645-52.
116. Caine, D. (1973) Psychological considerations affecting rehabilitation after amputation. *Medical Journal of Australia* **2**: 818-21.
117. Parkes, C.M. (1975) Psychosocial transitions: comparison between reaction to loss of a limb and loss of a spouse. *Journal of Pyschiatry* **127**: 204-10.
118. Kessler, H.H. (1951) Psychological preparation of the amputee. *Industrial Medicine and Surgery* **20**: 107-8.
119. Frank, R.G., Kashani, J.H., Kashani, S.R. *et al.* (1984) Psychological response to amputation as a function of age and time since amputation. *British Journal of Psychiatry* **144**: 493-7.
120. MacBride, A., Rogers, J., Whylie, B. and Freeman, S.J. (1980) Psychosocial factors in the rehabilitation of elderly amputees. *Psychosomatics* **21**: 258-65.
121. Caplan, L.M. and Hackett, T.P. (1963) Emotional effects of lower limb amputation in the aged. *New England Journal of Medicine* **269**: 1166-71.
122. Nichols, P.J.R. (1971) Some problems in the rehabilitation of the severely disabled. *Proceedings of the Royal Society of Medicine* **64**: 349-53.
123. Thompson, D.M. and Haran, D. (1984) Living with an amputation: what it means for patients and their helpers. *International Journal of Rehabilitation Research* **7**: 283-92.
124. Weiss, S.A., Fishman, S. and Krause, F. (1970) Symbolic impulsivity, Bender-Gestalt test and prosthetic adjustment in amputees. *Archives of Physical Medicine* **51**: 152-8.
125. Hunter, G.A. and Waddell, J.P. (1976) Management of patient requiring leg amputation for peripheral vascular disease. *Canadian Medical Association Journal* **115**: 634-8.
126. Rogers, J., McBride, A., Whylie, B. and Freeman, S.J. (1977-78) Use of groups in rehabilitation of amputees. *International Journal of Psychiatry* **8**: 243-55.
127. Kerstein, M.D. (1980) Group rehabilitation of vascular-disease amputee. *Journal of the American Geriatrics Society* **28**: 40-1.
128. May, C.H., McPhee, M.C. and Pritchard, D.J. (1979) Amputee visitor program as adjunct to rehabilitation of lower limb amputee. *May Clinic Proceedings* **54**: 774-8.
129. Harris, P.L., Read, F., Eardley, A. *et al.* (1974) The fate of elderly amputees. *British Journal of Surgery* **61**: 665-8.
130. Gonzalez, E.G., Corcoran, P.J. and Reyes, R.L. (1974) Energy expenditure in below knee amputees: correlation with stump length. *Archives of Physical Medicine and Rehabilitation* **55**: 111-19.
131. Traugh, G.H., Corcoran, P.H. and Reyes, R.L. (1975) Energy expenditure of ambulation in patients with above knee amputations. *Archives of Physical Medicine and Rehabilitation* **56**: 67-71.
132. Kihn, R.B., Warren, R. and Beebe, G.W. (1972) The 'geriatric' amputee.

Annals of Surgery **176**: 305–14.

133. DuBow, L.L., Witt, P.L., Kadaba, M.P. *et al.* (1983) Oxygen consumption of elderly persons with bilateral below knee amputations: ambulation *vs* wheelchair propulsion. *Archives of Physical Medicine and Rehabilitation* **64**: 255–9.

134. Huang, C.-T., Jackson, J.R., Moore, N.B. *et al.* (1979) Amputation: energy cost of ambulation. *Archives of Physical Medicine and Rehabilitation* **60**: 18–24.

135. Susak, Z., Gaspar, A. and Najenson, T. (1980) Arterial occlusive disease in amputee patients: assessment with the Doppler ultrasound flowmeter and correlation with rehabilitation. *Archives of Physical Medicine and Rehabilitation* **61**: 269–72.

136. McCollough, N.C., Jennings, J.J. and Sarmiento, A. (1972) Bilateral below knee amputation in patients over fifty years of age: results in thirty-one patients. *Journal of Bone and Joint Surgery* **54A**: 1217–23.

137. Weaver, P.C. and Marshall, S.A. (1973) A functional and social review of lower limb amputees. *British Journal of Surgery* **60**: 732–7.

138. Davis, W.C., Blanchard, R.S. and Jackson, F.C. (1967) Rehabilitation of the geriatric amputee: a plea for moderation. *Archives of Physical Medicine* **48**: 31–6.

139. Anderson, A.D., Cumming, V., Levine, S.L. *et al.* (1967) The use of lower extremity prosthetic limbs by elderly patients. *Archives Physical Medicine* **48**: 533–8.

140. Hamilton, E.A. and Nichols, P.J.R. (1972) Rehabilitation of the elderly lower limb amputee. *British Medical Journal* **2**: 2–3.

141. Steinberg, F.U., Garcia, W.J., Roettger, R.F. and Shelton, D.J. (1974) Rehabilitation of the geriatric amputee. *Journal of the American Geriatrics Society* **22**: 62–6.

142. Castronuovo, J.J., Deane, L.M., Deterling, R.A. *et al.* (1980) Below knee amputation: is the effort to save the knee justified? *Archives of Surgery* **115**: 1184–7.

143. Katrak, P.H. and Baggett, J.B. (1980) Rehabilitation of elderly lower extremity amputees. *Medical Journal of Australia* **1**: 651–3.

144. Steinberg, F.U., Sunwoo, I.-S. and Roettger, R.F. (1985) Prosthetic rehabilitation of geriatric amputee patients: a follow-up study. *Archives of Physical Medicine and Rehabilitation* **66**: 742–5.

145. Rosenthal, A.M. and Reddy, N.K. (1983) Revascularization surgery: impact on lower extremity amputations. *Archives of Physical Medicine and Rehabilitation* **64**: 125–6.

146. Mueller, M.J. and Delitto, A. (1985) Selective criteria for successful long-term prosthetic use. *Physical Therapy* **65**: 1037–40.

147. Clarke-Williams, M.J. (1969) The elderly double amputee. *Gerontologia Clinica* **11**: 183–92.

148. Brattgard, S.O., Grimby, G. and Höök, O. (1970) Energy expenditure and heart rate in driving wheel-chair ergometer. *Scandinavian Journal of Rehabilitation Medicine* **2**: 143–8.

149. Hilderbrandt, G., Voigt, E.-D., Bahn, D. *et al.* (1970) Energy costs of propelling wheelchair at various speeds: cardiac response and effect on steering accuracy. *Archives of Physical Medicine and Rehabilitation* **51**: 131–6.

150. Glaser, R.M., Edwards, M., Barr, S.A. and Wilson, G.H. (1975) Energy cost and cardiorespiratory response to wheelchair ambulation and walking. *Federal Proceedings* **34**: 461.

151. Wicks, J.R., Lymburner, K., Dinsdale, S.M. and Jones, N.L. (1977) Use of

multi-stage exercise testing with wheelchair ergotomy and arm cranking in subjects with spinal cord lesions. *Paraplegia* **15**: 252–61.

152. Sawka, M., Glaser, R.M., Laubach, L.L. *et al.* (1981) Wheelchair exercise performance in young, middle-aged and elderly. *Journal of Applied Physiology* **50**: 824–8.

9

Pressure sores

Introduction

The incidence of pressure sores on geriatric wards is between 20 and 50 per cent [1, 2] and on orthopaedic wards between 12 and 32 per cent [3-5], of which over two-thirds occur in those 70 years and over [3-5]. These are obviously ill patients who have required admission to hospital, but as many as half the pressures sores are managed at home [6]. The true prevalence is unknown, but levels of 43-86 patients per 100 000 of the population are quoted [7, 8].

In a review of 650 patients on a geriatric unit, 19 per cent had pressure sores on admission but 6 per cent developed them during the admission [9]; and higher figures of ulcer development in hospital have been reported [1, 10].

Aetiology

The cause of 'pressure' sores is not as straightforward as the name implies. It is impossible to apply uniaxial pressure to tissues without producing tissue distortion, deformation or shear forces [11]. It is this deformation which produces distortion of the cross-section of the capillaries, which in turn restricts the blood flow. Tissue deforms under its own weight at rest in a gravitational field unless immersed in a liquid of the same density as the tissue (Fig. 9.1). For instance, a deep-sea diver may spend two to three hours with pressure of up to 2025 mmHg pressure on the skin and yet does not develop pressure sores, probably because there is no deformation of the tissues [12]. This has some relevance to the discussion of flotation beds (see below).

Pressure, nevertheless, is an important factor irrespective of how it produces the ischaemia. On an ordinary hospital bed pressure on the skin may be as high as 150 mmHg [13]. Since the capillary pressure is about 12-33 mmHg [14, 15], and may be reduced even further in debilitated patients, anoxia is likely to develop if this pressure is

(a)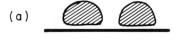

(b)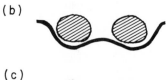

(c)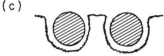

Fig. 9.1 Tissue deformity depending on surface: (a) firm surface; (b) soft surface; (c) flotation bed

maintained for long periods. About 70–80 per cent of externally applied pressure reaches the tissues [16], so a pressure of 40 mmHg on any area is likely to cause obstruction of the capillary network. It is unlikely that this is a sudden cut off point. Localized pressure of about 15 mmHg reduces the flow to about one-third of the non-load value, whereas between 15 and 30 mmHg there is little further change, after which blood flow progressively deteriorates to zero by about 120 mmHg pressure [17]. These measurements have been made on young people and may not be applicable to the elderly. For instance, blood flow over the ischial tuberosities was occluded in none of the young healthy men tested under 120 mmHg pressure, whereas some of the elderly occluded at a pressure as low as 20 mmHg [18]. This might relate to the weight of the patient, since thin patients show higher pressure and incidence of pressure sores over the bony prominences than do average-weight or obese subjects [19] (Fig. 9.2). With increasing body weight the maximum pressure occurred more frequently in soft-tissue areas.

Skin areas overlying bone are the most likely to develop pressure sores. However, although the ischial tuberosities bear the greatest weight during sitting [13, 14, 20] and can reach as high as 300 mmHg, only about 9 per cent of sores occur at this site whilst 43 per cent occur over the sacrum, 12 per cent on the trochanter, 11 per cent on the heel and 6 per cent on the lateral malleolus [21]. Pressure sores are, therefore, not directly related to the pressure levels. There is some evidence that different thresholds of pressure can be tolerated by various parts of the body [22, 23]. For instance, the coccyx can only tolerate about 14 mmHg, whereas the posterior part of the thighs can tolerate about

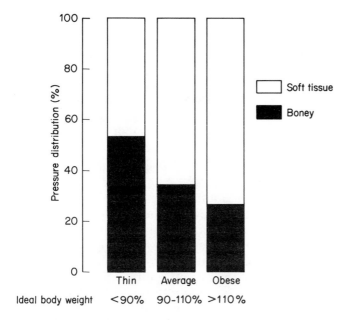

Fig. 9.2 Effect of body build on pressure distribution (after Garber and Krouskop [19])

80 mmHg. This may account for the observed distribution of pressure sores.

Pressure distributed over a large area is less damaging than localized pressure, while low pressure for a long period of time is more damaging to the tissues than high pressure for a short time. Animal experiments indicate that a constant pressure of 70 mmHg produces changes in the tissues within two hours, whereas there are minimal changes with intermittent pressure up to 240 mmHg [24].

Although the two most important factors in the development of pressure necrosis are the intensity and duration of the pressure [25, 26], other factors do play a part – such as shear forces between the patient and the support surface [26–33], friction [33–35], abrasion, temperature and moisture. The rate of development of pressure sores and their eventual severity depends largely on factors such as anaemia, protein deficiency and maceration from urinary and faecal incontinence [36]. For instance, incontinence in the immobile patient increases the risk of pressure sores around the pelvic area by about five times [37].

Shear forces generated by elderly hospital patients are about three times those of young healthy people [18]. With shear forces the collagen fibres begin to align, gradually occluding the blood vessels in the fibre matrix, and markedly reduce the pressure required to produce necrosis [33]. Friction seems to increase the susceptibility at pressures below 500 mmHg [33], probably by applying mechanical forces in the epidermis [24].

A rise in skin temperature is associated with an increase in metabolism [38], which is particularly relevant in the presence of anoxia at the pressure site. Elevated temperature also increases sweating, which in turn decreases the tensile strength in the skin [39], thus making it more vulnerable to shear stress.

It has been pointed out that amputated fingers routinely survive eight hours at room temperature without tissue breakdown [40], suggesting that transient ischaemia is unlikely to be the only factor in pressure sores. In experiments on pigs, muscle damage occurred at high pressure (500 mmHg) for a short duration (four hours), whereas skin destruction required higher pressure (800 mmHg) for a long duration (8 hours); skin breakdown did not occur with pressure at 200 mmHg which was sustained for 15 hours [40]. Daniel *et al.* postulated that normal tissue is far more resistant to pressure than is normally quoted and that pressure sores result from the threshold being lowered by changes in the soft tissues related to paraplegia, infection or repeated trauma.

There is some evidence that infections play an important part in starting the sore rather than being secondary to it [41]. This would certainly explain why some patients do not develop pressure sores although they remain immobile for long periods of time.

Types of pressure sore

Pressure sores are traditionally classified as superficial or deep. Superficial sores do not extend to the subcutaneous tissues or to muscle and normally heal quickly [42–44]. They will, however, progress to deep ulcers if the pressure is not relieved.

Using thermography [45] three types of pressure sore have been identified. The first type was associated with delayed healing and was the most common in geriatric units. Thermographically the temperature difference between the edge of the sore and the surrounding tissue was less than one Celsius degree. Most of these sores healed in four months. The second type usually healed in about six weeks and was found in otherwise healthy people who had lain in one position for too long or had an ill-fitting prosthesis. The temperature difference between the edge of the sore and the surrounding tissue was about 2.5 Celsius degrees. The third type was found in patients who were chronically ill or dying and was associated with alternative contraction and retraction of the margin of the sore at relatively short intervals. Satisfactory temperature differences were difficult to obtain because of the state of the patients.

Shea [46] subdivided pressure sores into four grades:

- Grade I – an acute inflammatory response involving all soft-tissue layers, producing an irregular, ill-defined area of soft-tissue swelling with erythema. At this level it is still a reversible condition.
- Grade II – an extension of Grade I leading to a fibroblastic response in all layers, presenting as a shallow, full-thickness ulcer with distinct edges and surrounding erythema.
- Grade III – progression into the subcutaneous fat, rapidly extending to undermine the ulcer edge. Although the muscle is not directly involved it becomes oedematous and inflamed. These wounds heal by secondary intention, leaving a thin avascular scar.
- Grade IV – pressure sores penetrating the deep fascia, damaging muscle and bone.

The closed pressure sore does not fit exactly into the above classification. It may have a small opening on the skin yet extend widely into the subcutaneous tissues. They are most common about the pelvis overlying boney prominences such as the ischial tuberosity or the greater trochanter.

Prevention

The scoring system described by Norton and her colleagues [1] (Table 9.1) is useful for identifying those patients at risk from pressure sores, although Welten [9] found that in spite of its use many patients still developed ulceration. The score gives a value to various aspects of general physical condition, mental state, activity, mobility and incontinence, giving a maximum score of 20. It was found that the incidence of pressure sores was inversely related to the score: 48 per cent of those with a score of less than 12, 32 per cent of those with scores between 12

Table 9.1 Pressure sore 'at risk' scale (Norton *et al.* [1])

A. GENERAL CONDITION	B. MENTAL STATE	C. ACTIVITY
4. Good	4. Alert	4. Ambulant
3. Fair	3. Apathetic	3. Walks with help
2. Poor	2. Confused	2. Chairbound
1. Very bad	1. Stupor	1. Bedfast
D. MOBILITY	E. INCONTINENCE	
4. Full	4. Not	
3. Slightly limited	3. Occasional	
2. Very limited	2. Usually of urine	
1. Immobile	1. Doubly	

and 14, 21 per cent of those with scores betweeen 15 and 17, and 5 per cent of those with scores of 18–20.

Those who do not move much are the most likely to develop sores, and certainly a low level of moving during sleep is associated with a high risk [47]. The cardinal prophylaxis is frequent change of posture, at least every two hours day and night [31]. This is very difficult to achieve. Patients do not always cooperate and are often upset over a change in position, wanting to return to the more stable position. The workload on nursing staff is great and turning as regularly as is pre-scribed, especially at night, is not always possible; and even when it is carried out it may still be insufficient to prevent pressure sores in very ill people.

One difficulty is for the patient to remember to move regularly. One way around this is to have a timing device fixed to the arm of the chair. Unfortunately the alarm needs resetting, though some automatically reset themselves either at specified times [48] or when the pressure is relieved if this is before the predermined time [49–53].

Attention should be given to the bed surface. Plastic coverings which are impermeable to water vapour should be removed unless they are an integral part of the mattress. The sheet covering the mattress, if rough, can become creased, producing both shear and local pressure. Sheepskin rugs overcome some of these problems, being soft, warm and wrinkle-proof [54] while allowing absorption of moisture, thus keeping the wound dry [55]. Sheepskin, however, soils easily and some patients are allergic to it; although man-made fibre 'sheepskin' rugs are more easily laundered and less allergenic. It must be recognized that sheepskin is ineffective if there is anything between the skin and the rug (e.g. a sheet or pyjamas).

Support surfaces

A variety of beds are available to prevent pressure sores. They are all based on the idea of distributing the body weight over as wide an area as possible. This is important since lying on a firm surface can produce local pressures as high as 300 mmHg [56], whereas if the body weight is well distributed the pressure can be as low as 17 mmHg [15]. Redfern *et al.* [57] investigated local pressure produced by ten diff-erent support surfaces (Fig. 9.3). The highest pressures were obtained from lying on a lino-covered floor and an operating table; moderate pressures (120–165 mmHg) on a 'Ripple' or a sprung mattress; lower levels (57–63 mmHg) on a water bed (not a flotation bed), foam mattress and the Stoke Mandeville bed; and the lowest pressures from a low-air-loss bed or feather pillows on 15 cm polyester foam blocks. The latter is obviously important since it is relatively cheap.

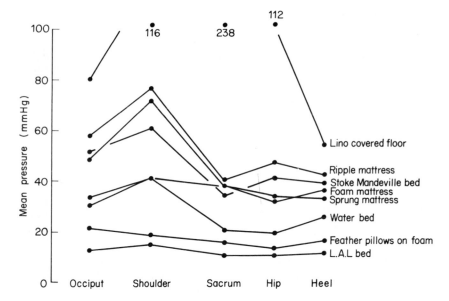

Fig. 9.3 Pressure on various parts of the body using different support surfaces

Static mattresses

Most hospital mattresses are too firm to prevent pressure sores. This may be one of the reasons why patients who are used to lying on soft beds at home suddenly develop pressure sores when admitted to hospital. It is not necessarily the hardness of the surface that is important, since the old-fashioned plaster of Paris moulded bed was very effective at preventing pressure sores because the support system fitted exactly to the contours of the patient, and although they prevented the patient changing position they kept the pressure per unit area to less than 25 mmHg.

Some of the simplest surfaces for pressure sore prevention include a microcellular sponge pad [58]; a gel pad support [27]; a foam mattress with wedges cut out to allow the foam to conform more closely to the body contours; the bead pillow mattress; and the vacuum pack (see Chapter 3). All of these claim to provide a reasonable redistribution of weight, although there have been no satisfactory comparative trials. They have the advantage that they are easy to clean and maintain and there are no working parts to go wrong.

Similarly, contour beds have been devised to prevent shear forces [59, 60]. These consist of beds made up of several sections which can be angulated to provide support whilst the patient is sitting up.

Alternating pressure mattresses

'Ripple' mattresses are a series of pillow-like cells arranged in parallel. Alternate cells are inflated while the adjacent cells are deflated. This pattern is reversed after a period of time, producing an alternating pressure system to relieve pressure from different parts of the body in cycles. Ripple mattresses have proved very successful [61–63], though they too have not been without their problems. The large-celled mattresses are probably more effective than those with small cells [63]. More recently an 'air-wave system' has been shown to be more effective than the traditional ripple mattress [64]. This consists of two layers of air cells rather than one and these are kept in register by moulds along each side. Pressure is alternated by deflating every third cell in turn in a cycle of 7.5 minutes. There is a gentle loss of air from the mattresses through numerous pin holes, which helps to keep the skin dry.

A variation of ripple mattresses consists of a honeycomb of small 4-inch cells which alternate in their level of inflation, although these have been shown not to be any more effective than a mattress composed of siliconized hollow fibres in an interwoven mesh, which helps to decrease friction [65].

Ripple mattresses are only effective when used correctly. Bliss [63] found that half of the mattresses in use were incorrectly installed: some were unplugged or not switched on; others had air tubes which were disconnected or kinked; in some the pressure had been incorrectly set; whilst others had foam pads or pillows between the patient and the mattress. In addition many of the beds had mechanical faults in either the mattress or the motor. These are all very important since a malfunctioning mattress results in local areas of pressure and therefore increases the risk of pressure sores.

Mechanical mattresses

More expensive is the tilting and turning bed which can be turned on its longitudinal angle to allow pressure to moved to a different part of the body. Since it is mechanical only one nurse is necessary to turn the patient, and it is therefore particularly useful for patients who have an impaired level of consciousness.

A different approach is shown in the hammock-style net bed, suspended from poles over the bed. These allow easy turning of the patient, and the net can be lowered to the bed proper for normal nursing procedures.

A more expensive, but very effective, patient-support system is the low-air-loss (L.A.L.) bed [66–70]. This is made up of a series of six groups of large, inflatable pillows. Since the pressure of the air in each group can be controlled separately, the force on different parts of the patient's body can be controlled as required. The bed can be tipped at the head or the foot, and it is also hinged at two places to allow the patient to sit up. Since the fabric of the pillows is permeable to water vapour the patient remains dry, although sweating can be induced if the air temperature is raised too high.

Water beds

There are several types of water bed available. By far the most success-ful is the flotation or immersion bed. This is a tank-like bed containing a large bag which is partially filled with water, so that when the patient lies on it he or she is suspended by the buoyancy of the water rather than by the tension of the bag. Since the patient is, in a sense, floating in the water there is much less deformation of tissues than on other surfaces (Fig. 9.1). This probably produces less distortion of the tissues which is such an important part of blood vessel occlusion. The temperature of the water must be well controlled, especially for the elderly who are vulnerable to hyper- or hypothermia [71].

Other types of water bed, whilst allowing some distribution of pressure, tend to form a hammock or 'bottom out' leaving the patient lying on a firm surface.

Another approach is shown in the fluidized bead bed system, which is a tank containing about 100 kg of glass microspheres through which air is blown, producing a fluid-like medium [72, 73]. The patient lies on a porous sheet on top of this 'fluid'. It has the advantage that the warm air keeps moisture to a minimum and helps to dry wounds, it has a bacteriocidal action [72], and is self-cleaning because the beads cling to any foreign matter entering the fluid. It also has the advantage that one nurse can move the patient easily, and when it is necessary to carry out nursing procedures the patient is moved into a suitable position and the pump switched off. The 'fluid' then sets, supporting the patient in the new position. It is easier for the patient to sit up on this type of bed than on a water bed. Its main disadvantage is its cost – about three times that of a Beaufort Winchester flotation bed, 50 per cent more than a low-air-loss bed, and 100 times the cost of a ripple mattress.

Wheelchair cushions

Disabled patients confined to a wheelchair are particularly at risk of developing pressure sores and a number of support systems are avail-able to help redistribute the pressure. These include foam [74, 75], gel [27, 76], water [77] and air cushions, as well as sheepskin rugs. For instance, a foam cushion only two inches thick will diminish the pressure under the ischial tuberosities by half [56].

There is probably not a lot of difference between the various types of cushion, though the gel type seems to create a higher pressure than most other systems [78, 79]. The types of cushion which come out well in studies of pressure relief are the pneumatic alternating pressure mattresses [79], static air cushions [79] and certain types of foam cushions [79]. However, in the same study another type of foam cushion had the worst pressure readings, so that care is required in the selection.

Pressure relief is, however, not the only important factor. For instance, those cushions containing foam tend to increase the skin temperature and sweating [79–81] since they are poor absorbers and conductors of heat. This is important especially in the presence of ischaemia. How much the moisture level rises will depend on the cover. Open cells are less likely to allow high humidity than those with a non-porous cover which prevents rapid diffusion [80, 81]. Gel pads show a considerably higher heat flux than foam [81] which helps to keep the temperature constant. After about two hours the temperature does begin to rise and the humidity begins to rise because of the non-porous nature of the gel. The patient should therefore restrict sitting to about two hours or change the cushion regularly.

Water flotation pads provide better control of skin temperature owing to the high specific heat of water combined with good conduction and mechanical circulation of the fluid [81].

It must be recognized that no cushion so far available can maintain the pressure below 50 mmHg when sitting [14, 56, 79, 80, 82, 83]. It has also been calculated that a pressure of 66 mmHg on the weight-bearing part of the sitting area is necessary to support a 72 kg man [56]. It is therefore unwise to rely on the cushion itself for protection, and the patient should still be encouraged or assisted to change position at regular intervals.

It has already been pointed out that various parts of the body have different thresholds of pressure, with the thigh tolerating greater pressures than the coccyx. This gives the opportunity to provide cushions with areas of differential pressure [23, 84], while a pre-ischial bar can help to redistribute the weight on to the thighs away from the ischial tuberosities.

Attempts have been made to reduce the pressure under the boney prominences by cutting, removing or inlaying the foam [85]. One of the problems is to identify the precise areas of the highest pressure. This can be done using a barograph [86], but the equipment is expensive and rarely available outside research centres. A simpler approach is a pressure-sensitive transducer system connected to a manometer

[80] which can be used to identify the areas of foam to be modified [87].

One important point which is not often recognized is that the cushions do deteriorate, become torn or damaged and this can make them ineffective. Quarterly assessment of cushions with correction of faults can markedly reduce the incidence of pressure sores [88]. Air cushions sometimes deflate slowly and this may not be noticed, though there are devices to give warning of such a failure [89].

Seating

Many elderly people will not be in a wheelchair and so there are other opportunities for distributing the pressure. For instance, a large armchair allows a greater amount of padding with pillows than does a wheelchair.

For those patients with severe deformities and immobility some

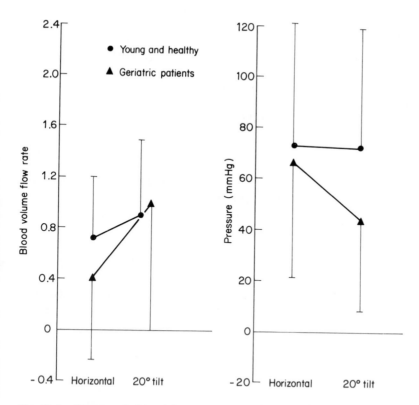

Fig. 9.4 Changes in blood flow and skin pressure on tilting to 20° from the horizontal position

system of moulded seating may be necessary. Apart from helping the deformities, comfort and functional ability may also improve [90]. The use of vacuum posture controllers has been described in Chapter 3.

Although use of the tip-back geriatric chair is generally dis-couraged, pressure sores may be one of the indications for its continuation. With the patient semi-recumbent (at 30°) the pressure on the buttock is about 40 mmHg, which rises to about 50 mmHg when sitting upright [70]. Tipping a chair backwards through 20° produced major benefits in elderly disabled people in terms of increased blood flow, lessening of pressure and lower shear forces [18] (Fig. 9.4).

Treatments

There is much controversy as to whether dressings should or should not be used on pressure sores; and if so which dressing.

The exposure method

As long as ulcers are kept clean and dry they will normally heal provided that pressure is relieved. The exposure method was suggested for burns in the 1940s [91] and gained other advocates throughout the world [92, 93]. This can be achieved by nursing the patient in an ambient temperature of 32–34°C with low humidity or by using an electric fan to keep the wound dry. This helps to reduce the exudation and usually provides some comfort to the patient. If the fan is too powerful the patient will feel cold and uncomfortable. Davis and Chu [94] have described the use of commercial hairdriers which have a long flexible tube as being ideal for this purpose.

Some units prefer to use oxygen rather than air, but there is no evi-dence that it is more effective and is probably based on the findings that hyperbaric oxygen can stimulate granulation tissue [95].

The value of heat in the treatment of pressure sores is uncertain. It did have its advocates during the 1950s and 60s who felt that it improved the circulation [96–98]. This is unlikely since blood vessels tend to maximally dilate in response to the trauma except in severe ischaemia, when heat would be contraindicated.

The occlusive method

Occlusive dressings are now recognized as being more effective in achieving wound healing than exposure [99–101]. They decrease wound pain and tenderness, decrease the inflammatory response, increase the rate of epithelization and increase collagen biosynthetic capacity. The main concern is that they may encourage infection. However, although bacteria are more numerous in wounds covered by dressings, most are normal flora from the adjacent skin and it is uncommon for the wound to become infected [102]. Indeed, some dressings may be effective at excluding infection [103–105] or at least not increase the bacterial count.

The ideal wound dressing [106] should:

- absorb excess exudate and toxic substances;
- maintain high humidity at the wound-dressing interface;
- allow gaseous exchange;
- demonstrate impermeability to micro-organisms;
- insulate the wound from low-temperature effects;
- show freedom from particles and other contaminants;
- allow removal without trauma at dressing change.

Non-adherent primary dressings

These include paraffin-impregnated gauze dressings, which have some degree of semi-occlusivity (e.g. Jelonet); open nylon fabric dressings (e.g. NA); and non-woven pads coated with aluminium and pierced with holes to allow fluid transmission (e.g. Metallinc).

Foam dressings

These have the advantages of conforming to the shape of the wound and being porous whilst providing insulation. They can absorb moisture while providing a moist interface. They are particularly useful for cavity dressings and allow removal of the dressing without adhesion for wound toilet.

Semi-permeable film dressings (e.g. Opsite)

These are transparent membranes (permeable to water vapour and oxygen but impermeable to water and bacteria) which are adhesive and cohesive. Their high flexibility allows them to conform to the shape of the area treated. They can also be used to protect vulnerable areas.

Paste dressings

Polysaccharide granular dressings (e.g. Debrisan or Bard) absorb exudate and macroparticles, including bacteria. They can be used as debriding agents and for cleansing the wound.

Debrisan, consisting of beads of dextran 0.1–0.3 mm in diameter, is effective in cleaning infected ulcers [107]. The powder can be used dry or as a paste mixed with oil. It is only necessary to dress the wound with Debrisan once, or rarely twice, a day for a few days; it is seldom necessary to continue for more than two weeks [108].

Hydrocolloids and hydrogels

These are compounds which are flexible, adhesive, impermeable to gas and moisture and absorb exudate. They swell when they absorb exudate and conform to the contours of the wound. Hydrogels swell three-dimensionally, whereas hydrocolloids swell in a linear fashion locally. Hydrogels are contraindicated in necrosis where anaerobic infections are suspected.

Biomaterials

These are natural, derived materials which may be modified for clinical use to act as hydrocolloids or hydrogels:

1. Alginates occur naturally in seaweeds and have been used (Sorbsan) in either a woven or non-woven fabric form for the treatment of wounds [109–111]. It is a highly absorbent, biodegradable hydrophilic gel which has the advantage that it is easily removed by washing in saline without damaging the surface of the wound [112]. It is not the product of choice for dry wounds or for those covered with eschar or slough, and these should be removed before using the dressing [112].
2. Sphagnum moss has been use for centuries for wound healing. It is highly absorbent and provides a good healing environment [113].
3. Karaya gum power sprinkled into the wound is claimed to have a beneficial effect on wound healing [114].

Enzymatic spray

An enzymatic spray that is water-dispersible and topically applied and contains trypsin, balsam peru and castor oil has been shown to increase the rate of healing of decubitus ulcers by a factor of 2.5 [115]. Balsam peru has a stimulating and bacteriocidal action; trypsin is used [116] to debride the eschar and necrotic tissue, while castor oil is said to improve epithelialization and probably also provides a protective covering.

The proteolytic enzymes help in the breakdown of fibrin, liquifaction of pus and removal of purulent exudate but do not help to remove necrotic tissue [117]. They have several disadvantages, including requiring frequent dressing, the inability to remove large amounts of slough, and causing local irritation [118] or allergic reactions [119].

Cleaning the ulcer

Sodium hypochlorite and boric acid (Eusol) is effective in cleaning the ulcer but also causes damage to the granulation tissue. It can also liberate endotoxin into the circulation owing to lysis of coliform organisms. If it is used it should be applied on a gauze swab at half strength and left for only half an hour. It certainly should not be used as a dressing left in the wound for longer periods. Barton and Barton [2] have suggested that its use can result in renal failure.

A whole host of other substances, for which there is no satisfactory evidence of their effect, have been used and include cetimide; preparations of benzoic, malic and salicylic acids; hydrogen peroxide; and iodine.

A simpler approach is to use dressings soaked in physiological saline to convert the grayish slough to healthy granulation tissue [43]. Others have recommended the use of 2 per cent sodium chloride solution or 20 per cent sodium sulphate solution to remove the slough [55].

Ionozone therapy

By passing steam over a mercury vapour arc a gaseous mixture of ionized water vapour, ozone and molecular and atomic oxygen is produced [120]. The ozone, being unstable, breaks down to atomic oxygen, which in turn further disintegrates releasing energy corresponding to the wavelength of ultra-violet light. In the laboratory the resulting vapour has a bacteriocidal effect and it is probably this effect which helps wound healing. There is some evidence from non-controlled trials [121, 122] and one controlled trial [120] that the rate of wound healing can be increased, and certainly patients benefit by relief of pain and discomfort.

There has been some concern that there are hazards in the use of any apparatus producing ozone [123]. Modern machines have a very low level of ozone concentration (less than 0.1 part per million), which is not regarded as hazardous even on prolonged exposure. It is also important that the machine be far enough away from the patient to avoid scalding from the steam.

Treating the infection

Most pressure sores will be infected but it is not too clear as to the necessity for antibiotic use. Topical antibiotics do decrease the number of bacteria in open wounds [124,125] but can produce local irritation and allergic reactions. The use of oral antibiotics in laboratory animals did not improve wound healing, probably because there was no decrease in the bacteria in the wound [126]. It seemed that the antibiotic was not reaching the granulating tissue, and the author's postulated that the fibrin in the wound was having an inhibitory effect.

Other agents have an antibacterial effect. Topical silver nitrate (0.5 per cent) has been shown to control infection sufficiently to decrease the mortality rate in elderly patients with burns involving less than 30 per cent of the body surface [127].

Nutritional supplementation

Pressure sores are often associated with a poor nutritional state. For instance, in a study of nursing home patients, all those with pressure sores had severe nutritional deficits [128]. This may be a contributory cause to the development of the sore, though as much as 50 g of protein can be lost from pressure sores in a day [129]. This suggests that protein supplementation is necessary in nearly all patients with open wounds.

Vitamin C supplementation has also been shown to increase collagen formation and increase wound healing [130]. The evidence for the use of zinc supplementation is less clear: in one uncontrolled trial there did seem to be some beneficial effect [131], but in double-blind controlled trials there was no conclusive evidence that healing was affected [132, 133].

Ultrasound

Ultrasound decreases the pain, bruising and swelling around surgical wounds [134] and increases the rate of healing of varicose ulceration [135, 136], probably because it increases fibroblast protein synthesis [137, 138]. It has also been shown to assist in the healing of pressure sores [139] and trophic ulcers [140].

Laser therapy

Laser light has a biostimulating effect on wound healing [141, 142] which seems to be independent of the wavelength. The reason for the effect is unknown, but it may be due to a direct effect on protein in the cell membranes [142].

Heel sores

Heel sores are particularly difficult to treat, largely because of the lack of underlying supportive tissues. There are several approaches to protecting the heels. A wedge-shaped foam pad can be used to keep the heels off the bed whilst distributing the weight over a larger area [143]. Other approaches include the use of foam rings which are strapped around the leg to suspend the heel above the bed; Plastazote splints with the area around the heel exposed; or sheepskin boots.

It is not clear whether it is better to remove the black dead skin or not. Taylor [144] found that massaging the intact skin area with a sponge after soaking the skin in warm saline was more effective than a dry gauze dressing. She found that improvement had occurred within seven days in the majority of the treated group, but in only 13 per cent of the control group; and 85 per cent of the treated group compared with 47 per cent of the control group were cured within three weeks.

Deep sores

In addition to the measures already described for superficial sores, a number of other measures are required for deep ulcers. The deep sore may have a wide mouth with easy drainage or a small opening with a large base, making drainage more difficult.

In an open wound the necrotic tissue should be removed, usually surgically, since its presence encourages infection, slows down the rate of healing and prevents the underlying tissue from proliferating [117].

There is a general tendency by nurses to pack wounds with gauze though this may well increase the local pressure. An alternative approach is to pack the wound with honey or a mixture of sugar and povidone–iodine 10% solution (Betadine) covered by a semi-permeable adhesive film dressing. This provides an occlusive dressing of a medium that moves when weight is placed on it, thereby redistributing the pressure within the wound. Sugar substances seem to improve the rate of formation of granulation tissue [96, 145] and its high osmotic pressure may have a bacteriostatic action.

One interesting case history has been described of an 86-year-old man with pressure sores which, in spite of intensive treatment, were not healing, but did so within four weeks of applying oxygen through a funnel fixed over the wound at a flow rate of 12–15 litres/minute for 15 minutes three to four times a day [146].

Closed wounds are more difficult to treat because of the problem of gaining access to the necrotic tissue. Many units use gauze ribbon soaked in antiseptic solutions. There is a great danger that this results in further pressure from the inside of the wound, thereby extending the area of necrosis. In this case packing with honey provides a more satisfactory and effective alternative, though it may be necessary to keep the surface open for drainage with a gauze strip or foam dressing.

Surgical management

When the ulcer involves the deep fascia, surgical management is the definitive treatment [46, 147]. In these cases plain radiography will help to show osteomyelitis is present and whether there is ectopic bone adjacent to the pressure sore, and to define the extent of the pressure sore [148]. Sinography is indicated when there is uncertainty about the size of the lesion, especially those with undermined margins and those having sinus tracts [148]. Computer tomography (CT) is claimed to be useful for pressure sores larger than 5 cm which are complicated by sinus tracts and/or extensive undermined margins [148]. Whereas sinography demonstrates the internal size of the pressure sore cavity, CT can also define the external margin of the lesion. It also has the advantage that it is more likely than other radiological approaches to detect intra-and extra-pelvic abscesses [149].

Where there is protrusion of bony prominences into the ulcer, these may need to be pared down [150], and in deep ulcers a muscle rotation flap may be necessary [151–153] following complete excision of the ulcer, surrounding scar and underlying bursa [147, 150]. One of the problems is to get the wound clean enough for surgery and this may take several weeks of careful nursing care. One way around this has been to use carbon dioxide laser debridement; this allows the dead material to be removed easily and can then be followed by immediate rotation flap closure [154].

It has been suggested that, although the surgical treatment of pressure sores is fairly well standardized, the final result is directly proportional to the motivation of the patient and the ability of the rehabilitation team to train the patient to keep pressure off the area.

The diabetic foot

The progressive angiopathy, neuropathy and deformity of the diabetic foot leave it particularly prone to ulcers which are difficult to heal. This is largely due to the small-vessel disease with thickening of the basement membrane [155], which probably leads to a perfusion defect affecting the nutrition of the tissues [156]. The larger vessels are no more affected than for a matched population [157, 158]. Nevertheless, diabetic neuropathic ulcers do occur in the foot where there is severe sensory impairment in the presence of a good blood supply [159]. They are often associated with abnormal foot alignment which forces the body weight to be borne by areas not originally designed for the purpose. The ulcers then occur at the site of maximal vertical loading [160] and horizontal shear forces [161]. The local treatment requires controlling infection, improving the circulation and protecting the hypoaesthetic areas [162].

Protecting the hypoaesthetic area

A well-lined, moulded, below-knee plaster cast can be used to protect the hypoaesthetic area while the wound is healing [161, 162]. The main purpose is to decrease the vertical and shearing forces acting on the foot [161, 163] as well as distributing the weight over as large an area as possible and protecting the most vulnerable areas. Although the wound heals no quicker than with bed rest, at least the patient can maintain mobility [161]. This type of boot is often too heavy for the elderly, and simple polypropylene or Plastazote footwear usually gives satisfactory protection if moulded to take the pressure away from the ulcerated area.

Advice to patients at risk

The feet should be washed daily in warm water (40°C) and the skin dried with a soft towel by dabbing, not by vigorous rubbing. If the skin is very dry with a tendency to crack, it should be massaged with a lanolin cream; if moist, then it can be kept reasonably dry by applying surgical spirit and talcum powder. The aim is to prevent infection which tends to occur at the extreme degrees of dryness or moistness. The feet should be kept warm and the patient should avoid walking around with bare feet since this increases the risk of trauma.

The patient should examine the feet carefully at regular intervals. A mirror on a long handle or resting on the floor will be required for many elderly patients to carry this out.

Toenails should be kept short but not too short. It is usually easier for the hard nails associated with peripheral vascular disease to be cut (preferably by a chiropodist) after soaking. The corners of the nail should not be cut down since this is a common cause of ingrowing toe nails.

It is essential that the diabetic patient wears footwear that is comfortable and well-fitting. It is important to avoid tight shoes – many fashionable women's shoes, especially, give little support. Ideally flat shoes, with good support so that the heel is kept in the heel-well when walking, should be worn. It may be necessary to use a Plastazote inlay which has been moulded to relieve pressure on the most vulnerable areas. If insoles are used it is important to wear shoes that have enough depth to accommodate them.

Foot abnormalities such as corns and callosites should be treated carefully on the advice of a chiropodist. The hard skin should not be pared down with a razor or file since these are likely to produce tissue damage.

The patient should be advised to avoid tight garments and elastic supports, which will compromise a vulnerable circulation. One point that is often missed is that holes in stockings produce local pressure. Since patients nearly always present to the clinician well-dressed, this point is too easily forgotten.

Stopping smoking is an essential ingredient in decreasing the rate of progress of the arteriopathy. This is one of the few indications for being strict about smoking in the elderly.

Conclusions

The vast number of treatments and the lack of good research makes it difficult to recommend the 'best buy' in the management of pressure sores. The most important guideline is to avoid prolonged pressure on vulnerable areas. Those patients who are frail, ill or disabled, especially if there is mental disturbance, should be turned at least every two hours. Pressure relief can be assisted by a number of surfaces: those which simply redistribute pressure over a wider area will still require the patient to be turned at regular intervals; those which alternate the pressure mechanically will also require regular, though not as frequent, changes of position; whereas those which provide very good redistribution of body weight – such as the flotation bed, the low-air-loss bed or the fluidized bead beds, will required much less frequent turning.

Occlusive and semi-occlusive dressings are now recognized as providing the optimal healing environment, though there is, at the moment, little to choose between the different types. There is rarely any need to add other potions, ointments or medications.

References

1. Norton, D., Exton Smith, A.N. and McLaren, R. (1962) *An Investigation of Geriatric Nursing Problems in Hospital.* National Corporation for the Care of Old People, London. (Reprinted by Churchill Livingstone, London: 1975).
2. Barton, A.A. and Barton, M. (1981) *The Management and Prevention of Pressure Sores.* Faber, London.
3. Jordon, M.M. and Clark, M.O. (1977) *Report on the Incidence of Pressure Sores in the Patient Community of the Glasgow Health Board Area.* Bioengineering Unit. University of Strathclyde, and the Glasgow Health Board.
4. Jordon, M.M., Nichol, S.M. and Melrose, A.L. (1977) *Report on the Incidence*

of *Pressure Sores in the Patient Community of the Borders Health Board Area on 13th October 1976.* Bioengineering Unit, University of Strathclyde, and the Borders Health Board.

5. Versluysen, M. (1985) Pressure sores in elderly people: the epidemiology related to hip operations. *Journal of Bone and Joint Surgery* **67B**: 10–13.

6. Editorial (1973) The cost of pressure sores. *Lancet.* **ii**: 309.

7. Petersen, N.C. and Bittman, S. (1971) The epidemiology of pressure sores. *Scandinavian Journal of Plastic and Reconstructive Surgery* 5: 62–6.

8. Barbel, J.C., Jordon, M.M. and Clark, M.O. (1979) Incidence of pressure sores in the Greater Glasgow area. *Lancet* **ii**: 548–50.

9. Welten, J.B.V. (1973) Pressure sores, prevention and treatment. *Gerontologia Clinica* **15**: 234–46.

10. Irvine, R.E., Memon, A.H. and Shera, A.S. (1961) Norethandrolone and prevention of pressure sores. *Lancet* **ii**: 1333–4.

11. Chow, W.W., Juninall, R.C. and Cockrell, J.L. (1976) In: *Bed Sore Biomechanics*, pp. 95–102 (Eds: Kenedi, R.M., Scales, J.T. and Cowden, J.M.). Macmillan, London.

12. Neumark, O.W. (1981) Deformities, not pressure, is the cause of pressure sores. *Care, Science and Practice* **1**: 41–5.

13. Lindan, O., Greenway, R.M. and Piazza, J.M. (1965) Pressure distribution on surface of the human body. *Archives of Physical Medicine and Rehabilitation* **46**: 378–85.

14. Houle, R.J. (1969) Evaluation of seat devices designed to prevent ischaemic ulcers in paraplegic patients. *Archives of Physical Medicine and Rehabilitation* **50**: 587–94.

15. Siegel, R.J., Vistnes, L.M. and Laub, D.R. (1973) Use of water beds in the prevention of pressure sores. *Journal of Plastic and Reconstructive Surgery* **47**: 31–7.

16. Kosiak, M. (1961) Etiology of decubitus ulcers. *Archives of Physical Medicine and Rehabilitation* **42**: 19–29.

17. Holloway, G.A., Daly, C.H., Kennedy, D. and Chimoskey, J. (1976) Effects of external pressure loading on human skin blood flow measured by ^{133}Xe clearance. *Journal of Applied Physiology* **40**: 597–600.

18. Bennett, L., Kavner, D., Lee, B.Y. *et al.* (1981) Skin blood flow in seated geriatric patients. *Archives of Physical Medicine and Rehabilitation* **62**: 392–8.

19. Garber, S.L. and Krouskop, T.A. (1982) Body build and its relationship to pressure distribution in the seated wheelchair patient. *Archives of Physical Medicine and Rehabilitation* **63**: 17–20.

20. Kosiak, M., Kubicek, W.G., Olson, M. *et al.* (1958) Evaluation of pressure as a factor in production of ischial ulcers. *Archives of Physical Medicine and Rehabilitation* **39**: 623–9.

21. Petersen, N.C. (1976) The development of pressure sores during hospitalisation. In: *Bed Sore Biomechanics*, pp. 219–24 (Eds: Kenedi, R.M., Cowden, J.M. and Scales, J.T.). Macmillan, London.

22. Annual Report of Progress, Ranchos Los Amigos Hospital, Downey, California. December 1973 to November 1974.

23. Spinal Cord Injury Service (1979) *Seating Systems for Body Support and Prevention of Tissue Trauma: Progress Report No. 2.* V.A. Hospital, Palo Alto, California. 9 May.

24. Dinsdale, S.M. (1973) Decubitus ulcers in swine: light and electron microscopy study of pathogenesis. *Archives of Physical Medicine and Rehabilitation* **54**: 51–6.

25. Trumble, H.C. (1930) The skin tolerance for pressure and pressure sores. *Medical Journal of Australia*: 724-6.
26. Lowthian, P.T. (1970) Bed sores – the missing link. *Nursing Times*: 1454-8.
27. Spence, W.R., Burk, R.D. and Rae, J.W. (1967) Gel support for prevention of decubitus ulcers. *Archives of Physical Medicine and Rehabilitation* **48**: 283-8.
28. Cochrane, G.V. and Slater, G. (1973) Experimental evaluation of wheelchair cushions. *Bulletin of Prosthetics Research*: 10-19, 29-61.
29. Dawson, R.L.G. (1974) Treatment of pressure sores. *Nursing Times*: 1108-10.
30. Stark, H.L. (1977) Directional variations in the extensibility of human skin. *British Journal of Plastic Surgery* **30**: 105-14.
31. Guttmann, L. (1955) The problem of the treatment of pressure sores in spinal paraplegics. *British Journal of Plastic Surgery* **8**: 196-213.
32. Elson, R.A. (1965) Anatomical aspects of pressure sores and their treatment. *Lancet* **i**: 884-7.
33. Dinsdale, S.M. (1974) Decubitus ulcers: role of pressure and friction in causation. *Archives of Physical Medicine and Rehabilitation* **55**: 147-52.
34. Sulzberger, M.B., Cortese, T.A., Fishman, L. *et al.* (1966) Studies on blisters produced by friction: results of linear rubbing and twisting techniques. *Journal of Investigational Dermatology* **47**: 456-65.
35. Naylor, P.F.D. (1955) Experimental friction blisters. *British Journal of Dermatology* **67**: 327-42.
36. Moolten, S.E. (1972) Bedsores in chronically ill patients. *Archives of Physical Medicine and Rehabilitation* **53**: 430-8.
37. Lowthian, P.T. (1976) Pressure sores: practical prophylaxis. *Nursing Times* **72**: 295-8.
38. Brown, A.C. and Brenglemann, G. (1965) Energy metabolism. In: *Physiology and Biophysics*, pp. 1030-79 (Eds: Ruch, R.C. and Patton, H.D.). W.B. Saunders: Philadelphia.
39. Wildnauer, R.H., Bothwell, J.W. and Douglass, A.B. (1971) Stratum coreum biomechanical properties. I: Influence of relative humidity on normal and extracted human stratum corneum. *Journal of Investigative Dermatology* **56**: 72-8.
40. Daniel, R.K., Priest, D.L. and Wheatley, D.C. (1981) Etiological factors in pressure sores: an experimental model. *Archives of Physical Medicine and Rehabilitation* **62**: 492-8.
41. Robson, M.C. (1979) Difficult wounds: pressure ulcerations and leg ulcers. *Clinics in Plastic Surgery* **6**: 537-40.
42. Bliss, M.R. and McLaren, R. (1967) Preventing pressure sores in geriatric patients. *Nursing Mirror* **123**: 434-7.
43. Weiss, A.A. (1960) Management of decubitus ulcers. *New York State Journal of Medicine* **60**: 79-82.
44. Edberg, E.L., Cerny, K. and Stauffer, E.S. (1973) Prevention and treatment of pressure sores. *Physical Therapy* **53**: 246-52.
45. Barton, A.A. and Barton, M. (1973) The clinical and thermographical evaluation of pressure sores. *Age and Ageing* **2**: 55-9.
46. Shea, J.D. (1975) Pressure sores: classification and management. *Clinical Orthopaedics and Related Research* **112**: 89-100.
47. Exton-Smith, A.N. and Sherwin, R.W. (1961) Prevention of pressure sores – significance of spontaneous bodily movements. *Lancet* **ii**: 1124-6.
48. Klein, R.M. and Fowler, R.S. (1981) Pressure relief training device: the microcalculator. *Archives of Physical Medicine and Rehabilitation* **62**: 500-1.
49. Chawla, J.C., Andrews, B. and Bar, C. (1978/79) Using warning devices to improve pressure-relief training. *Paraplegia* **16**: 413-19.

50. Fordyce, W.E. and Simons, B.C. (1968) Automated training system for wheelchair pushups. *Public Health Report* **83**: 527-8.
51. Malament, I.B., Dunn, M.E. and Davis, R. (1975) Pressure sores: operant conditioning approach to prevention. *Archives of Physical Medicine and Rehabilitation* **56**: 161-5.
52. Patterson, R.P. and Stradal, L.C. (1973) Warning devices for prevention of ischaemic ulcers in patients who have injured spinal cord. *Medical and Biological Engineering* **11**: 505-7.
53. Temes, W.C. and Harder, P. (1977) Pressure relief training devices. *Physical Therapy* **57**: 1152-3.
54. Davis, L. (1959) Sheepskins and decubitus ulcers. *Journal of Medical Association of Alabama* **29**: 165-6.
55. Walker, K.A. (1971) In: *Pressure Sores: Prevention and Treatment*, pp. 7-75. Butterworth, London.
56. Kosiak, M. (1976) Mechanical resting surface: its effect on pressure distribution. *Archives of Physical Medicine and Rehabilitation* **57**: 481-4.
57. Redfern, S.J., Janeid, P., Gillingham, M.E. and Lunn, H.F. (1973) Local pressures with ten types of patient support systems. *Lancet* **ii**: 277-80.
58. Wigzell, F.W. and Connon, A. (1975) First impression of a microcellular sponge pad in the prevention of bed sores. *Gerontologia Clinica* **17**: 230-5.
59. Gainsborough, H. (1967) My second best bed. *British Hospital Journal Social Services Review* **77**: 859.
60. Andrews, J. (1971) Hospital beds. *Lancet* **i**: 442.
61. Bliss, M.R., McLaren, R. and Exton-Smith, A.N. (1966) Mattresses for preventing pressure sores in geriatric patients. *Monthly Bulletin of the Ministry of Health* **25**: 238-67.
62. Bliss, M.R., McLaren, R. and Exton-Smith, A.N. (1967) Preventing pressure sores in hospital: a controlled trial of a large celled ripple mattress. *British Medical Journal* **i**: 394-7.
63. Bliss, M.R. (1981) Clinical research in patient support systems. *Care, Science and Practice* **1**: 17-27.
64. Exton-Smith, A.N., Overstall, P.W., Wedgwood, J. and Wallace, G. (1982) Use of the 'air wave system' to prevent pressure sores in hospital. *Lancet* **i**: 1288-90.
65. Daechsel, D. and Conine, T.A. (1985) Special mattresses: effectiveness in preventing decubitus ulcers in chronic neurologic patients. *Archives of Physical Medicine and Rehabilitation* **66**: 246-8.
66. Scales, J.T. and Hopkins, L.A. (1971) Patient-support system using low-pressure air. *Lancet* **ii**: 885-8.
67. Scales, J.T. (1972) The L.A.L. patient support system. *Proceedings of the Royal Society of Medicine* **65**: 1065-6.
68. Greenfield, R.A. (1972) The L.A.L. bed system. *Nursing Times* **68**: 1192-4.
69. Scales, J.T., Lunn, H.F., Janeid, P.A. *et al.* (1974) Prevention and treatment of pressure sores using air support systems. *Paraplegia* **12**: 118-31.
70. Jeneid, P. (1976) Static and dynamic support systems – pressure differences on the body. In: *Bed Sore Biomechanics*, pp. 287-99 (Eds: Kenedi, R.M., Cowden, J.M. and Scales, J.T.). Macmillan, London.
71. Brydon, J. (1977) Making heated water beds work. *British Journal of Hospital Equipment* **2**: 29.
72. Hargest, T.S. (1976) Problems of patient support: the air fluidised bed as a solution. In: *Bed Sore Biomechanics*, pp. 269-75 (Eds: Kenedi, R.M., Cowden, J.M. and Scales, J.). Macmillan, London.
73. Taylor, C.W., Ryan, D.W., Dunkin, L.J. *et al.* (1980) Fluidised bead bed in the

intensive therapy unit. *Lancet* **i**: 568–70.
74. Koreska, J. and Albisser, A.M. (1975) A new foam for support of the physically handicapped. *Biomedical Engineering* **10**: 56–62.
75. Ma, D.M., Chu, D.S. and Davis, S. (1970) Pressure relief under the ischial tuberosities and sacrum using a cut board. *Archives of Physical Medicine and Rehabilitation* **57**: 352–4.
76. Paradis, R., Williams, M., Manthey, A. *et al.* (1975) Floatation pad therapy for decubitus ulcers. *Archives of Physical Medicine and Rehabilitation* **56**: 40–3.
77. Weinstein, J.D. and Davidson, B.A. (1966) Fluid support system in the prevention and treatment of decubitus ulcers. *American Journal of Physical Medicine* **45**: 283–90.
78. Palmieri, V.R., Haelan, G.T. and Cochran, G.V. (1980) Comparison of sitting pressures on wheelchair cushions as measures by air cell transducers and miniature electronic transducers. *Bulletin of Prosthetics Research* **10–33**: 10–30.
79. Seymour, R.J. and Lacefield, W.E. (1985) Wheelchair cushion effect on pressure and skin temperature. *Archives of Physical Medicine and Rehabilitation* **66**: 103–8.
80. Mooney, V., Einbund, M.J., Rogers, J.E. and Stauffer, E.S. (1971) Comparison of pressure distribution qualities in seat cushions. *Bulletin of Prosthetics Research* **10–16**: 129–43.
81. Stewart, S.F.C., Palmieri, V., Cochrane, G.Van B. (1980) Wheelchair cushion effect on skin temperature, heat flux, and relative humidity. *Archives of Physical Medicine and Rehabilitation* **61**: 229–33.
82. Souther, S.G., Carr, S.D. and Vistnes, L.M. (1974) Wheelchair cushions to reduce pressure under bony prominence. *Archives of Physical Medicine and Rehabilitation* **55**: 460–4.
83. De Lateur, B.J., Berni, R., Hongladarom, T. and Giaconi, R. (1976) Wheelchair cushions designed to prevent pressure sores: an evaluation. *Archives of Physical Medicine and Rehabilitation* **57**: 129–35.
84. Key, A.G., Manlet, M.T. and Wakefield, E. (1978–79) Pressure redistribution in wheelchair cushions for paraplegics: its application and evaluation. *Paraplegia* **16**: 403–12.
85. Garber, S.L. (1979) Classification of wheelchair seating. *American Journal of Occupational Therapy* **33**: 652–4.
86. Mayo-Smith, W. and Cochrane, G.V.B. (1981) Wheelchair cushion modification: device for locating high pressure regions. *Archives of Physical Medicine and Rehabilitation* **62**: 135–6.
87. Peterson, M.J. and Adkins, H.V. (1982) Measurement and redistribution of excessive pressures during wheelchair sitting. *Physical Therapy* **7**: 990–4.
88. Ferguson-Pell, M., Wilkie, I.C. and Barbenel, J.C. (1980) Pressure sore prevention for the wheelchair user. *Proceedings of the International Conference on Rehabilitation Engineering, Toronto*, pp. 167–71.
89. Werner, P. and Perkash, I. (1982) Warning mat to signal air seat cushion failure. *Archives of Physical Medicine and Rehabilitation* **63**: 188–90.
90. Bardsley, G.I. (1984) The development of body support systems. *International Journal of Rehabilitation Research* **7**: 88–9.
91. Wallace, A.B. (1949) Treatment of burns: a return to basic principles. *British Journal of Plastic Surgery* **2**: 232–4.
92. Barr, P.O., Birke, G., Liljedahl, S. *et al.* (1968) Oxygen consumption and water loss during treatment of burns with warm dry air. *Lancet* **1**: 164–8.
93. Sorenson, B. and Thomson, M. (1968) The burns unit in Copenhagen. III: Treatment and mortality. *Scandinavian Journal of Plastic and Reconstructive Surgery* **2**: 16–23.

94. Davis, S.W. and Chu, D.S. (1974) Air-current treatment for decubitus ulcers. *Archives of Physical Medicine and Rehabilitation* **55**: 138-9.
95. Rosenthal, A.M. and Schurman, A. (1971) Hyperbaric treatment of pressure sores. *Archives of Physical Medicine and Rehabilitation* **52**: 413-15.
96. Smigel, J.O. and Russell, A. (1962) The do's and don'ts of therapy for decubitus lesions, with emphasis on the use of the electric lamp. *Journal of the American Geriatrics Society* **10**: 975-85.
97. Nyquist, R.H. (1959) Brine bath treatments for decubitus ulcers. *Journal of the American Medical Association* **169**: 927-32.
98. Williams, R.W. (1968) Report on the W.R.P.T. investigation into the treatment of pressure sores. *Physiotherapy* **54**: 288-9.
99. Winter, D.G. (1962) Formation of the scab and the rate of epithelialisation of superficial wounds in the skin of the young domestic pig. *Nature* **193**: 293-4.
100. Hinman, C.D. and Maibach, H. (1963) Effect of air exposure and occlusion on experimental skin wounds. *Nature* **200**: 377-8.
101. Alvarez, O.M., Mertz, P.M. and Eaglstein, W.H. (1983) The effect of occlusive dressings on collagen synthesis and the re-epithelization of superficial wounds. *Journal of Surgical Research* **35**: 142-8.
102. Eaglstein, W.H. (1985) The effect of occlusive dressings on collagen synthesis on re-epithelialization in superficial wounds. In: *An Environment for Healing: The Role of Occlusion* (Ed: Ryan, T.J.). Royal Society of Medicine International Congress and Symposia Series No. 88.
103. Easmon, C.S.F. (1985) Skin flora under chest dressings. In: *An Environment for Healing: The Role of Occlusion* (Ed: Ryan, T.J.). Royal Society of Medicine International Congress and Symposia Series No. 88.
104. Shuck, J.M., Pruitt, B.A. and Moncrief, J.A. (1969) Homograft skin for wound coverage: a study of versatility. *Archives of Surgery (Chicago)* **98**: 472-9.
105. Rappaport, I., Pepino, A.T. and Dietrick, W. (1970) Early use of xenografts as a biological dressing in burn trauma. *American Journal of Surgery* **120**: 144-8.
106. Turner, T.D. (1985) Current and future trends in wound management: modern surgical dressings. *Pharmacy International*, June: 131-4.
107. Jacobsson, S., Rothman, U. and Arturson, G. (1976) A new principle for the cleansing of infected wounds. *Scandinavian Journal of Plastic and Reconstructive Surgery* **10**: 65-72.
108. Mummery, R.C. (1981) Bacteriological aspects of wound management. *Care, Science and Practice* **1**: 37-40.
109. Blaine, G. (1947) Experimental observation on absorbable alginate products in surgery. *Annals of Surgery* **125**: 102-14.
110. Gilchrist, T. and Martin, A.M. (1983) Wound treatment with Sorbisan - an alginate fibre dressing. *Biomaterials* **4**: 317-20.
111. Fraser, R. and Gilchrist, T. (1983) Sorbsan calcium alginate fibre dressing in footcare. *Biomaterials* **4**: 222-4.
112. Thomas, S. (1985) Use of calcium alginate dressing. *The Pharmaceutical Journal* **235**: 188-90.
113. Barnett, S. and Varley, S. (1985) Research into the medical uses of sphagnum moss. In: *Bayer Prize Entries 1985*. Tissue Viability Society, Wessex.
114. Wallace, G. and Hayter, J. (1974) Karaya for chronic skin ulcers. *American Journal of Nursing* **74**: 1094-8.
115. Yucel, V.E. and Basmajian, J.V. (1974) Decubitus ulcers: healing effect of an enzymatic spray. *Archives of Physical Medicine and Rehabilitation* **55**: 517-19.
116. Hisplop, H.H. and Pritchard, J.C. (1962) A clinical trial of creams for the prevention and treatment of pressure sores in geriatric patients. *British Journal of Clinical Practice* **16**: 409-12.

117. Kahn, S. (1960) A guide to the treatment of decubitus ulcers in paraplegia. *Surgical Clinics of North America* **40**: 1657–75.
118. Guthrie, R.H. and Goulian, D. (1973) Decubitus ulcers: prevention and treatment. *Geriatrics* **28**: 67–71.
119. Fisher, A.A. (1971) The role of topical medications in the management of stasis ulcers. *Angiology* **22**: 206–10.
120. Ahtmann, V. (1967) Ionozone irradiations. *Zeitschrift fur Haut-und Geschlechstrankhein* **42**: 723–8.
121. Dolphin, S. and Walker, M. (1979) Healing accelerated by Ionozone therapy. *Physiotherapy* **65**: 81–2.
122. Church, L. (1980) Ionozone therapy for skin lesions in elderly patients. *Physiotherapy* **66**: 50–1.
123. King, G. (1972) Home made ozone – a case for control. *New Scientist* **56**: 146.
124. Shuck, J.M. and Moncrief, J.A. (1969) The management of burns. I: General considerations and the sulfamylon method. *Current Problems in Surgery*: 3–52.
125. Krizek, T.J. and Cossman, D.V. (1972) Experimental burn wound sepsis: variation in response to topical agents. *Journal of Trauma* **12**: 553–62.
126. Robson, M.C., Edstrom, L.E., Krisek, T.J. and Groskin, M.G. (1974) The efficacy of systemic antibiotics in the treatment of granulating wounds. *Journal of Surgical Research* **16**: 299–306.
127. Hartford, C.E. and Ziffren, S.E. (1971) Improved survival of burned aged patients treated with 0.5% silver nitrate. *Journal of the American Geriatrics Society* **19**: 833–9.
128. Pollard, J.P. and Le Quesne, L.P. (1983) Method of healing diabetic foot ulcers. *British Medical Journal* **286**: 436–7.
129. Guttman, L. (1976) The prevention and treatment of pressure sores. In: Bed Sore Biomechanics, pp. 153–9 (Eds: Kenedi, R.M., Cowden, J.M. and Scales, J.T.). Macmillan, London.
130. Taylor, T.V., Rimmer, S., Day, B. *et al.* (1974) Ascorbic acid supplementation in the treatment of pressure sores. *Lancet* **ii**: 544.
131. Cohen, C. (1968) Zinc sulphate in bedsores. *British Medical Journal* **2**: 561 (letter).
132. Brewer, R.D., Milhaldzic, N. and Dietz, A. (1967) The effect of oral zinc sulfate on the healing of decubitus ulcers in spinal cord injured patients. *Proceedings Annals of Clinical Spinal Cord Injuries Conference* **17**: 70–2.
133. Norris, J.R. and Reynolds, R.E. (1971) The effect of oral zinc sulfate therapy on decubitus ulcers. *Journal of the American Geriatric Society* **19**: 793–7.
134. Ferguson, H.N. (1981) Ultrasound in the treatment of surgical wounds. *Physiotherapy* **67**: 43.
135. Dyson, M., Franks, C. and Suckling, J. (1976) Stimulation of healing of varicose ulcers by ultrasound. *Ultrasonics* **14**: 232–6.
136. Dyson, M. and Suckling, J. (1978) Stimulation of tissue repair by ultrasound: a survey of the mechanisms involved. *Physiotherapy* **64**: 105–8.
137. Dyson, M., Pond, J.B. Joseph, J. and Warwick, R. (1968) The stimulation of tissue regeneration by means of ultrasound. *Clinical Science* **35**: 273–85.
138. Dyson, M. and Pond, J.B. (1970) The effect of pulsed ultrasound on tissue regeneration. *Physiotherapy* **56**: 136–42.
139. Paul, B.J., LaPratta, C.W., Dawson, A.R. *et al.* (1980) Use of ultrasound in the treatment of pressure sores in patients with spinal cord injury. *Archives of Physical Medicine and Rehabilitation* **41**: 438–40.
140. Galinsky, A.B. and Levina, S.I. (1964) Vascular origins of trophic ulcers and applications of ultrasound on pre-operative treatment to plastic surgery. *Acta Chirgurica Plastica* **6**: 271–8.

141. Mester, E. (1980) Laser application in promoting wound healing. In: *Lasers in Medicine* (Ed: Koebner, H.K.). John Wiley, Chichester.
142. Fenyo, M. (1984) Theoretical and experimental basis of biostimulation. *Optics and Laser Technology* **16**: 209–15.
143. Brocklehurst, J.C. (1964) Preventing pressure sores on the heels. *Nursing Times* **60**: 1249–50.
144. Taylor, V. (1979) Intact heel decubitus: an innovative treatment with a special cleansing sponge. *Archives of Physical Medicine and Rehabilitation* **60**: 283–5.
145. Adams, L.A. and Bluefarb, S.M. (1968) How we treat decubitus ulcers. *Postgraduate Medicine* **44**: 269–71.
146. Gorecki, Z. (1964) Oxygen under pressure applied directly to bedsores: case report. *Journal of the American Geriatrics Society* **12**: 1147–8.
147. Griffith, B.H. (1963) Advances in the treatment of decubitus ulcer. *Surgical Clinics of North America* **43**: 245–60.
148. Hendrix, R.W., Calenoff, L., Lederman, R.B. and Neiman, H.L. (1981) Radiology of pressure sores. *Diagnostic Radiology* **138**: 351–6.
149. Firooznia, H., Rafii, M., Golimbu, C. *et al.* (1982) Computed tomography of pressure sores, pelvic abscecss, and osteomyelitis in patients with spinal cord injury. *Archives of Physical Medicine and Rehabilitation* **63**: 545–8.
150. Herceg, S.J. and Harding, R.L. (1978) Surgical treatment of pressure ulcers. *Archives of Physical Medicine and Rehabilitation* **59**: 193–200.
151. Ger, R. (1971) The surgical management of decubitus ulcers in muscle transposition. *Surgery* **69**: 106–10.
152. Griffith, B.H. and Schultz, R.C. (1961) The prevention and surgical treatment of recurrent decubitus ulcers in patients with paraplegia. *Plastic and Reconstructive Surgery* **23**: 248–60.
153. Sanchez, S., Eamegdool, S. and Conway, H. (1969) Surgical treatment of decubitus ulcers in paraplegics. *Journal of Plastic and Reconstructive Surgery* **43**: 25–8.
154. Stellar, S., Meijer, R., Walia, S. and Mamoun, S. (1973) Carbon dioxide debridement of decubitus ulcers followed by immediate rotation flap or skin graft closure. *Annals of Surgery* **179**: 230–7.
155 Aagenes, O. and Moe, H. (1961) Light- and electron-microscope study of skin capilaries in diabetics. *Diabetes* **10**: 253–9.
156. Ismail, A.A., Khalifa, K. and Medwar, K.R. (1965) Capillary loss of radio-iodinated serum albumin in diabetics. *Lancet* **ii**: 810–13.
157. Conrad, M.C. (1967) Large and small artery occlusion in diabetics and non-diabetics with severe vascular disease. *Circulation* **36**: 83–91.
158. Kelly, P. and James, J.M. (1970) Criteria for determining the proper level of amputation in occlusive vascular disease. *Journal of Bone and Joint Surgery* **52A**: 1685–8.
159. Ellenberg, M. (1968) Diabetic neuropathic ulcer. *Journal of Mount Sinai Hospital, New York* **35**: 585–94.
160. Ctercteko, G.C., Dhanendran, Hutton, W.C. and Le Quesne, L.P. (1981) Vertical forces acting on the feet of diabetic patients with neuropathic ulceration. *British Journal of Surgery* **68**: 609–14.
161. Pollard, J.P., Le Quesne, L.P. and Tappin, J.W. (1983) Forces under the foot. *Journal of Biomedical Engineering* **5**: 37–40.
162. Meggitt, B. (1976) Surgical management of the diabetic foot. *British Journal of Hospital Medicine* **26**: 227–32.
163. Tappin, J.W., Pollard, J. and Beckett, E.A. (1980) Method of measuring 'shearing' forces on the sole of the foot. *Clinical Physics and Physiological Measurement* **i**: 83–5.

10

Oedema and venous conditions

Oedema

Oedema is generally thought to be due to venous stasis associated with incompetence of the valves in the small veins connecting the superficial and deep venous channels. Normally the muscle pump of the leg muscles reduces the venous pressure from about 130 cm of water to about 50 cm, but only to about 100 cm when the veins are incompetent [1]. However, it has been pointed out that even when the saphenous veins have been stripped, and all the visible perforating veins tied, that the superficial system continues to drain satisfactorily [2]. Moreover, many perforating veins are valveless and others have their valves pointing in the opposite direction.

Oedema is likely to occur if there is a rise in the capillary pressure, a decrease in the interstitial fluid pressure, a rise in the osmotic pressure in the interstitial fluid or a decrease in the osmotic pressure of the plasma.

Increase in the capillary pressure occurs with heart failure, incompetence of the valves of the deep veins or with venous obstruction. When this occurs the high venous pressure is not lowered efficiently by the calf muscle pump [3], resulting in extravasation of macromolecules from distended capilliaries [4] and presenting as lipodermatosclerosis.

There is, however, an even larger increase in the capillary pressure when erect, which accounts for the dependent oedema associated with inactivity or standing for long periods of time.

Normally there is an increase in the precapillary resistance in the foot on standing which protects against excessive capillary rise in pressure [5, 6] This vasoconstriction is often lost in diabetics [7], probably accounting for the oedema commonly found associated with diabetic neuropathy [5, 8].

Dependent oedema is the commonest cause of ankle swelling in the elderly. The danger is that diuretics are prescribed unnecessarily because it is diagnosed as being due to failure. Some argue that it is worth while giving a course of diuretics to assist the removal of the fluid, since the longer the oedema is present the more likely it is to become permanent owing to inflammation of the subcutaneous tissues, subsequent fibrosis and lymphatic blockage by macroglobulins. Long-term diuretics should not be required, the treatment being to correct the cause (i.e. the dependent nature of the legs).

An increase in the osmotic pressure of the interstitial fluid occurs in damage to the capillary wall from infection or trauma. It is also possible that lymphatic obstruction produces oedema owing to the high osmotic pressure from the protein accumulation. A decrease in the osmotic pressure is seen in hypoproteinaemic states, such as protein-losing nephropathy or malnutrition.

Management of oedema

Leg elevation

The pressure in the legs is directly related to their vertical distance from the heart (Fig. 10.1); the pressure at the ankle when standing is higher than when sitting, which in turn is higher than when lying with the feet elevated.

Although it is generally thought that elevation of the leg improves venous drainage, this is probably not true [2]. There is an increase in blood flow in the veins on elevating the leg, but this very rapidly slows

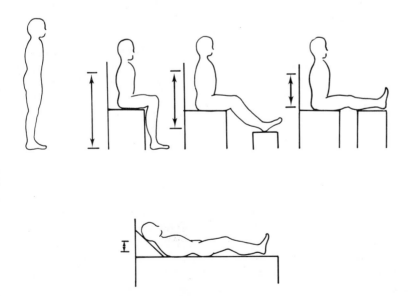

Fig. 10.1   Ankle venous pressure in different positions

to a level lower than that when dependent, probably due to a decrease in the amount of blood in the veins. The reason that elevation helps in oedema is probably more related to the decrease in the intracapillary pressure which slows the formation of more oedema and encourages reabsorption of that oedema present.

Oedema fluid moves around the body to settle in the most dependent area, although this might not be obvious clinically. A reduction in leg oedema may merely redistribute the fluid, which then returns when the legs are again dependent.

Patients should be encouraged to walk regularly to take advantage of the muscle pump in the calf muscles. They should preferably wear well-fitting shoes since loose slippers encourage shuffling which produces less effective muscle pumping action. When sitting the patient should keep the feet elevated, preferably to the horizontal.

Compression bandages

There is evidence that compression bandaging decreases the oedema [9] and increases the velocity of venous flow in the legs [10–12], probably by increasing the interstitial pressure. There is a great danger of the bandages being misapplied to an extent that the microcirculation is compromised.

There is a popular view that the pressure provided by the bandaging should not be greater than 10 mmHg if the patient is on bed rest – corresponding to moderate stretch on a new crêpe bandage with 50 per cent overlap. At full stretch a crêpe bandage can exert up to five times this pressure, though the tension does ease off after application [2]. However, if the patient is mobile then higher bandage pressure (up to 80–90 mmHg) produces a greater venous pumping [2, 13–15]. If high-pressure bandaging is used then it is important that the patient removes the bandage at night, otherwise the drop in the perfusion pressure associated with elevation of the legs will result in ischaemia and pain. If pain does develop then the patient should walk around for a few minutes to increase the capillary pressure in the feet.

It is normal practice to graduate the tension of the bandage as the dressing proceeds up the leg. There is probably little point in doing so for a patient at rest; but for those who are more mobile the pressure at the ankle is likely to be about twice that at the groin and therefore this would seem logical advice. However, Johnsone and Pflug [2] have pointed out that the compression exerted by an elastic bandage not only varies with the tension but also inversely with the radius of curvature of the bandage surface. Thus, even if the bandage is applied at even tension, the compression forces will decrease from foot to groin as the circumference of the leg increases.

Graduated elasticated stockings

The general belief that graduated compression is important has resulted in the manufacture of graduated elastic stockings. Those with a pressure of 18 mmHg at the ankle and 8 mmHg at mid-thigh have been shown to produce a fall in the venous pressure when walking [16] and the compensate for venous hypertension [12] by raising the interstitial pressure and decreasing the ambulatory venous pressure [16–18]; to increase the flow through unocculuded veins resulting in an improvement of the venous return [10, 14, 17]; and to improve the capillary clearance [15].

All of these positive effects may be more due to the compression than to the fact that the pressure is graduated, since in the majority of fittings graduated compression in not actually achieved [19].

Scott (20) recommends that elastic stockings should be stout, seamless, below-knee, one-way stretch and with heels. The reason for recommending below-knee stockings is that varicose and gravitational oedema is confined to below the knee: varicose ulcers are never seen on the thigh; stockings around the knee and thigh produce constriction of venous drainage from the rest of the leg; and stout above-knee stockings are difficult to keep up – to which might be added that long, stout stockings are very difficult for elderly people to put on. The reason for advising that the stockings have heels is to avoid local areas of pressure which develop at the edge of heel-less stockings.

Patients often complain of the tightness of stockings, though it has been suggested that this is pathognomic for patients in whom the venous component is only a minor factor in their symptoms [14]. Those with severe venous states frequently demand firm compression stockings.

Pneumatic intermittent compression

There are a number of reports that pneumatic intermittent compression (see Chapter 3) can be of help in the treatment of oedema [2, 21–23]. The effect of compression is to squeeze the blood in both the arterial and venous trees. However, at the pressures used in the splints this will have little, if any, effect on the large arteries, and thus the effect is greater in the veins. The blood, therefore, empties from the veins during the compression phase, and because of the venous valves, retrograde filling does not take place. Therefore any filling of the veins will be from the periphery, with decrease in the capillary pressure allowing reabsorption of fluid.

Lipodermatosclerosis

High venous pressure results in the exudation of macromolecules, leading to the development of lipodermatosclerosis. Elastic stockings help to enhance the release of plasminogen activator locally [24], which by helping to break down the extravasated pericapillary fibrin deposits may account for the healing of the lipodermatosclerosis seen with graduated stocking use [25].

In intractable cases of liposclerosis with induration and pigmentation, stanozol, an anabolic steroid, is claimed to be of some help. Most of the evidence for this comes from uncontrolled trials [26, 27], whereas the same authors in a controlled trial found no difference between the treated and control groups [25]. Stanozol tends to produce fluid retention which counteracts the effect of compression stockings: and liver function tests may also become abnormal, though they usually return to normal when treatment is discontinued.

Varicose ulceration

Varicose ulcers are areas of gangrene of the skin and subcutaneous tissue near to the ankle. They rarely penetrate to muscle or bone. Most patients who develop these ulcers have usually had a deep-vein thrombosis [28], although the ulcer may take a decade or two to develop. It is possible that the underlying disturbance is one deposition of an impermeable fibrin cuff around the dermal capillaries [29, 30].

The type of ulcer seen in the elderly is more common in females than males (ratio of 4:1) and is less often associated with obesity as in those occurring in the younger patient.

Varicose ulcers are often recurrent and difficult to heal. Prolonged rest is probably the most effective treatment; however, this is rarely possible and even when healed in this way they often return. Exercise is probably as important as rest since the area of ulceration depends on the ability of the calf muscles to reduce vein pressure [31]. Patients should either walk around or sit with their feet elevated; they should not stand for long periods.

Several dressings have been used for varicose ulcers. These include zinc oxide 10% impregnated cotton bandage (Viscopaste PB7), a combination of zinc paste, calamine and clioquinol bandage (Quinaband), or zinc oxide 6% and ichthammol paste impregnated bandage (Ichthopaste). These all have the advantages of requiring dressing only twice a week and, because they set quite firm, prevent the patient from interferring with the ulcer. It is important that these dressings are placed tangentially up the leg, since as they dry they contract and this can cause vascular insufficiency if placed around the circumference of the leg. There is little to chose between these different dressings, though Ichthopaste is often better when there is pruritis.

It has already been indicated above that the use of oral zinc sulphate in the healing of wounds is debatable. Zinc is a component of the enzyme system which is necessary for replication of epithelial cells. Several authors have felt that it is an important factor in healing of varicose ulcers [32–35]. The plasma zinc concentrations of patients with venous ulcers is unrelated to the rate of healing [32, 36]. However, the concentration in the skin may be more important than the blood levels [32]. The accidental addition of zinc to the diet of rats was found to increase the rate of healing of thermal burns and excised wounds [35]. This was confirmed in other animal experiments and then in healing granulating wounds following excision of pilonidal sinus in young men [35] using zinc sulphate 200 mg three times a day.

Ultrasound has also been shown in a controlled trial of ultrasound versus 'mock' ultrasound (the machine used but not switched on) to have a marked effect on the healing of varicose ulceration [37].

One of the most distressing features of leg ulcers, and for that matter pressure sores, is the pungent smell associated with a green exudate. There have been reports that topical 1% metronidazole can help to eliminate the foul smell and promote healing [38, 39]. This requires further verification since the trial was poorly controlled and the treatment always followed the control period.

Activated charcoal cloth (Actisorb) is used by some clinicians as a deodorizer. Some nurses find that placing yoghurt in the wound decreases the odour, probably by replacing one set of bacteria with another. Sugar or honey is said to have a similar effect on odour.

Sores appearing on the lower leg are not necessarily due to varicose ulceration. Other types are: ischaemic, vasculitis (tend to be multiple and painful), neurotrophic, haemolytic ulcer (usually associated with infection), pressure sores, traumatic, pyogenic or malignant.

Skin laceration

Lacerations over the skin may take months to heal in the elderly, especially those with thin skin or those receiving steroids. Simple suturing often fails because the skin is so fragile and oedematous, and it may result in infection and delayed healing [40]. A simpler method is to ensure that the edges of the wound are in apposition, fix them with adhesive strips and provide further protection by means of an elastic or zinc paste bandage [41]. A few patients may require a split skin graft [42, 43].

It is probably wise to have a skin biopsy from the ulcer if it fails to heal within four months [44], to avoid missing the diagnosis of a malignant ulcer.

References

1. Lofgen, K.A. (1954) Measurement of ambulatory venous pressure in the lower extremity. *Surgical Forum* **5**: 163–8.
2. Johnson, H.D. and Pflug, J. (1975) In: *The Swollen Leg: Cause and Treatment*. Heinemann, London.
3. Burnand, K.G., O'Donnell, T.F. and Lea Thomas, M. (1979) The relative importance of incompetent communicating veins in the production of varicose veins and venous ulcers. *Surgery* **82**: 9–14.
4. Burnand, K.G., Whimster, I., Naidoo, A. and Browse, N.L. (1982) Pericapillary fibrin in the ulcer-bearing skin of the leg: the cause of lipodermatosclerosis and venous ulceration. *British Medical Journal* **285**: 1071–2.
5. Hendriksen, O. (1976) Local reflex in microcirculation in human subcutaneous tissue. *Acta Physiologica Scandinavica* **97**: 447–56.
6. Levick, J.R. and Michael, C.C. (1978) The effects of position and skin temperatures on the capillary pressure in fingers and toes. *Journal of Physiology (London)* **274**: 97–109.
7. Rayman, G., Hassan, A. and Tooke, J.E. (1986) Blood flow in the skin of the foot related to posture in diabetes mellitus. *British Medical Journal* **292**: 87–90.
8. Williamson, J.R. and Kilo, C. (1977) Current status of capillary basement membrane disease in diabetes mellitus. *Diabetes* **26**: 65–73.
9. Beninson, J. (1961) Six years of pressure gradient therapy. *Angiology* **12**: 38–45.
10. Meyerovitz, B.R. and Nelson, R. (1965) Measurements of the velocity of blood in the lower limb veins with and without compression. *Surgery* **56**: 481–6.
11. Makin, G.S., Mayes, F.B. and Holyroyd, A.M. (1969) Studies on the effect of 'Tubigrip' on flow in the deep veins of the calf. *British Journal of Surgery* **56**: 369–72.
12. Stemmer, R., Marescaux, J. and Furderer, C. (1980) Compression treatment of the lower extremities particularly with compression stockings. *The Dermatologist* **31**: 355–65.
13. Curwen, I.H.M. and Scott, B.O. (1952) The ambulant treatment of complications resulting from varicose veins and allied conditions. *Annals of Physical Medicine* **1**: 17–25.
14. Partsch, H. (1984) Do we need compression stockings exerting high pressure? *VASA* **13**: 52–7.
15. Jones, N.A.G., Webb, P.J., Rees, R.I. and Kakkar, V.V. (1980) A physiological study of elastic compression stockings in venous disorders of the leg. *British Journal of Surgery* **67**: 569–72.
16. Sigel, B., Edelstein, A.L., Savitch, L., Hasty, J.H. and Felix, W.R. (1975) Types of compression for reducing venous stasis. *Archives of Surgery* **110**: 171–5.
17. Sigel, B., Edelstein, A.L., Felix, W.R. and Memhardt, C.R. (1973) Compression of the deep venous system of the lower leg during inactive recumbency. *Archives of Surgery* **106**: 38–43.
18. Horner, J., Fernandes, E., Fernandes, J. and Nicolaides, A.N. (1980) Value of graduated compression stockings in deep venous insufficiency. *British Medical Journal* **280**: 820–1.
19. Swain, I., Williamson, H., Forder, F. *et al.* (1985) *Assessment of Anti-Embolism*

Stockings. Report of the Wessex Regional Research Committee.

20. Scott, B.O. (1983) The management of stasis ulceration of the skin. In: *Peripheral Vascular Disease in the Elderly*, pp. 178-180 (Ed: McCarthy, S.T.). Churchill Livingstone, Edinburgh.

21. Pflug, J.J. (1975) Intermittent compression in the management of swollen legs in general practice. *Practitioner* 215: 69-76.

22. McColloch, J.M. (1981) Intermittent compression for the treatment of chronic stasis ulceration. *Physical Therapy* 61: 1452-3.

23. Zelikovski, A., Deutsch, A. and Reiss, R. (1983) The sequential pneumatic compression device in surgery for lymphoedema in the limbs. *Journal of Cardiovascular Surgery* 24: 122-6.

24. Clarke, R.L., Orandi, A. and Cliffton, E.E. (1960) Tourniquet induction of fibrinolysis. *Angiology* 11: 367-70.

25. Burnand, K.G., Clemenson, G., Morland, M., Jarrett, P.G.M. and Browse, N.L. (1980) Venous lipodermatosclerosis: treatment of fibrinolytic enhancement and elastic compression. *British Medical Journal* 280: 7-11.

26. Browse, N.L., Jarrett, P.E.M., Moreland, M. and Burnand, K. (1977) Treatment of liposclerosis of the leg by fibrinolytic enhancement: a preliminary report. *British Medical Journal* 2: 434-5.

27. Burnand, K.G., Pattison, M. and Browse, N.L. (1982) In: *Anabolic Steroids: 6th International Congress on Fibrinolysis*, pp. 526-8 (Eds: Davidson, J.F., Bachman, F., Bouvier, C.A. and Kruitof, E.K.O.). Churchill Livingstone, Edinburgh.

28. Dodd, H. and Crockett, S.B. (1956) In: *The Pathology and Surgery of Veins of the Leg*. Longman, Edinburgh.

29. Browse, N.L., Gray, L., Jarrett, P.E.M. and Morland, M. (1977) Blood and vein wall fibrinolytic activity in health and vascular disease. *British Medical Journal* 1: 478-81.

30. Jarrett, P.E.M., Burnand, K.G., Morland, M. and Browse, N.L. (1976) Fibrinolysis and fat necrosis in the lower leg. *British Journal of Surgery* 63: 157.

31. Burnand, K.G., Whimster, I., Clemenson, G. *et al.* (1981) The relationship between the number of capillaries in the skin of the venous ulcer-bearing area of the lower leg and the fall in foot venous pressure during exercise. *British Journal of Surgery* 68: 297-300.

32. Greaves, M.W. and Skillen, A. (1970) Effects of long-continued ingestion of zinc sulphate in patients with venous leg ulceration. *Lancet* ii: 889-91.

33. Sarjeant, G.R., Galloway, R.E. and Gueri, M.G. (1970) Oral zinc sulphate in sickle-cell ulcers. *Lancet* ii: 891-2.

34. Husain, S.L. (1969) Oral zinc sulphate in leg ulcers. *Lancet* i: 1069-71.

35. Pories, W.J., Lewis, R.G., Plecha, F.R. *et al.* (1968) Delayed wound healing in surgical patients due to zinc deficiency. *Journal of the American Medical Association* 204: 533.

36. Myers, M.B. (1970) Zinc and healing. *Lancet* ii: 1253-54 (letter).

37. Dyson, M., Franks, C. and Suckling, J. (1976) Stimulation of healing of varicose ulcers by ultrasound. *Ultrasonics* 14: 232-6.

38. Jones, P.H., Willis, A.T. and Ferguson, I.R. (1978) Treatment of anaerobically infected pressure sores with topical metronidazole. *Lancet* i: 214 (letter).

39. Baker, P.G. and Haig, G. (1981) Metronidazole in the treatment of chronic pressure sores and ulcers. *Practitioner* 225: 569-73.

40. Rozner, L. and Ashby, E.C. (1965) Anatomical and physiological factors in below knee wounds. *Lancet* i: 1362-5.

41. Crawford, B.S. and Gibson, M. (1977) The conservative management of pre-tibial lacerations in elderly patients. *British Journal of Plastic Surgery* 30: 174-6.

42. Gaze, N.R. (1978) Early mobilization in the treatment of shin injuries. *Injury* **10**: 209–10.
43. Ramni, S.R. and Weston, P.A.M. (1980) Pretibial flap wounds: early grafting under regional anaesthesia as an outpatient procedure. *Injury* **12**: 360–4.
44. Ackroyd, J.S. and Young, A.E. (1983) Leg ulcers that do not heal. *British Medical Journal* **286**: 207–8.

11

Foot disorders

Introduction

The foot is particularly susceptible to trauma because it has to bear pressure and shear forces associated with carrying the weight of the body. The elderly foot is particularly susceptible to such trauma owing to a combination of poor blood supply, thinning of the skin, neuropathic disorders and neglect of foot care not only in old age but over a lifetime. Foot disorders are not only common in the elderly but are often accepted as a part of growing old. Williamson [1] found that about one-third of elderly people at home had foot disorders which they had not reported to their family doctor. In spite of this high prevalence there is very little written in the geriatric literature on foot disorders.

In a study of foot disorders on a geriatric rehabilitation unit, only one patient had no problems with her feet. [2] The commonest disorders present were (figures in per cent): toenails needing cutting (66), pitting oedema (49), toe deformities (39), onychogryphosis (38), corns/callosities (30), bunion complex (29), and maceration between the toes (27).

Nail disorders

Onychogryphosis

Onychogryphosis, the grossly thickened hypertrophic nail plate, is common in the elderly, probably being due to a combination of trauma over the years and systemic disease. A similar picture is seen in onychomycosis, a fungal infection, where the nail is thick and crumbly.

Treatment requires cutting the nail with heavy-duty clippers and then using an electric burr-drill to pare the remaining nail plate.

Onychocryptosis

Ingrowing toe nail (onychocryptosis) is a painful condition where the borders of the nail are excessively curved, grow into the toe and may become infected. A number of causes have been suggested, including trauma, tight shoes, toe deformity and careless cutting of the toenails.

Treatment is best undertaken by a trained chiropodist who will remove the offending part of the nail and provide appliances to 'train' the growing nail into a more normal shape. Alternatively a partial nail avulsion can be performed under local anaesthesia, which will provide permanent removal of the involuted portion.

Hyperkeratoses

Thickened skin, in the form of corns or callosities, occurs at several sites, usually in response to pressure or shearing forces. On the sole of the foot they are usually found over the metatarsal heads and weight bearing becomes very painful.

Management is primarily by control of the causitive factors, usually biomechanical dysfunction. The hyperkeratosis is pared away and pressure-relieving padding applied. This is achieved by an 'in-shoe' device to correct or compensate for biomechanical problems. These relieve pressure by providing shock absorption by creating local moulding in the foam substance corresponding to the high-pressure areas.

Corns and callosities often occur on the tops of the toes and may be caused by local pressure – usually from ill-fitting shoes, often in combination with deformed joints and/or abnormal foot function. They appear as a hard cornified lesion, usually with a particularly hard central core. The treatment is initial enucleation and paring of the corn, protecting the area with padding to deflect the pressure, and providing advice on skin care and footwear (see below).

Metatarsalgia

Pain in the metatarsal joints can be due to a wide variety of conditions, including arthritis, disordered foot function, skin atrophy, displacement of the plantar fibro-fatty pad, and obesity. People of all ages often complain of foot pain when first getting up and about after a long period in bed. This is thought to be due to disuse weakness of the intrinsic foot muscle. It can be prevented by foot exercises in bed and gradual introduction of weight bearing.

Hallux valgus as a cause of metatarsalgia is discussed below.

Hallux rigidus, due to osteoarthrosis of the first metatarsophalangeal joint, restricts the dorsiflexion of the toe. Management consists of preventing further damage by avoiding unnecessary dorsiflexion of the toe. This can be achieved by stiffening the sole of the shoe or by providing a metatarsal bar (to lie behind the metatarsal heads) to the shoe. Since these tend to weaken the shoe and rapidly wear down, it is more satisfactory to provide rocker soles.

Loss of the plantar fibro-fatty pad is common in old age, though particularly so in rheumatoid arthritis. Since the pad acts as a shock-absorber it is not surprising that pain develops in the underlying tissues, especially at the heel and the metatarsal heads. Treatment is by a replacement pad in the form of a soft insole.

Excessive pronation of the foot creates disturbance of the joint and tendon functions, resulting in abnormal forces through the ankle and subtalar joints 'unlocking' the midtarsal joint and creating pressure on the second, third and fourth metatarsal heads. Management includes correction of the cause of the excessive pronation. 'In-shoe' devices which stabilize the heel and support the inner longitudinal arch are usually helpful. Traditionally soft pads have been used to help redistribute the pressure by correcting the foot deformity. Unfortunately in the elderly these sometimes create further localized pressure and skin atrophy. For this reason it is preferable to use a Plastazote insert. The thermoplastic material is first softened by heating, and then the patient stands on it while the foot is in its optimal position; the material is allowed to set and is then inserted into the shoe. As with all inserts it is important to ensure that there is sufficient room for both the insert and the foot; a larger size shoe may be required.

Since walking requires a hinge action at the level of the metatarsal heads, pressure is created on the skin by shearing forces. One way of overcoming this is to provide the rotation on the sole of the shoe, rather than in the foot, by using shoes with a rocker sole. These should preferably have rubber heels since a hard heel increases the heel pressure significantly [3]. They do, however, decrease the range of movement required at the ankle equivalent to the angle built into the rocker [3]. Rocker shoes are also useful in hallux rigidus and claw toes.

Hallux valgus

Hallux valgus is common at all ages and may not cause symptoms until old age, when the deformity may worsen or an ulcer develops owing to a combination of thinning of the skin and arterial or neuropathic dysfunction.

Hallux valgus is a common cause of chronic foot pain [4, 5]. This may be due to the deranged mechanics of the foot, though some of the pain may arise in the abductor hallucis muscle [4, 6, 7], possibly due to reflex spasm associated with irritation arising from the metatarsopha-langeal joint [8].

The treatment is basically one of pressure relief, either by padding to redistribute the pressure, cutting away an area of the shoe, or providing moulded shoes. The shoes require extra width with a soft area overlying the deformity. This can be achieved by cutting out an area overlying the deformity and replacing it with a softer material of similar colour. Other techniques are described below.

Claw toes

Claw toes are caused by a number of factors, including biomechanical dysfunction and tight shoes. The deformity results in the metatarsal heads becoming more prominant on the plantar surface and callosities developing on the dorsum of the toes. Treatment essentially involves pressure-relieving padding. The shoes will require extra depth and a soft toecap.

Heel pain

Pain in the heel has a number of causes, including loss of the fatty pad, a calcanean spur, arthritis, callosities, rheumatoid nodules or inflammed bursae.

For the calcanean spur the symptoms usually settle if the foot can be rested. The usual appoach is to provide a soft insert to relieve pressure. In difficult cases special shoes may be required which provide elevation of the arch by producing heel inversion, thus relieving pressure on the plantar fascia [9]. Anti-inflammatory drugs, local steroid injection or ultrasound have also been used.

Oedema of the feet

Swelling of the feet is not uncommon in the elderly, especially towards the end of the day. Where this is troublesome, shoes are available which have fastenings extending to the toes. This allows the shoes to be loosened as required while still being supportive.

Appropriate shoes

Shoes should have sufficient space to accommodate the foot under dynamic as well as static conditions. The foot changes its shape during walking and this is the reason why shoes made from a plaster cast of the foot do not necessarily produce full relief of pressure.

Ideally there should be about 1.5–2 cm between the end of the longest toe and the tip of the shoe; and there should be no compression of the toes. If deformities make it difficult to relieve pressure using simple padding, then pressure can be relieved by stretching local areas of the shoe using proprietary leather expanders, cutting an area from the shoe or providing specialized shoes. Cheap and quickly made Plastazote shoes are available for persistent problems.

Specially made shoes need to meet certain criteria:

1. They must be supportive without being tight. Shoes that are too loose will also cause problems, either by slipping off or by increasing shear forces and friction. Similarly backless shoes are not helpful in preventing frictional forces and do not give support. Loose slippers result in a large amount of movement within the shoe and do not support the internal structure of the foot.
2. They must be able to accommodate the changes in foot volume which occur throughout the day.
3. They need to accommodate the changes in foot shape which occur in different positions.
4. There should be good support on those areas that are normally not weight bearing, so that the weight can be distributed over as wide an area as possible, preventing stresses leading to further deformity. This equalization of forces can be achieved, for instance, with a Plastazote insert.
5. They should be able to substitute for loss of normal joint movement. An example of this is the rocker shoe.

Where the deformity is severe there are a number of approaches. Soft felt boots can be provided which generally give comfort, though they may not be able to relieve pressure at all points unless they are too loose to be practicable. Modern thermoplastics provide the opportunity to make lightweight shoes which can be moulded to the most deformed foot. These are really only practicable for indoor use. If outdoor shoes are required, then more heavy-duty leather shoes designed especially for the patient will be necessary. These are very expensive and unnecessary for the majority of disabled elderly people. However, they are more likely to be worn and be comfortable than the Plastazote or extra-depth shoes [10], though this finding may be due to the selection procedure for the more expensive shoes. The fact that one-third of patients are still uncomfortable in special shoes and one-sixth never wear them [10] does suggest that insufficient attention is being paid to the prescription, design and provision of shoes.

To give sufficient support the shoes should be firmly, not tightly, laced. This creates problems for many patients who have arthritis of the hands. In this case the use of Velcro fittings is appropriate.

Whatever the design, shoes can only relieve pressure on the top and side of the foot. If a moulded insert is required it is important to take this into account when designing the shoe.

In milder cases of foot disorder the patient should be advised to wear well-supporting shoes. It is important for them to understand that the width of the heel is as important as its height. The narrower the heel the less the support and, therefore, the greater the degree of instability; which in turn causes pressure within the foot and against the shoe.

In summary, then, most foot disorders can be controlled by appropriate padding, and redistribution or removal of pressure. In many cases this requires simple inserts, though some will require specialized orthoses and provision of well-designed shoes.

References

1. Williamson, J. (1964) Old people at home: their unreported needs. *Lancet* i: 1117-21.
2. Ebrahaim, S.B.J., Sainsbury, R. and Warton, S. (1981) Foot problems of the elderly: a hospital survey. *British Medical Journal* **283**: 949-50.
3. Peterson, M.J., Perry, J. and Montgomery, J. (1985) Walking patterns of healthy subjects wearing rocker shoes. *Physical Therapy* **65**: 1483-9.
4. Travell, J. and Rinzler, S.H. (1952) The myofascial genesis of pain. *Postgraduate Medicine* **11**: 425-34.
5. Cailliet, R. (1968) *Foot and Ankle Pain*. F.A. Davis Co., Philadelphia.
6. Melzack, R., Stillwell, D.M. and Fox, E.J. (1977) Trigger points and acupuncture points for pain: correlations and indications. *Pain* **3**: 3-23.
7. Cailliet, R. (1977) *Soft Tissue Pain and Disability*. F.A. Davis Co., Philadelphia.
8. Durant, R., Galletti, R. and Pantaleo, T. (1985) Electromyographic observations in patients with foot pain syndromes. *American Journal of Physical Medicine* **64**: 295-303.
9. Campbell, J.W. and Inman, V.T. (1974) Treatment of plantar fasciitis and calcaneal spurs with the UC-BL shoe insert. *Clinical Orthopaedics* **103**: 57-62.
10. Klenerman, L. and Hughes, J. (1986) Surgical footwear: an assessment of the place of ready-made extra-depth shoes. *Health Trends* **18**: 45-6.

12

Respiratory disorders

General features

A number of changes occur in the respiratory system with advancing age. There is a general decrease in the flexibility in the chest wall [1] owing to a combination of kyphosis, calcification of the costal cartilages [2] and decrease in the effectiveness of the muscles of respiration. At the alveolar level there is a decrease in the surface area [3–5] and extensibility [6] of the wall with a decrease in elastic recoil and an associated increase in the duct space leading to the alveoli. Even in non-smokers there is a decrease in the forced expiratory volume in one second and the forced vital capacity with advancing age [7, 8]. There is a progressive decrease in the arterial pO_2 with advancing age, though the pCO_2 remains relatively constant, while the response to anoxia [9, 10] and hypercapnoea are both decreased with advancing age.

Chronic bronchitis, with or without emphysema, is the major respiratory condition likely to require the help of the rehabilitation team. About 3–4 per cent of disability in the United States is due to chronic lung disease [11]. Although the incidence of chronic bronchitis decreases in old age, the prevalance continues to rise with as many as 40 per cent of elderly men and 20 per cent of elderly women being symptomatic [12]. The prognosis is similar in elderly and younger groups [13]; indeed the elderly seem to develop less hypoxia or hypercapnoea.

Management of chronic obstructive airways disease

Management should include advice to decrease, and preferably stop, smoking. Even for the ederly this can reduce the mortality rate [14]. It can decrease the amount of sputum being produced and lower the risk of further chest infections.

Chest physiotherapy

The benefits of chest physiotherapy are unclear. One of the problems is that, though the patients may subjectively feel better after physiotherapy, there are few changes on laboratory and spirometric testing. Physiotherapy does seem to improve the expectoration of sputum and increase blood oxygenation [15]. On the other hand it does not seem to alter the course of the illness in acute exacerbations in terms of length of pyrexia, length of hospital stay or radiological changes [16].

During acute phases or in the presence of pneumonia, steam inhalation produces symptomatic improvement; but there seems to be no evidence that blood gases or spirometric testing are altered. It seems to be particularly helpful when the patient is not expectorating.

In respiratory failure chest physiotherapy may be required every two or three hours, to be continued throughout the night. There is little evidence, however, that physiotherapy is of help in chronic states. Water or saline nebulizers seem to help to moisten the secetions, and for patients at home pouring boiling water over Friar's Balsam and inhaling the steam can produce symptomatic relief.

Activity in the chronic bronchitic tends to decrease below optimal levels, with associated general decrease in fitness and wellbeing. Exercise programmes do make the patient feel better even when there is no objective evidence of improved respiratory function [17], and exercise tolerance may be increased [18, 19].

A number of studies have described rehabilitation programmes [20–28]. These have included postural drainage, exercises, breathing instructions and education, with beneficial effects on outcome in terms of subjective improvement, decreased admission rate to hospital and improvement in exercise tolerance in spite of very little change in pulmonary function tests. There has, however, been a report of improvement in blood gases over a period of one and two years [29]: this was not a controlled trial, but since the patients could be expected to deteriorate rather than improve over this period, circumstantial evidence is for the benefit of a rehabilitation programme.

These studies are counterbalanced by others which have not shown benefit from breathing exercises. In comparing a rehabilitation programme with placebo controls using ultra-violet light [30] or with chloramphenicol and a placebo (potassium iodide) [31], no difference was demonstrated in any of the parameters measured.

There are few studies primarily of rehabilitation programmes for elderly people with chronic chest disease. In one study using a programme of thorough assessment, education of patient and carers, instruction of techniques for breathing, a graded exercise programme, control of weight and prevention of infection, 97 per cent of elderly patients gained subjective improvement, 83 per cent improved their physical endurance, 11 per cent showed an improvement on pulmonary function tests, whilst there was an increase in daily activities and chest expansion and a reduction in the use of corticosteroids and the hospital admission rate [28].

The aims of chest physiotherapy (32) are to:

- promote, where possible, a normal relaxed pattern of breathing;
- teach controlled breathing with the minimum of effort;
- assist with the removal of secretions;
- aid re-expansion of the lung tissue;
- mobilize the thoracic cage;
- prevent over-expansion of the lungs in emphysema.

Improving diaphragmatic breathing

Limitation of movement of the chest cage means that the elderly depend on greater use of diaphragmatic breathing. Training is aimed at minimizing the work of breathing, improving ventilation of the lung bases and controlling breathing during exertion.

There have been several reports of the beneficial effects of diaphragmatic training in chronic obstructive airways disease, with a reduction in the minute ventilation and decrease in respiratory rate [33–35], though there is no effect on blood gases [33, 36, 37]. Others have been unable to show improvement in lung volume [36, 38] or regard the benefit as being due to an 'indirect form of psychotherapy' [39]. Slowing of the respiratory rate may result in a decrease in the ratio of dead space to tidal volume, thus providing benefit as has been shown for emphysematous patients [40].

Even when there is a demonstrable increase in diaphragmatic movement following training, it is not necessarily associated with improvement in lung function tests [30, 31], nor is improvement in lung function necessarily associated with an increase in diaphragmatic movement [31]. The latter may not be a real change but may be due to diminished vertical movement of the chest wall without true alteration in the diaphragmatic excursion [35].

A technique to improve diaphragmatic breathing has the patient sitting with the back and head supported so that the muscles of the abdominal wall area relaxed. The patient then breathes in and out gently, preferably through the nose, with the chest relaxed, action of the accessory muscles of respiration and upper chest being controlled. Forced or prolonged expiration should be discouraged since these result in further narrowing of the bronchi.

There are problems in emphysema since the diaphragm is depressed by the increased lung volume; it therefore contributes only about 30 per cent of the effort of breathing compared with about 65 per cent in the normal individual. Some patients find that they breathe better if they breathe in quickly and then breathe out slowly through pursed lips to delay airway closure.

Improving thoracic cage movement

There are a number of exercises which can be used to improve the movement of the thoracic cage. These generally require the patient to expand the chest wall against pressure provided either by an attendant or against self-administered resistance. The patient practises breathing gently without the resistance and is then instructed to expand the chest against gentle resistance at a level that does not restrict the chest wall movement. The pressure is maintained throughout the inspiratory phase but is removed for the expiratory phase.

Increasing expiration

One problem in emphysema is that the lungs become over-inflated owing to difficulty in breathing out. Traditional training, which emphasizes expiration, does not seem to be particularly effective and can make the patient more anxious. The classical picture of emphysema is a person who is anxious, tense and making noisey attempts to breathe. The chest seems rigid and the accessory muscles of respiration obviously very active. One approach, contrary to normal teaching, is to encourage the patient to take a deep breath in and to stop breathing out earlier than normal: although this might be expected to encourage further trapping of air in the chest, what probably happens is that the pressure rise during expiration requires active muscle activity to expire the air and this in effect compresses the bronchial tree – effectively producing bronchoconstriction and air trapping. By stopping the expiratory phase early this excess intrathoracic pressure is avoided, thereby preventing further disruption of the alveoli and allowing a greater movement and exchange of air.

Increasing sputum expectoration

Although it was emphasized above that the patient should not carry out forced expiration since this tends to further increase the obstruction, the technique of short, forced expiratory phases often helps to remove sputum. Even in asthmatic patients this does not seem to increase bronchospasm [41].

The main use of postural drainage is to assist secretion removal from specific lobes or segments. It is most effective in bronchiectasis and therefore more useful in the younger population. There is very little good scientific evidence available on the effectiveness of postural drainage in chronic obstructive lung disease, and the available information is contradictory. Some have found no change in pulmonary function tests [42–45] and little or no change in sputum volume [42, 45, 46], duration of fever or gas exchange [47] after postural drainage, while others have found an improvement in vital capacity [48–50], sputum viscosity and blood gases [48], though this is not necessarily associated with the volume of sputum expectorated [51]. It has been shown by Maloney *et al.* [45] that, although the amount of sputum expectorated over 24 hours does not alter, the amount produced during the period of postural drainage is much increased, which probably makes it easier and more comfortable for the patient.

The value of mucolytic agents in improving the flow of mucus during postural drainage is also doubtful. In one study of patients with chronic obstructive airways disease, postural drainage preceded by a mucolytic agent was compared with drainage preceded by a brochodilator – the latter was the most effective in improving pulmonary function tests [52].

Postural drainage requires the patient to lie with the foot of the bed elevated to assist drainage from various lobes. This position is not applicable for the posterior and anterior segments of the upper lobes and the anterior segment of the lower lobe, where flat lying is required. Although some patients can tolerate this, unfortunately chronic airways disease in the elderly is often complicated by heart failure, which may make it impossible to maintain the necessary positions. The conditions limiting positioning for postural drainage include orthopnoea, heart failure, pulmonary oedema, recent haemoptysis, moderate to severe hypertension, dysrhythmias and regurgitation [32].

Postural drainage involves more than passive lying; it needs assitance from the therapist with percussion, shaking of the chest wall as well as coughing and forced expiration on the part of the patient [41]. Some studies have found that percussion and vibration increase mucus clearance [51, 53, 54]. This does not seem to occur in normal subjects [55, 56] but may require a larger volume of mucus to be effective. Some care is required in the elderly who are also prone to osteoporosis if fractures are to be avoided. There is also some evidence that percussion increases bronchoconstriction [57], and so it may be necessary to precede the treatment with bronchodilators.

There are limitations to the use of postural drainage. Few elderly patients can tolerate lying in the necessary positions long enough for the mucus to move far in the bronchial tree. This is especially relevant when the sputum is thick and tenacious. The best results are obtained with the greater amount of head-down posture, and this is certainly not tolerated by many elderly patients. The amount of flow at the levels of inclination used is probably very slight. Theoretically the mucus will flow faster if there is high pressure above it with a low pressure below; unfortunately the absorption of air in the distal bronchial tree produces a partial vacuum which tends to resist mucus drainage.

Some of the benefit of postural drainage may be due to the improved function of the diaphragm which is known to occur when the patient is lying in the head-down position [58, 59].

If nurses and family talk with the patient from the bottom of the bed or from a distance, this necessitates the reply to be spoken loudly. This additional exercise often encourages coughing and improved ventilation. Since the activity is not thought of as 'exercise' the patient is usually more relaxed, and this in turn assists breathing.

Positioning

Many bronchitics, especially where there is associated emphysema, hold the chest in a permanent state of inspiration. This limits the amount of air being moved and produces a raised intrathoracic pressure, which further obstructs the airways. There are several techniques which can be used to overcome or compensate for these difficulties.

Many patients learn to purse the lips and therefore increase the pressure throughout the airways, thereby delaying closure. This is particularly helpful during periods of dyspnoea. The technique helps to reduce the minute volume and respiratory rate whilst increasing the tidal volume and improving the blood gases [60, 61].

The use of diaphragmatic breathing was discussed above.

Positioning at rest

When in bed the patient should lie on the side with the head and shoulders elevated by four or five pillows (i.e. the equivalent of sitting up but side lying).

When sitting, two good poses are the following:

- Lean forward on pillows placed on a table with the arms abducted and elevated to shoulder level.

- Sit leaning forwards with the forearms resting on the thighs (this is a more relaxing position than gripping the knees, when the shoulder girdle is held rigid).

Leaning forward has long been accepted as an important method of improving breathing in patients with chronic obstructive airways disease [62]. It has the effect of decreasing dyspnoea, decreasing the use of accessory muscles of respiration and improving diaphragmatic action whilst decreasing the minute ventilation and lung volume in emphysematous patients [63–65]. Thus bending forward 30–40° from the erect position, by allowing relaxation of the abdominal muscles, produces less resistance to the diaphragm descending during inspiration whilst providing no prolongation of expiration.

Standing

When standing the patient should avoid tense rigid poses. Two possibilities are the following:

- Lean against a wall with the feet slightly apart and about 30 cm from the wall. The arms should hang down loosely to relax the shoulder girdle.
- Lean forward against a wall with the arms resting on a surface which is just below shoulder level. Again the aim is to relax the shoulder girdle.

Walking

When walking the patient should attempt to control breathing in a rhythmical way. Some patients find it helpful to breath in for two or three steps and then breath out over the next two or three steps.

Some patients also find it helpful to walk with a high gutter or pulpit frame which allows the arms to be supported with a relaxed shoulder girdle. Ideally the frame should have wheels.

Bending

When bending forward to pick up an object or to put on shoes and stockings, it is usually helpful to take a breath and then exhale whilst bending down. This prevents the discomfort of the raised abdominal pressure being transmitted to an already full intrathoracic cage.

Improving exercise tolerance

Exercise tolerance can be improved by graduated increases in exercise [21, 24, 25, 66, 67], even when there are no objective changes on blood gas analysis and spirometry [68–72]; and it is thought that exercise also helps to mobilize the secretions [73]. In one controlled trial using a rehabilitation programme of relaxation exercises [74], positional postural drainage preceded by heated aerosols or bronchodilators and exercises (including level walking at various speeds, cycling against a load and stair climbing supplemented by oxygen therapy), those in the rehabilitation group improved in exercise tolerance with less oxygen cost though with no significant change in spirometric or other laboratory tests.

For the elderly exercise can be simply graduated by increases in walking distance [75], static cycling [72] or climbing a number of stairs [67]. The distance should start off quite short and be carried out twice a day, both distance and frequency being increased at weekly intervals. The distance, the time frequency and rate of increase will obviously vary between individuals.

Rehabilitation in a physiotherapy department using a treadmill is also effective in reducing the post-training oxygen consumption, minute ventilation, heart rate and respiratory rate, as well as producing improvement in dyspnoea levels and activities of daily living [76]. In nearly all patients with lung disease there is a fall in the arterial oxygen levels during the exercise programme [76–78], and this must be relevant in elderly patients with increased risk of heart disease. There does not seem to be any effective way of identifying the likely level of the fall in PaO_2 prior to the exercise [76], and so treadmill patients should ideally be monitored throughout by electrocardiography, blood pressure and blood gases analysis. This is rarely practicable in the average rehabilitation unit. There should, however, be oxygen available, and there is evidence that this is effective in improving exercise tolerance during hypoxia [79–81].

Assessing the effect of training programmes is difficult. From the discussion above it is obvious that pulmonary function tests and blood gas analysis are unreliable indices of improvement since there may well be increased tolerance to exercise and a subjective feeling of improved wellbeing in the absence of significant objective changes. The 12-minute walking test (TMWT) used for younger patients with chronic respiratory problems is limited by other factors such as arthritis, Parkinsonism and balance disturbances in the elderly. In the TMWT the distance walked on the level in 12-minutes is measured, though the patient may stop for a rest during this time [82]. Attempts have been made to use a 2-minute walking test, but this offers insufficient information. A 6-minute walking test has been shown to give equivalent information to the TMWT [83].

Some patients benefit from portable oxygen cylinders which can increase exercise tolerance [84, 85]. Both of these studies showed that a wheeled walking aid on which the patient leans on forearm supports can also increase walking tolerance. A combination of both oxygen and walking aid produced a three- to sixfold increase in walking tolerance.

Environmental and psychological factors

Home environmental reorganization is important. The bed can be brought downstairs and a commode used if the toilet is too far or inaccessible. Oxygen cylinders placed at strategic points may assist the exercise tolerance.

Common experience indicates that patients with chronic airways obstruction breathe better in warm, moist conditions and less well in cold air. Avoidance of outside activity during weather which exacerbates the dyspnoea is common sense.

It is also important to advise about smoking, dirty atmospheres and rapid changes in temperature or humidity which tend to aggravate breathing difficulties. Advice is also required of the need to maintain adequate hydration to lessen the viscosity of the sputum.

As with all rehabilitation programmes, education of the patient and relatives is important in management. They all need to understand the basic concept of the lung pathology and physiology and what the rehabilitation programme is trying to achieve. This is particularly important since there is a large element of anxiety associated with dyspnoea, especially when the patient is required to continue exercises over the long term without the benefit of professional supervision.

Anxiety is indeed, such a common finding in patients with dyspnoea [86] that it warrants special attention. Although psychotherapy or physical therapy alone can help to improve the patient psychologically, the latter was required to improve functional ability [86]. A number of studies have shown that psychological wellbeing and decrease in anxiety occurs with a comprehensive rehabilitation programme in chronic respiratory disease.

The methods of education include individual teaching, group sessions or information booklets, all of which seem to achieve the same effect on anxiety levels. Most exercise programmes show a significant effect on anxiety levels, and so a combination of the educational and physical approaches should be used for as optimal outcome.

Pre- and postoperative chest physiotherapy

The elderly are particularly prone to chest infection following operations, especially those involving the abdomen or thorax.

Whether there is any real benefit from breathing exercises before and after surgery is still debatable. There is evidence that atelectasis is least common in those patients who have physiotherapy before and after surgery [87–89]. However, in the absence of a previous history of chest infection, preoperative chest physiotherapy has no effect on the postoperative complications [90]. Those most likely to develop post-operative chest complications are those with a previous history of respiratory problems, and smokers [90]. The site of the operation is also significant, with abdominal operations, especially upper abdomen, having a high incidence and orthopaedic disorders a lower incidence [90].

The techniques used are basically deep-breathing exercises and training in coughing and emphasis on sustained inspiration [89]. Post-operatively, incision-supporting techniques are also useful.

References

1. Turner, J.M., Mead, J. and Wohl, M.E. (1968) Elasticity of human lungs in relation to age. *Journal of Applied Physiology* **25**: 664–71.
2. Semine, A.A. and Damon, A. (1975) Costochondrial ossification and ageing in five populations. *Human Biology* **47**: 101–16.
3. Mauderly, J.L. (1978) Effect of age on pulmonary structure and function of immature and adult animals and man. *Federation Proceedings* **38**: 173–7.
4. Niewoehner, D.E. and Kleinerman, J. (1964) Morphological basis of pulmonary resistance in the human lung and effects of ageing. *Journal of Applied Physiology* **36**: 412–18.
5. Thurlbeck, W.M. and Angus, G.E. (1975) Growth and ageing of normal human lung. *Chest* **67** (Suppl.): 3–7.
6. Sugihara, T., Martin, C.J. and Hildebrandt, J. (1971) Length–tension properties of alveolar wall in man. *Journal of Applied Physiology* **30**: 874–8.
7. Morris, J.F., Koski, A. and Johnson, L.C. (1971) Spirometric standards for healthy nonsmoking adults. *American Review of Respiratory Diseases* **103**: 57–67.
8. Milne, J.S. (1978) Longitudinal respiratory studies in older people. *Thorax* **33**: 547–54.
9. Kronenberg, R.S. and Drage, C.W. (1973) Attenuation of the ventilatory and heart rate responses to hypoxia and hypercapnia with aging in normal man. *Journal of Clinical Investigation Pathology, Research and Practice* **52**: 1812–19.
10. Freeman, E., Sutton, R.N.P. and Cevikbas, A. (1982) Respiratory infections on long stay wards. *Journal of Infection* **4**: 237–42.
11. Tager, I.B. and Speizer, F. (1975) The role of infection in chronic bronchitis. *New England Journal of Medicine* **292**: 563–71.
12. Caird, F.I. and Akhtar, A.J. (1972) Chronic respiratory disease in the elderly. *Thorax* **27**: 764–8.
13. Burrows, B., Niden, A.H., Barclay, W.R. and Kajik, J.E. (1965) Chronic obstructive lung disease. *American Review of Respiratory Diseases* **91**: 521–40.
14. Gentleman, J.F., Brown, K.S. and Forbes, W.F. (1978) Smoking and its effect on mortality of the aged. *American Journal of the Medical Sciences* **276**: 173–83.
15. Holody, B. and Goldberg, H.S. (1981) The effect of mechanical vibration on arterial oxygen in acutely ill patients with atelectasis or pneumonia. *American Journal of Respiratory Diseases* **124**: 372–5.

16. Graham, W.G.B. and Bradley, B.S. (1978) Efficacy of chest physiotherapy and intermittent positive-pressure breathing in the resolution of pneumonia. *New England Journal of Medicine* **299**: 624–7.
17. Brundin, A. (1974) Physical training in severe chronic obstructive lung disease. *Scandinavian Journal of Respiratory Diseases* **55**: 25–36.
18. Cockcroft, A.E., Saunders, M.J. and Berry, G. (1981) Randomised controlled trial of rehabilitation in chronic respiratory disability. *Thorax* **36**: 200–3.
19. McGavin, C.R. (1977) A place for physical rehabilitation in the management of chronic bronchitis. *The Journal of the Chest, Heart and Stroke Association* **2**: 19–21.
20. Petty, T.L., Nett, L.M., Finnegan, M.M. *et al.* (1969) A comprehensive care program for chronic airway obstruction. *Annals of Internal Medicine* **70**: 1109–20.
21. Petty, T.L., Brink, G.A., Miller, M.W. *et al.* (1970) Objective functional improvement in chronic airway obstruction. *Chest* **57**: 216–23.
22. Fishman, D.B. and Petty, T.L. (1971) Physical, symptomatic and psychological improvement in patients receiving comprehensive care for chronic airway obstruction. *Journal of Chronic Disease* **24**: 775–85.
23. Miller, W.F. (1971) Useful methods of therapy. *Chest* **60** (Suppl.): 2–5.
24. Kimbel, P., Kaplan, A.S., Alkalay, I. *et al.* (1971) An in-hospital program for rehabilitation of patients with chronic obstructive airways disease. *Chest* **60** (Suppl.): 6S–10S.
25. Neff, T.A. and Petty, T.L. (1971) Outpatient care for patients with chronic airways obstruction – emphysema and bronchitis. *Chest* **60**: 11S–17S.
26. Farrington, J.F. (1971) Rehabilitation of the pulmonary cripple in private practice. *Chest* **60** (Suppl.): 18S–20S.
27. Burrows, B. and Petty, T.L. (1971) Long-term effects of treatment in patients with chronic airways obstruction. *Chest* **60** (Suppl.): 25S–27S.
28. Obley, F.A. and Preiser, F.M. (1972) Comprehensive outpatient respiratory care: a program conducted in a suburban private practice. *Journal of the American Geriatrics Society* **22**: 521–4.
29. Guthrie, A.G. and Petty, T.L. (1970) Improved exercise tolerance in patients with chronic airway obstruction. *Physical Therapy* **50**: 1333–7.
30. McNeil, R.S. and McKenzie, J.M. (1955) An assessment of the value of breathing exercises in chronic bronchitis and asthma. *Thorax* **10**: 250–5.
31. Petersen, E.S., Essmann, V., Honcke, P. and Munkner, C. (1967) A controlled study of the effect of treatment on chronic bronchitis: an evaluation using pulmonary function tests. *Acta Medica Scandinavica* **182**: 293–305.
32. Gaskell, D.V. and Webber, B.A. (1980) *The Brompton Hospital Guide to Chest Physiotheraphy*. Blackwell Scientific Publications, Oxford.
33. Campbell, E.J.M. and Friend, J. (1955) Action of breathing exercises in pulmonary emphysema. *Lancet* **1**: 325–9.
34. Miller, W.F. (1954) A physiologic evaluation of the effects of diaphragmatic breathing training in patients with chronic pulmonary emphysema. *American Journal of Medicine* **17**: 471–7.
35. Sinclair, J.D. (1955) Effect of breathing exercises in pulmonary emphysema. *Thorax* **10**: 246–9.
36. Beckdale, M.R., McGregor, M., Goldman, H.I. and Braudo, J.L. (1954) A study of the effects of physiotherapy in chronic hypertrophic emphysema using lung function tests. *Disease of the Chest* **26**: 180–4.
37. Sackner, M.A., Silva, G., Banks, J.M., Watson, D.D. and Smoak, W.M. (1974) Distribution of ventilation during diaphragmatic breathing in obstructive lung disease. *American Review in Respiratory Disease* **109**: 331–7.

38. Cole, M.B., Stansky, C., Roberts, F.E. and Hargen, S.M. (1962) Studies in emphysema: long-term results of training in diaphragmatic breathing on the course of obstructive emphysema. *Archives of Physical Medicine and Rehabilitation* **43**: 561-6.
39. Donald, K.W. (1953) Definitions and assessment of respiratory function. *British Medical Journal* **1**: 415-22, 473-8.
40. Motley, H.L. (1963) Effects of slow deep breathing on blood gas exchange in emphysema. *American Review of Respiratory Disease* **88**: 485-92.
41. Pryor, J.A. and Webber, B.A. (1979) An evaluation of the forced expiration technique as an adjunct to postural drainage. *Physiotherapy* **65**: 304-7.
42. March, H. (1971) Appraisal of postural drainage for chronic obstructive pulmonary disease. *Archives of Physical Medicine and Rehabilitation* **52**: 528-30.
43. Emirgil, C., Sobol, B.J., Norma, J. *et al.* (1969) Study of the long term effect of therapy in chronic obstructive pulmonary disease. *American Journal of Medicine* **47**: 367-77.
44. Haas, A. and Luxzak, A. (1961) Importance of rehabilitation in treatment of chronic pulmonary emphysema. *Archives of Physical Medicine and Rehabilitation* **42**: 733-9.
45. Maloney, F.P., Fernandez, E. and Hudgel, D.W. (1981) Postural drainage effect after bronchodilator inhalation in patients with chronic airway obstruction. *Archives of Physical Medicine and Rehabilitation* **62**: 452-5.
46. Kang, B., Rogers, W.L., Niederhuber, S.S. *et al.* (1974) Evaluation of postural drainage with percussion in chronic obstructive lung disease. *Journal of Allergy and Clinical Immunology* **53**: 109.
47. Anthonisen, P., Rus, P. and Sogaard-Andersen, T. (1964) The value of lung physical therapy in the treatment of acute exacerbations of chronic bronchitis. *Acta Medica Scandinavica* **175**: 715-19.
48. Pham, Q.T., Peslin, R., Puchelle, E. *et al.* (1973) Respiratory function and the rheological status of bronchial secretions collected by spontaneous expectoration and after physiotherapy. *Bulletin of Respiration (Nancy)* **9**: 293-314.
49. Shapiro, B., Vostinak-Foley, E., Hamilton, B. and Buehler, J. (1977) Rehabilitation in chronic obstructive pulmonary disease: a two year prospective study. *Respiratory Care* **22**: 1045-57.
50. Bateman, J., Newman, S., Daunt, K., Pavia, D. and Clarke, S. (1979) Regional lung clearance of excessive bronchial secretions during chest physiotherapy in patients with chronic airways obstruction. *Lancet* **1**: 294-7.
51. Clarke, S.W., Cochrane, G.M. and Webber, B. (1973) The effects of sputum on pulmonary function. *Thorax* **28**: 262.
52. Tecklin, J. and Holsclaw, D. (1976) Bronchial drainage with aerosol medications in cystic fibrosis. *Physical Therapy* **56**: 999-1004.
53. Denton, R. (1962) Bronchial secretions in cystic fibrosis: the effects of treatment with mechanical percussion vibration. *American Review of Respiratory Disease* **86**: 41-6.
54. Thomson, M., Pavia, D., Jones, C. and McQuiston, T. (1975) No demonstrable effect of s-carboxymethylcystein on clearance of secretion from the human lung. *Thorax* **30**: 669-73.
55. Rivington-Law, B., Epstein, S. and Thompson, G. (1979) The effects of chest wall vibration on pulmonary function in normal subjects. *Physiotherapy Canada* **31**: 319-22.
56. Pavia, D., Thompson, M. and Phillipakos, D. (1976) A preliminary study of the effect of a vibrating pad on bronchial clearance. *American Review of Respiratory Disease* **113**: 92-6.

57. Campbell, A., O'Connell, J. and Wilson, F. (1975) The effect of chest physiotherapy upon the FEV1 in chronic bronchitis. *Medical Journal of Australia* **1**: 33–5.
58. Gayrard, P., Becker, M. and Bergofsky, E.H. (1968) Effects of abdominal weights on diaphragmatic position and excursions in man. *Clinical Science* **35**: 589–601.
59. Barach, A.L. and Beck, G.J. (1954) The ventilatory effects of head down position in pulmonary emphysema. *American Journal of Medicine* **16**: 55–60.
60. Thorman, R.L., Stoken, G.L. and Ross, J.C. (1966) Efficacy of pursed lips breathing in patients with chronic obstructive airway disease. *American Journal of Respiratory Disease* **93**: 100–5.
61. Mueller, R.E., Petty, T.L. and Filley, G.F. (1970) Ventilation and blood gas changes induced by pursed lip breathing. *Journal of Applied Physiology* **28**: 784–9.
62. Barach, A.L. (1955) Breathing exercises in pulmonary emphysema and allied chronic respiratory disease. *Archives of Physical Medicine and Rehabilitation* **36**: 379–90.
63. Barach, A.L. and Dulfano, M.J. (1968) Effect of chest vibration on pulmonary emphysema. *Annals of Allergy* **26**: 10–17.
64. Barach, A.L. (1974) Chronic obstructive lung disease: postural relief of dysponea. *Archives of Physical Medicine and Rehabilitation* **55**: 494–504.
65. Petty, T.L. and Guthrie, A. (1971) The effects of augmented breathing manoeuvres on ventilation in severe chronic airway obstruction. *Respiratory Care* **16**: 104–8.
66. Pierce, A.K., Taylor, H.F., Archer, R.K. *et al.* (1964) Responses to exercise training in patients with emphysema. *Archives of Internal Medicine* **113**: 36–8.
67. McGavin, C.R., Gupta, S.P., Lloyd, E.L. and McHardy, G.J.R. (1977) Physical rehabilitation for the chronic bronchitic: results of a controlled trial of exercises in the home. *Thorax* **32**:: 307–11.
68. Petty, T.L., Hudson, L.D. and Neff, T.A. (1973) Methods of ambulatory care. *Medicine Clinics of North America* **57**: 751–62.
69. Burrows, B. and Earle, R.H. (1969) Course and prognosis of chronic obstructive lung disease. *New England Journal of Medicine* **280**: 397–404.
70. Renzitti, A.D., McClement, J.H. and Litt, R.D. (1966) Veterans Administration–Army cooperative study of pulmonary functions. 3: Mortality in relation to respiratory function in chronic obstructive pulmonary disease. *American Journal of Medicine* **41**: 115–29.
71. Howard, P. (1967) Evaluation of the ventilatory capacity in chronic bronchitis. *British Medical Journal* **3**: 392–5.
72. Alison, J.A., Samios, R. and Anderson, S.D. (1981) Evaluation of exercise training in patients with chronic airway obstruction. *Physical Therapy* **61**: 1273–7.
73. Thacker, E. (1971) *Postural Drainage and Respiratory Control.* Lloyd-Luke Ltd., London.
74. Haas, A. and Cardon, H. (1969) Rehabilitation in chronic obstructive pulmonary disease: a 5-year study of 252 male patients. *Medical Clinics of North America* **53**: 593–606.
75. Woolf, C.R. (1972) A rehabilitation program for improving exercise tolerance of patients with chronic lung disease. *Canadian Medical Association Journal* **106**: 1289–92.
76. Moser, K.M., Bokinsky, G.E., Savage, R.T. *et al.* (1980) Results of a comprehensive rehabilitation program: physiologic and functional effects of

patients with chronic obstructive pulmonary disease. *Archives of Internal Medicine* **140**: 1596–1601.

77. Nicholas, J.J., Albert, R., Gabe, R. *et al.* (1970) Evaluation of an exercise program for patients with chronic obstructive lung disease. *American Review of Respiratory Diseases* **102**: 1–9.

78. Jones, N.L. (1960) Pulmonary gas exchange during exercise in patients with chronic airways obstruction. *Clinical Science* **31**: 39–50.

79. Cotes, J.E. and Gilson, J.C. (1956) Effect of oxygen on exercise ability in chronic respiratory insufficiency. *Lancet* **2**: 872–5.

80. Pierce, A.K., Paez, P.N. and Miller, W.F. (1965) Exercise therapy with the aid of a portable oxygen supply in patients with emphysema. *American Review of Respiratory Diseases* **91**: 653–7.

81. Block, A.J., Castle, J.R. and Keith, A.S. (1974) Chronic oxygen therapy: treatment of chronic obstructive lung disease at sea level. *Chest* **65**: 279–86.

82. McGavin, C.R., Gupta, S.P. and McHardy, G.J.R. (1976) Twelve minute walking test for assessing disability in chronic bronchitis. *British Medical Journal* **1**: 822–3.

83. Butland, R.J.A., Pang, J.A., Gross, E.R., Woodcock, A.A. and Geddes, D.M. (1981) Two, six and twelve minute walks compared. *Thorax* **3**: 225.

84. Campbell, E.J.M. (1957) Portable oxygen equipment and walking-aid in pulmonary emphysema. *British Medical Journal* **2**: 1518–21.

85. Grant, B.J.B. and Capel, L.H. (1972) Walking aid for pulmonary emphysema. *Lancet* **2**: 1125–7.

86. Lustig, F.M., Haas, A. and Castillo, R. (1972) Clinical and rehabilitation regime in patients with chronic obstructive pulmonary diseases. *Archives of Physical Medicine and Rehabilitation* **53**: 315–22.

87. Thoren, L. (1954) Postoperative pulmonary complications: observations on their prevention by means of physiotherapy. *Acta Chirgura Scandinavica* **107**: 193–205.

88. Palmer, K.N.V. and Sellick, B.A. (1953) The prevention of postoperative pulmonary atelectasis. *Lancet* **1**: 164–8.

89. Grimwood, M. and Warren, C.P.W. (1981) Physiotherapy and pulmonary complications following cholecystectomy. *Physiotheraphy Canada* **33**: 217–20.

90. Nichols, P.J.R. and Howell, B. (1970) Routine pre- and post-operative physiotherapy: results of a trial. *Rheumatology and Physical Medicine* **10**: 321–36.

13

Deafness and hardness of hearing

General features

Hearing almost universally declines with advancing age [1-3]. About one-third of people 65 years and over, and 60 per cent of those over 70 years [4], have impairment which can make communication difficult [5-9]. It must, however, also be recognized that some people in their eighties have near-perfect hearing. Elderly males are affected more often than women [3, 10], although there is evidence that for those 75 years and over the rate of hearing loss is greater for women than men [2]. In spite of the high incidence of hearing problems only a small proportion seek help, have a hearing test or are willing to participate in an aural rehabilitation programme [11-14]. This is one potential area for effective screening to prevent disability, though the difficulty is to find a suitable screening test.

Speech consists of a wide range of sound frequencies (100-10 000 Hz), the vowels being of low frequency while consonants are weaker and of high frequency. Ordinary speech at one metre has a sound level of about 65 dB which decreases by about 10 dB with each trebling of the distance the source moves away. This is influenced by age with the ability to repeat word lists at a 50 per cent intelligibility rate requiring a sound intensity of 19 dB for young people (18-24 years) but 42 dB for people 69-79 years [15]. Much also depends on the type of room in which a conversation is taking place: bare, empty rooms result in reverberation and the imposition of other background noises, whereas a room with a lot of soft furnishings helps to cut down on the reflected sounds.

Classification

The severity of hearing difficulties has been classified by Fisch [7] as follows:

- *Normal hearing.*
- Slight impairment, where there are some difficulties but a louder voice is heard well.
- *Moderate impairment*, where there are difficulties hearing a quiet voice or hearing normal speech when the conditions are not favourable.
- *Moderately severe impairment*, where there are considerable difficulties in hearing normal conversation but speech can be heard when the voice is moderately loud or when combined with lip reading.
- *Severe impairment*, where it is impossible to hear voices even in the best conditions and there is difficulty in understanding even a loud voice without lip reading.
- *Very severe impairment*, where normal voices are not heard at all, although very loud voices are heard, they cannot be understood and communication is difficult even with lip reading.

This classification is not all-embracing and has its limitations. For this reason audiometry has been used to define the severity of hearing loss. Guidelines have been set [16] whereby: with a hearing loss of 0–25 dB there is no need for a hearing aid; for loss of 25–40 dB a hearing aid will be required part of the time under certain circumstances; for a loss of 40–55 dB there will be a need for frequent use of the aid; for 55–80 dB loss the hearing aid will be useful; and for over 80 dB loss there is a great need for the aid but it will be of limited value. Unfortunately pure tone loss on audiometric testing does not give a complete picture of the amount of functional hearing loss [2]. There are several reasons for this, including the time taken and the concentration required to carry out the test, the acoustic properties of the surroundings, the difficulty in real life of discriminating between the noises which are meant to be heard and the background noise, and the effect of poor vision on compensating for speech loss [17–19]. Many elderly people have greater difficulty in understanding speech when there is background noise or poorer acoustic conditions than the audiometry tests imply.

To a large extent reliance is placed on self-reporting of deafness or specific questioning as part of a general interview. Unfortunately patients' assessment of their hearing loss is likely to result in misclassification of a large number of people as deaf who have little disability, and a small number with hearing difficulties would be missed [20], there being about a 70 per cent correlation between self-assessment and audiometric testing [21]. Nevertheless a combination of self-assessment and the clinician's impression of the hearing loss is probably a more sensitive guide than a formal hearing test for the elderly.

Hearing is such a complex process that simple laboratory tests are likely to be of limited value. There have been attempts to develop broader measuring scales which take into account both speech and non-speech hearing, emotional response to hearing loss, distortion of speech, localization of the sound, personal opinion of hearing and tinnitus [22, 23].

In general, higher frequencies are more affected than lower ones. The importance of this is that the high-frequency consonants are lost whereas the lower-frequency vowels are retained, making speech difficult to understand. Thus the patient may give contrary advice of 'speak up, I can't hear' and 'don't shout, I'm not deaf'. Both are actually true: he cannot hear the high frequencies, but shouting simply increases the volume of the low frequencies which can then become uncomfortable. This is also exacerbated by 'loudness recruitment' in which there is a disproportionate increase of loudness after a certain threshold of sound volume. This has a major disadvantage in that unwanted sounds such as dogs barking, children shouting and doors banging are heard at the expense of wanted information such as speech. The elderly are also less able than younger people to cope with fast speech [24]. Another problem is the difficulty in localizing the sound from the background noise.

Consequences of hearing loss

There is no doubt that deafness causes a lot of unhappiness both for the individual and for those around him. Depression is twice as common in elderly people with hearing problems than in those without [25]. Deafness is also one of the least tolerated forms of impairment and causes a tremendous amount of irritation and frustration. The deaf person subsequently becomes left out of discussions and not surprisingly begins to develop paranoid feelings that others are talking about him, with resulting social isolation and anxiety. This may take on the appearance of dementia, and there is some evidence that hearing loss may contribute to the cause of the dementia [26–29]; though others have been unable to find such a correlation [25, 30]. This could be because of the strong association between the degenerative disorders with advancing age. Jones *et al.* [9] found that, although confusion was associated with hearing loss, the correlation disappeared when adjusted for other disabilities. They similarly found that anxiety and depression were more closely corre-lated with general disability than with hearing loss. These views are supported by Powers and Powers [8] who found that 'elderly persons reporting hearing difficulties do not experience disruptions in their social world, or problems of adjustment that are much different from those encountered by elderly persons reporting no hearing problems'. Contrary to popular belief they found that those who were hard of hearing received more, not less, support from their families and that they were less likely, not more likely, to feel lonely.

The reaction of society to the deaf is entirely different from the reaction to the blind. There is a general tendency to assist the blind person who declares his disability with a white stick and dark glasses, whereas most will admit to avoiding the frustrations of helping the deaf person who responds by trying to hide the disability. This is seen in the demand for smaller and smaller hearing aids.

One of the major roles of the rehabilitation team is to achieve acceptance by the patient of the deafness and the hearing aid. Without this, no amount of assessment or prescription is of help [31].

Hearing aids

The methods of amplifying sound to improve hearing fall into two main groups, acoustic and electronic.

Simple acoustic aids

These are the old-fasion hearing trumpets – the simplest being made by cupping the hand around the ear. Hearing tubes are not popular with the elderly but are effective in that they provide amplification without distortion. Modern collapsible tubes are available and are particularly useful on wards since they can be used by any patient with a hearing disorder.

Electronic aids

Electronic aids simply amplify sound and are sufficient to overcome the majority of communication barriers in elderly people [32]. Although the basic concept is to amplify sound, electronic aids are complex instruments which require some understanding by patient, relatives and staff. They consist of three major components: the *microphone* which converts sound into electrical activity, the *amplifier* which controls and increases the power output to the *receiver*, which converts the electrical activity back to sound waves.

The ear mould is often overlooked but is a vital part of the aid. It has to be a good fit, because when it is too tight pressure can result in soreness, and when too loose amplified sound escapes, creating a whistling from feedback.

Many staff are puzzled by the three operations marked O, T, and M on the amplifier. O is the on-off switch; T is for 'Telecoil', for use with an induction coil on telephones and other electronic devices, including some lecture halls and adapted televisions; and M is for microphone, for use in normal conversation. It is important that the aid be switched to the appropriate operation for effective communication.

Several types of electronic hearing aid are available. The ideal aid will [34]:

- cover the whole speech range;
- provide selective amplification for areas where there is selective hearing loss;
- selectively amplify the quieter elements of speech (consonants) to the level of the more audible vowels;
- iron out the extremes of variation in intensity;
- protect the wearer from the amplification of loud environmental noise.

Types of electronic aid

The *body-worn aid* consists of a microphone, an amplifier and battery in a case worn at chest level. The amplifier and microphone are in a comparatively large box which is worn clipped into a pocket or in a container hung from the neck. This requires a long wire to the earpiece. It has the disadvantages that it picks up the sound of clothes rubbing against the microphone container and is more conspicious than the other types of aid. It is particularly useful where high-frequency amplification is required, since the distance between amplifier and receiver reduces the amount of feedback, which is the cause of unwanted whistling noise.

The *behind-the-ear aid* consists of a microphone, amplifier and battery in a small container which lies behind the ear, and which is attached to the earpiece by a small length of tubing. The controls on this are very small and other disabilities may prevent the elderly person manipulating them. The main advantage is that of cosmesis, and this probably accounts for the greater compliance for use [33]. They are, however, less effective than the body-worn aids when a large amount of high-frequency amplification is required.

In *spectacle hearing aids* the components are incorporated into the 'arms' of the spectacles.

Finally, with *in-the-ear aids* all the components fit into the external ear. Advances in microelectronics now allow a reasonably good frequency response and have reduced the problems of acoustic feedback. The controls are very small and particularly difficult to manipulate.

Whichever aid is used, the sound can be transmitted by bone or by an ear insert.

Problems with hearing aids

Amplification of sound is only part of the solution for the hard of hearing since it also produces distortion of the sound and amplifies all components, not only of speech but also of background noise, which may become unbearable or even painful. Even with amplification the consonants may not be heard clearly, and therefore speech remains unintelligible.

The clinician is often faced with the problem of the hard of hearing patient who does not have a hearing aid, which makes taking a case history difficult. There are several potential aids for the clinician. McArdle [35] reviewed three types: (a) the simple speaking tube (an acoustic aid); (b) a communicator (an electronic aid with a microphone connected to an amplifier leading to an earpiece which the patient holds to the ear); and (c) a 'converser' which has a pair of earphones connected to an amplifier in a box. The speaking tube is cheap but patients liked it the least of the three types. The more cumbersome converser was preferred by two-thirds of the patients.

Non-wearing of hearing aids

Simply providing a hearing aid does not guarantee its use. The prevalence of non-wearing is quite high, with about 40 per cent of people not wearing them for personal reasons [36].

To some extent the wearing of aids depends on their availability and cost. For instance, the number of people having hearing aids increases proportionally with the economic status of a country as measured by its Gross National Product. The highest number of hearing aid users is where there is state provision of the aids [37]. However, in Britain, with its state provision, between 10 and 20 per cent of those with hearing aids never use them [38, 39]. This is not necessarily because of over-provision or because aids are less appreciated when they are free than when they are paid for. Denmark has a similar free provision, and at a higher rate than in Britain, but a non-use of only 2–6 per cent [40–42]. This is probably due to a well-organized educational programme in Denmark where patients who have been prescribed a hearing aid receive four weekly 2-hour sessions of training [43]. The introduction of a training scheme in Britain has been shown to improve the use of hearing aids [44]. A further factor in improving the use is the amount of follow-up with the provision of a maintenance service for the hearing aid. This is more effective than waiting for the patient to self-report difficulties [45].

Whether age is a factor in non-use of hearing aids is debatable. Some studies have reported low compliance in old age [46–48], but others have found no relationship between non-use and age [39, 42,

49]. There are, however, a number of elderly people who will not comply with hearing aid use. For this reason there has been an attempt to predict those likely to wear a hearing aid by developing a scale which incorporates the degree of hearing loss, the patient's own assessment, age, physical disability of the hands and eyes, motivation to hear better and the attitude to hearing aids [50].

It is important that the patient understands that an aid will not reproduce normal hearing. Many patients, not understanding what the aid is designed to do, become disillusioned and do not wear it. One other misconception is that the hearing aid will increase the rate of further hearing loss. The cosmetic element is also important in that many people do not like to advertise that they are deaf. This is not surprising when we consider the negative attitudes of society to the deaf person.

There are a number of other reasons why aids are not worn. One is the lack of understanding on how to use the aid, which results in an unpleasant whistling sound – audible to all around. Rehabilitation staff should understand the causes and techniques of overcoming this problem (see below). Other causes of non-wearing of aids are:

1. The electronic mechanism may be defective. This requires expert advice.
2. Wax may have built up in the ear, thereby creating further deafness.
3. Wax may have blocked off the end of the earpiece. This is common and should be checked regularly.
4. The ear may have become sore owing to irritation from the earpiece.
5. There my be difficulty in adapting to hearing amplified background noises. The technique to help overcome this is to persuade the patient to concentrate on specific background noises in an attempt to re-educate the brain to accepting the signals as background noise. It is also worth while emphasizing that the volume should be kept at the lowest which allows speech to be heard. Many patients turn up the volume to a level that is beginning to become difficult to tolerate. Unfortunately this produces distortion of sound as well as amplifying unwanted background noises.

The whistling aid

The high-pitched whistle emitting from a hearing aid is painful to the patient and irritating to all around. There are several possible causes for the noise:

1. The ear mould may be too loose, allowing feedback of the amplified sound. Carers should ensure that the earpiece is fitting snugly.
2. The volume control could be turned up too high.
3. Leakage of sound from the tube or connections somewhere between the receiver and the earpiece might be the problem.
4. In the case of body-worn amplifiers, the amplifier may be too near to the receiver – move it to a more distal position.
5. There may be wax in the ear, or condensation in the tube.

Other aids to independence

Telephone modifications

A number of adaptations to telephones are available. This may involve replacing the conventional receiver with one that has a special amplifier, or providing an additional earpiece to allow both ears to be used.

If an induction loop system is installed then the conversation can be heard directly through the hearing aid. Many modern public telephones have these. It is important to switch the hearing aid to the T operation.

Difficulties in hearing the telephone ring can be overcome by a louder bell or by using a flashing light. The latter has the disadvantage that the person must be in the room where the light is flashing, but this can be overcome by adapting the lighting system so that all the house lights flash on and off when the phone rings.

Electronic devices are already available which allow handwriting converted into electronic signals to be transmitted down the telephone line and reconverted into handwriting on a special pad at the receiving end. These are expensive but are likely to become cheaper and more readily available in the future.

Radio and television

These are an important feature of modern society. They have the advantage that the volume can be controlled, though this may cause distress to other members of the family with normal hearing. There are ways around this. A small extension loudspeaker, for example, can be used as an earpiece. The use of induction coils can also allow the television or radio to be heard directly through the hearing aid without having to increase the volume or disturbing other listeners. It can also be used by several hard of hearing people in the room at the same time.

Many television programmes now carry captions to help those who are hard of hearing. In the United Kingdom these can be provided for certain programmes by tuning into the Ceefax (BBC) or Oracle (ITV) subtitles. Similar systems are available in other countries and have been shown to be of great benefit for the deaf [51].

Doorbells and alarm clocks

The deaf person can be alerted to the ringing of a doorbell by having amplified extension bells or by attaching the system to the house lights. Similar warning can be given by using a pressure-sensitive door mat which alerts the deaf person to someone coming into the house.

Alarm clocks may not be heard, and so, again, a light flashing alarm clock or one that produces vibration in the pillow may be more effective. For those with only some difficulty in hearing, standing the alarm clock on a biscuit tin may amplify the noise sufficiently to be heard.

Advice to carers

There are a number of simple steps carers can take to improve communication. For example, when speaking to a hard of hearing person first of all make sure that the hearing aid is being worn and is switched on – they rarely are. Then make sure that the speaker's face is in a good light and that words are clearly spoken with good lip movements. Fortunately consonants, which are largely lost in presbycusis, are relatively easy to pick up by lip reading and therefore help to compensate for the deafness. In view of the difficulties of recruitment and distortion of sound, the speaker should speak loudly but not shout. In view of the difficulty in understanding rapid speech, the speaker should talk relatively slowly and leave a longer interval between sentences. Wherever possible conversation should take place in an area where there is little distraction by other background noises.

When in a group make sure that the deaf person has his back to the window (so that the light falls on the other speaker's face) and that he can see as many faces as possible. If the group is sympathetic to the deaf person they can help tremendously by using non-verbal cues such as indicating who is going to speak next or is doing so at the time – this is particularly relevant when conversation is moving around the group or several people attempting to speak at the same time.

Speech should be neither too slow nor too fast – both make it difficult to grasp the context of the speech. If a patient does not understand, rephrasing the question may help to provide further clues which were missed in the first approach, largely owing to the ability to lip-read only certain words.

Speech therapy

One of the many disconcerting problems with deafness is the tendency for the deaf person to shout owing to lack of auditory feedback. Speech therapists can help to train the person to modify the voice level and improve the quality of speech, since it often becomes slurred and monotonous.

References

1. Hinchcliffe, R. (1959) The threshold of hearing as a function of age. *Acoustica* **9**: 303–8.
2. Eisdorfer, C. and Wilkie, F. (1972) Auditory changes on the aged: a follow-up study. *Journal of the American Geriatrics Society* **20**: 377–82.
3. Siegelaub, B., Friedman, G.D., Adnour, K. and Seltzer, C.C. (1974) Hearing loss in adults: relation to age, sex, etc. *Archives of Environmental Health* **29**: 107–9.
4. Herbst, K.G. and Humphrey, C. (1981) Prevalence of hearing impairments in the elderly living at home. *Journal of the Royal College of General Practitioners* **31**: 155–60.
5. Townsend, P. and Wedderburn, D. (1965) *The Aged in the Welfare State.* Occasional Papers in Social Administration No. 14. Bell, London.
6. Goldberg, E.M. (1970) *Helping the Aged: A Field Experiment in Social Work*, pp. 66. George Allen & Unwin, London.
7. Fisch, L. (1985) The ageing auditory system. In: *Textbook of Geriatric Medicine and Gerontology*, 3rd Edn. (Ed: Brocklehurst, J.C.). Churchill Livingstone, London.
8. Powers, J.K. and Powers, E.A. (1978) Hearing problems of elderly persons: social consequences and prevalence. *Journal of the American Speech and Hearing Association*, February: 79–83.
9. Jones, D.A., Victor, C.R. and Vetter, N.J. (1984) Hearing difficulty and its psychological implications for the elderly. *Journal of Epidemiology and Community Health* **38**: 75–8.
10. Schein, J.D. and Delk, M.T. (1974) *The Deaf Population in the United States.* National Association of the Deaf, Silver Spring, MD.
11. Rassi, J. and Harford, E. (1968) An analysis of patient attitudes and reactions to a clinical hearing aid selection program. *The Journal of the American Speech and Hearing Association* **10**: 283–90.
12. Northern, J.L. and Sanders, D.A. (1972) Philosophical considerations in aural rehabilitation. In: *Handbook of Clinical Audiology* (Ed: Katz, J.). Williams & Wilkins, Baltimore.
13. Oyer, E.J. (1976) Exchanging information within the older family. In: *Aging and Communication* (Eds: Oyer, H.J. and Oyer, E.J.). University Park Press, Baltimore.
14. Alpiner, J.G. (1973) The hearing aid in rehabilitation for adults. *Journal of the Academy of Rehabilitative Audiology* **6**: 55–7.
15. Corso, J.F. (1977) Auditory perceptions and communication. In: *The*

Handbook of Pyschology of Aging, pp. 475-551 (Eds: Birren, J.E. and Shaie, N.). Litton, New York.

16. Hodgson, W.R. (1977) Clinical measures of hearing performance. In: *Hearing Aid Assessment and Use in Audiologic Habilitation* (Eds: Hodgson, W.R. and Skinner, P.H.). Williams & Wilkins, Baltimore.

17. Carhart, R. and Tillman, T. (1970) Interaction of competing speech signals with hearing loss. *Archives of Otolaryngology (Chicago)* **91**: 273-9.

18. Nabelek, K.A. and Pickett, J.M. (1974) Monaural and binaural speech perception through hearing aids under noise and reverberation with normal and hearing impaired listeners. *Journal of Speech and Hearing Research* **17**: 724-39.

19. Tonning, F.-M. (1978) Evaluation of hearing aid fitting based on the patients' experiences from everyday listening conditions. *Scandinavian Audiology* **7**: 13-17.

20. Milne, J.S. (1976) Hearing loss related to some signs and symptoms in older people. *British Journal of Audiology* **10**: 65-73.

21. High, W.S., Fairbanks, G. and Glorig, A. (1964) Scale for self-assessment of hearing handicap. *The Journal of Speech and Hearing Disorders* **29**: 215-30.

22. Atherley, G.R.C. and Noble, W.G. (1971) Clinical picture of occupational hearing loss obtained with hearing measurement scale. In: *Occupational Hearing Loss* (Ed: Robinson, D.W.). Academic Press, London.

23. Thomas, A. and Ring, J. (1981) A validation study of the hearing measurement scale. *British Journal of Audiology* **15**: 55-60.

24. Calearo, C. and Lazzaroni, A. (1957) Speech intelligibility in relation to the speed of the message. *Laryngology* **67**: 410-19.

25. Herbst, K.G. and Humphrey, C. (1980) Hearing impairment and mental state in the elderly living at home. *British Medical Journal* **281**: 903-5.

26. Kay, D.W.K., Beamish, P. and Roth, M. (1964) Old age mental disorders in Newcastle-upon-Tyne. *British Journal of Psychiatry* **110**: 668-82.

27. Hodkinson, H.M. (1973) Mental impairment in the elderly. *Journal of the Royal College of Physicans of London* **7**: 305-17.

28. Maule, M.M., Milne, J.S. and Williamson, J. (1984) Mental illness and physical health in older people. *Age and Ageing* **13**: 349-56.

29. Uhlmann, R.F., Larson, E.B. and Koepsell, T.D. (1986) Hearing impairment and cognitive decline in senile dementia of the Alzheimer's type. *Journal of the American Geriatrics Society* **34**: 207-10.

30. Thomas, P.D., Hunt, W.C., Garry, P.J. *et al.* (1983) Hearing acuity in a healthy elderly population: effects on emotional, cognitive and social status. *Journal of Gerontology* **38**: 321-5.

31. Ramsdell, D.A. (1978) The psychology of the hard-of-hearing and deafened adult. In: *Hearing and Deafness*, 4th Edn. H. Davis.

32. Hall, M.R.P. (1973) The assessment of the value of three types of hearing aid to overcome the communication barrier of deafness in the elderly patient in the hospital setting. *Age and Ageing* **2**: 125-7.

33. Haggard, M.P., Foster, J.R. and Iredale, F.E. (1981) Use and benefit of postaural aids in sensory hearing loss. *Scandinavian Audiology* **10**: 45-52.

34. Mills, R. (1985) The auditory system. In: *Principles and Practice of Geriatric Medicine* (Ed: Pathy, M.S.J.). John Wiley, Chichester.

35. McArdle, C. (1975) Communicating with hard of hearing patients. *Age and Aging* **4**: 116-18.

36. Watson, L.E. and Tolan, T. (1967) *Hearing Tests and Hearing Instruments*. Hofner, New York.

37. Stephens, S.D.G. (1977) Hearing aid use by adults: a survey of surveys. *Clinical Otolaryngology* **2**: 385-402.

38. Brooks, D.N. (1972) The use and disuse of Medresco hearing aids. *Sound* **6**: 80–5.
39. Carstairs, V. (1973) Utilization of hearing aids issued by the National Health Service. *British Journal of Audiology* **7**: 72–6.
40. Jordon, O., Greisen, O. and Bentzen, O. (1967) Treatment with binaural hearing aids. *Archives of Otolaryngology* **85**: 319–26.
41. Frederiksen, E., Blegvad, B. and Rojskjoer, C. (1974) Binaural hearing aid treatment of presbycusus patients 70 to 80 years. *Scandinavian Audiology* **3**: 83–6.
42. Ewertsen, H.W. (1974) The use of hearing aids (always, often, rarely, never). *Scandinavian Audiology* **3**: 173–6.
43. Ewertsen, H.W. (1974) Hearing rehabilitation in Denmark. *Hearing Instruments* **25**: 21–4.
44. Brooks, D.N. (1979) Counselling and its effect on hearing aid use. *Scandinavian Audiology* **8**: 101–7.
45. Ward, P.R. (1981) Effectiveness of aftercare for older people prescribed a hearing aid for the first time. *Scandinavian Audiology* **10**: 99–106.
46. Bicknell, M.R. and Davies, M.K. (1968) A survey of Medresco hearing aids issued at a provincial centre. *Journal of Laryngology and Otology* **82**: 529–36.
47. Kodieck, J. and Garrad, J. (1955) The hearing aid in use: a survey of 1459 patients. *Journal of Laryngology and Otology* **69**: 807–16.
48. Surr, R.K., Schuchman, G.I. and Montgomery, A.A. (1979) Factors influencing use of hearing aids. *Hearing Instruments* **30**: 19–21.
49. Jensen, P.A. and Funch, E. (1968) The results of hearing aid treatment of geriatric patients. In: *Geriatric Audiology*, p. 110 (Ed: Liden, G.). Almqvist & Wiksell, Stockholm. p 110.
50. Rupp, R.R., Higgins, J. and Maurer, J.F. (1977) A feasibility scale for predicting hearing aid use (FSPHAU) with older individuals. *Journal of the Academy of Rehabilitative Audiology* **10**: 81–104.
51. Schein, J.D. (1980) From zero to line 21: closing the TV gap for deaf viewers. *Journal of Educational Technology Systems* **9**: 241–5.

14

Visual impairment

General features

One-third of identified handicapped people have visual problems [1], 80 per cent of whom are over retirement age, 79 per cent have at least one other major disability, and 62 per cent need the help of another person in travelling beyond their home [2].

Accurate figures are available for the number of people registered blind, but this is not the full representation of those whose eyesight is poor enough to effect their quality of life. There are about 23 blind people in a population of 10 000 [3], although this is probably an underestimation by about 30 per cent [4]. The partially sighted prevalence rate is about 11 per thousand of the population [3], but this again is probably under-reported by about 50 per cent [5].

Under-reporting is particularly common in old age [1], with only about a half of those with visual disturbance having the disorder diagnosed [2]. It seems that after the age of 75 years about 90 per cent of individuals will have some disorder which puts them at risk of losing their vision. However, even when elderly people are known to be blind detailed information about their needs has been less well defined than for younger people [6].

Disturbances of vision increases with advancing age [7–11], with about 5 per cent of those 85 years and over being registered blind [3], while most of those being registered as partially blind (70 per cent) or blind (85 per cent) are over 65 years [10, 12]. The figures for the United States [13] and Iceland [14] have varied between three and eight blind people per thousand of population, much depending on the definition of blindness and the design of the study.

The main causes of visual impairment in the elderly are cataract, macular degeneration, glaucoma, diabetes mellitus and vascular disease. In the elderly several different causes may be present at the same time, which adds complications when considering surgery.

Cataracts

Opacity of the lens increases with advancing age [9, 15, 16], being common after the age of 50 and present to some degree in nearly all people over the age of 75 [17, 18]. Significant cataract resulting in visual impairment has been found in 19 per cent of elderly males and 32 per cent of elderly females [9], increasing from about 5 per cent of those 52–64 to 20 per cent in those 65–74 and nearly 50 per cent in those 75–85 years.

Cataracts do not necessarily cause any symptoms since the visual disturbances depend on the size, site and density of the cataract. The decrease in light reaching the retina results in increasing degrees of blurred vision, colours appear more dull, and there may be monocular double vision, Reading, especially smaller print, becomes more difficult.

The effect of light on vision depends on the site of the cataract. When it is at the front of the lens it produces glare; if in the nucleus, vision is not altered by different intensities of light.

Glare becomes greater with an increase in the brightness of the light, and so many people with cataracts prefer to be in subdued lighting. One way around this is to diffuse the light by using a lamp cover to enlarge the light source. Multiple small light sources are more effective than one large bright light for the same reason. Some patients who are affected by glare benefit from photochromic lenses which react to the amount of light, becoming darker as the light intensity increases.

Blindness from cataract can be prevented by surgery. This is so successful (95–98 per cent of cases) that 'it (surgery) should not be withheld from any elderly person regardless of age or physical disability' [19].

Surgical removal of the lens results in long-sightedness and the need for a replacement lens, which may be intraocular, a contact lens or thick spectacles. Thick spectacles for unilateral removal of the lens cannot produce binocular vision even if there is good vision in the other eye since the lens produces a difference of image size between the two eyes of 20–30 per cent. Contact lenses produce about 20 per cent magnification whereas the intraocular lens produces very little magnification. Contact lenses are not well-tolerated by the elderly owing to the tendency to drier eyes and the difficulty in manipulating the lens on to the cornea. Soft extended-wear contact lenses may be of some help to some patients, though they are more expensive. Operation for unilateral cataract is unlikely to be beneficial if the patient will not wear a contact lens or if it is not possible to provide an intraocular lens.

Many elderly people find it very difficult to wear thick-lens spectacles since the magnification makes objects appear closer than they actually are and makes straight lines distorted, especially on peripheral vision. The distortion can be minimized by telling the patient to turn the head, rather than the eyes, when looking to the side to keep vision in the central field. Unless the patient adapts then he or she is at risk from falls.

The intraocular lens is easier to adapt to but has a higher complication rate from the additional surgical manipulation [20, 21] and damage to the corneal endothelium from the implant [22, 23].

Many patients are told that the cataract needs to 'ripen' before it can be removed. This used to be true when cataract extraction was extracapsular, when it was important to allow the lens to become opaque so that the lens material could be washed out, leaving behind the posterior capsule. Modern intracapsular extraction allows the lens to be removed in its capsule.

Macular degeneration

Macular disease is the second commonest cause of visual impairment in the elderly. The picture seen through the ophthalmoscope is of small patches (Drusen or colloid bodies) around the macula. These may be asymptomatic in elderly people – visual disturbance arises as they enlarge, to lift up and disrupt the pigment cells associated with atrophy of the retina and pigment epithelium. This affects the central fine vision used for reading and for detection of colour. Since peripheral vision is not affected the person can still see but is unable to enjoy reading or watching television. The earliest symptoms are a loss of fine discrimination. Later there is a distortion of straight lines in central vision. Gradually the area of central visual loss increases: at first only small print cannot be read, but this then progresses to larger print. Because of the differential rate of degeneration between the two eyes, symptoms may not become obvious until relatively late owing to compensation by the better eye. The macula is also liable to be damaged in hypertension, renal disorders and diabetes mellitus.

Attempts to improve vision largely involve improving illumination and using magnifying aids. These vary from simple magnifying glasses to miniature telescopes. The latter are particularly useful for seeing distant objects such as bus numbers or the television. Some patients can develop the technique of seeing objects by looking slightly away from them, i.e. using peripheral vision. For this reason it is worth reassessing the patient for new spectacle lenses. There is hope that laser therapy will be able to slow down the rate of deterioration of vision due to macular degeneration [24, 25].

Glaucoma

In chronic simple (open-acute) glaucoma there is resistance to the outflow of fluid from the eye and the intraocular pressure rises. In the elderly, field loss may occur at pressures lower than for younger people, probably because of concomitant arteriosclerosis.

Glaucoma is especially common among those over 70 years of age [26–28]. There is an association between diabetes mellitus and open-angle glaucoma [29–32]; indeed the probability of having an abnormal glucose tolerance test increases as the depth of the anterior chamber decreases [32], probably because the lens of a diabetic is larger than in non-diabetics [31].

Increased intraocular pressure results in compression of the optic nerve affecting capilliary nutrition. The early changes are upper and lower scotomas extending out from the blind spot which progressively constrict the visual field as the condition deteriorates. Once the damage has occurred treatment is ineffective, though early diagnosis and treatment may prevent deterioration.

Treatment involves instilling pilocarpine drops into the eye to miose the pupil, changing the pattern of the trabecular network which is blocking drainage. Compliance tends to be poor since some patients find the miosis unpleasant. This can be overcome by prescribing timolol which has no effect on pupil size but acts on aqueous secretion. Instillation of drops may be a difficult task for elderly people with poor coordination. It is important for the rehabilitation team to ensure that the patient understands the need to use the drops, that he or she can manage to do so or that some arrangement can be made for a relative, neighbour or other person to do this regularly.

Surgical treatment provides an alternative drainage pathway, although the tendency of the operation to increase the rate of cataract development makes medical management the preferred treatment.

Diabetic retinopathy

Visual disturbance due to diabetes mellitus tends to occur in middle age. This is especially true of proliferative retinopathy, which is more common in the younger insulin-dependent diabetic; there is a proliferation of new vessel growth into the vitreous and a tendency to rupture, which results in a sudden loss of vision in that eye. More common in the elderly later-onset diabetic is the development of microaneurysms and the ophthalmological appearance of exudates and haemorrhages.

Symptoms depend on which part of the eye is affected. If the macula is affected there are early symptoms of loss of vision; otherwise there is patchy loss of vision corresponding to the parts of the retina damaged by the exudates.

Vascular disorders

These often produce a central field loss owing to lesions around the macula. Sudden loss of vision is usually due to vascular occlusion, either within the eye or on the visual cortex. Transient loss of vision occurs with transient ischaemic attacks within the carotid artery territory.

Psychological responses

There is a large psychological component to poor vision. Many elderly patients will not agree to an operation for cataracts because they fear that if the operation fails they will be permanently blind or that they are too old for an operation [34].

Although vision is not directly required for communication, non-blind people tend to assume that the blind person is deaf as well (he may be) and talk through the accompaning person. This causes important effects on the role the individual plays in society [35] and produces social handicap.

Prognosis

Most forms of visual disturbance in the elderly tend to deteriorate with time. Milne [36] found that if cataract was present the visual acuity deteriorated by about 24 per cent over a period of 5 years and by about 10 per cent in those without cataracts. However, there was an improvement in the visual acuity of 15 per cent of men and 10 per cent of women over a 5-year period.

The elderly person with visual disturbances becomes markedly handicapped owing to a combination of multiple pathology and difficulty in learning new tasks. There seems to be a correlation between visual loss and dementia [37], which is likely to complicate management further.

The amount of functional ability does not correlate directly with the degree of visual impairment, and much depends on social and psychological factors [38–40]. In one study only 56 per cent of visually disabled people regarded poor sight as one of their greatest problems [10].

The presence of other disorders obviously influences the outcome. Vision is important for the control of balance, especially in the absence of or decrease in other forms of feedback about position (see Chapter 15).

Aids to living

General measures

Registration

Registration on the partially sighted or blind register with the local authority is important so that the patient can have full access to the local facilities for the visually handicapped and can obtain 'talking' books and newspapers. In the United Kingdom, tax payers who are registered as blind have their personal tax-free allowance increased and those on supplementary pensions can receive higher benefits. Registration will also ensure that the elderly person has the services of a social worker for the blind, who can provide information on benefits, services and aids available for improving the quality of life; this includes travel concessions, holidays and access to 'talking' library facilities.

Lighting

Lighting in the homes of elderly people is very often below optimal levels [10] and correction of this results in a marked improvement in visual acuity [41].

Appropriate lighting means more than just brightness: it also involves lack of glare and good colour. Filament bulbs which produce light with a wide colour spectrum are preferable to sodium lamps, which are limited to the red–yellow part of the spectrum. This is especially important if colour discrimination is affected.

Spectacles

Many elderly people have not had their eyesight tested for many years. A new prescription for simple corrective lenses may make all the difference in deteriorating vision. Good care of the spectacles is also important, because dirty or scratched lenses seriously impair vision.

Low-vision aids

Low-vision aids produce mainly magnification. Large lenses are of low magnification, and so the patient should be advised to try out a few lenses first since a smaller lens may be more effective for his or her needs.

A number of modifications to lenses are available. For instance, some magnifiers have a light source attached to assist with illumination and cut down shadows, while others are attached to a stand for those patients who are unable to hold a lens steadily or without tiring.

For those with some residual vision, large-print books, available from most libraries, may be sufficiently clear to make reading possible.

Guide aids

The correct term for the white walking stick should be a 'symbol' stick/cane, since its main use is to inform others of the disability of the blind person. It does, however, have a use in providing the blind person with information about the position of objects around him and is used as an extension of the arm and hand. It does not, however, warn about the drop of a curb and does not detect objects at head height. Ideally it should be long enough to reach the sternum when placed on the ground.

Sonic pathfinders are available which provide auditory warning of changes of object distance by creating varying tone sounds. They obviously depend on good hearing ability. In one study of blind adults (age not stated) the use of a long stick/cane with and without the use of a sonic pathfinder was compared: there was no significant difference between the two for the productive walking index (time spent walking to the total time taken), the amount of veering whilst walking or the incidents of tripping or colliding with objects [42]. The use of the sonic pathfinder did, however, significantly improve the awareness of pavement position, decreased the number of contacts with walls, helped to maintain a central position on the pavement, and gave better warning of objects obstructing the path.

Braille

Although Braille is probably the best known communication aid for the blind, it has limited use for the elderly who become blind late in life. This is mainly because of difficulties in learning new techniques and the sensitivity of the fingers required to read the six dots which make up the letters. Other difficulties include the weight of Braille books, which have to be about twenty times larger than conventional texts.

Other special equipment

Entertainment and information

Reading is obviously difficult, but there are now a large number of 'books on tape' available for blind people. Some areas have a local 'talking newspaper' which provides up-to-date local news items on audio tape. The Royal National Institute for the Blind (RNIB) has produced information tapes covering air, rail and coach travel, gas and electricity supplies, National Savings, postal and telephone services and shopping – which over 80 per cent of the blind members of the RNIB Talking Book Library have found to be useful [6]. Radios and televisions are obviously also useful. In the United Kingdom a receiver is available which will pick up only the sound of television programmes – this does not require a television licence since no picture is received.

Clocks

Clocks with raised numbers are available so that the time can be 'felt'. Many of these have raised dots (two at three, six and nine o'clock positions, three dots at the twelve o'clock position and single dots for other intervening numbers). There are wrist watches with similar methods of displaying the time.

Card and table games

A number of games have had the cards adapted, usually in Braille, so that the face value can be read. There are also playing cards with large printed symbols for those with limited vision.

There are now adapted pieces and boards for chess, draughts, dominoes, crosswords, Scrabble, Othello, Ludo and Solitaire, as well as many other table games. Dice with raised numerals are available.

Sound beacons

These are pocket-size electronic devices which emits sounds. They can be used as markers so that the blind person can find the way back to a specific spot such as a seat on the lawn.

Signature templates

Plastic guides for signatures on cheque, pension and allowance books are available. Simple templates are also available to assist in the addressing of envelopes.

Measuring devices

These include rulers and tape measures with tactile markings to indicate either inches or centimetres.

Knitting

Aids are available to assist the blind knitter, including gauges for the knitting needles, a counter to keep an account of the number of rows already knitted, needle threaders and sock darning mushrooms.

Rain alerts

These are electronic devices sensitive to moisture which warn the blind person by an audible signal that the atmosphere is too moist, or that it is raining, when the washing is hanging out to dry.

Money counters

These are devices for keeping an account of money spent when shopping.

Cooking

A large number of aids are available for the blind cook. For example, one device holds a loaf of bread, the knife being held in a guide to provide control of the bread slice thickness. There are measuring jugs with raised markings on the inside.

Liquid level indicators are electronic devices consisting of two wires suspended over the side of a cup or glass; when the liquid reaches the level of the wires an electric circuit is completed and an audible bleep is emitted. The device has long and short arms to cope with different amounts of liquids.

Medication

A dispenser is available which fits on to a standard medicine bottle and dispenses 5 ml doses of liquid accurately and without mess. A number of containers are available which have specific compartments for the different times of day when medication is to be taken. Tablets are placed in these by a carer. Some of these containers have braille markings for easy identification of the time of day when the tablets should be taken. For those with limited vision the labels on the bottles are more likely to be read if the instructions are typed, preferably in large print [43].

Climbing stairs

A raised area or a notch on the hand rail near the top and bottom of stairs helps to warn the blind person when they are approaching a different level.

Advanced high-technology aids

A number of devices are becoming available using closed-circuit television. This allows good and variable magnification on to a television set, providing facilities both for enhancing the contrast and for image reversal (i.e. turning the black-on-white print of a book into a white-on-black image on the television screen). These aids are expensive and cannot be moved easily because of their bulk and weight. They nevertheless have a use for a small number of patients who wish to read a lot.

Reading machines which convert the written word into synthetic speech are becoming available. At present they are very expensive (about £20 000), but as with most electronic equipment they are likely to decrease in price over the next few years.

Advice to carers

Those working with blind people can help by understanding a few simple principles:

- When speaking to a blind person speak to him or her by name (so that he or she knows that they are being spoken to), and introduce yourself.
- Tell the blind person when you are leaving – it is unpleasant to find that you have been talking to empty space.
- Be clear in your comments – do not rely on facial expressions.
- Leave everything in its place. Moving furniture can be dangerous and moving objects from their normal positions means that they will not be found.

References

1. Warren, M.D. (1985) The Canterbury studies of disablement in the community: prevalence, needs, and attitudes. *International Journal of Rehabilitation Research* **8**: 3–18.
2. Cullinan, T.R. (1977) *The Epidemiology of Visual Disability: Studies of Visually Disabled People in the Community.* University of Kent, Health Services Research Unit Report No. 28.
3. Royal National Institute for the Blind (1984) *Initial Demographic Study: Report of RNIB.* Shankland Cox, London.

4. Graham, P.A., Wallace, J., Welsby, E. and Grace, H. (1968) Evaluation of postal detection of registerable blindness. *British Journal of Preventive and Social Medicine* **22**: 238–41.
5. Page, J. (1974) Definitions of blindness and partial sight. In: *Technological Prosthetics for the Partially Sighted* (Ed: Graham, M.D.). IIASA.
6. Hall, L. (1983) Who are Britain's blind people? – Report of a survey carried out for the Royal National Institute for the Blind, United Kingdom, in 1981. *International Journal of Rehabilitation Research* **6**: 349–50.
7. Kornzweig, A.L., Feldstein, M. and Schneider, J. (1957) The eye in old age. *American Journal of Ophthalmology* **44**: 29–37.
8. Gordon, D.M. (1967) Visual impairment of the older patient. *Journal of the American Geriatrics Society* **15**: 1025–30.
9. Milne, J.S. and Williamson, J. (1972) Visual acuity in older people. *Gerontologia Clinica* **14**: 249–56.
10. Cullinan, T.R. (1978) Visually disabled people at home. *Health Trends* **10**: 90–2.
11. Stone, D.H. and Shannon, D.J. (1978) Screeing for impaired visual acuity in middle age and general practice. *British Medical Journal* **2**: 859–63.
12. Department of Health and Social Security (1979) *Blindness and Partial Sight in England 1969–1976*, Report on Public Health and Medical Subjects No. 129, HMSO.
13. Goldstein, H. (1972) Demography of blindness. In: *Science and Blindness*. American Foundation for the Blind, New York.
14. Bjornsson, G. (1955) Prevalence and causes of blindness in Iceland. *American Journal of Ophthalmology* **39**: 202–8.
15. Kornzweig, A.L. (1964) Ocular conditions of the aged. *Geriatrics* **19**: 24–34.
16. Elwood, J.H. (1967) A survey of eyes in the elderly. *Journal of the Irish Medical Association* **60**: 369–72.
17. Cinotti, A.A. and Patti, J.C. (1968) Lens abnormalities in an ageing population of non-glaucomatous patients. *American Journal of Ophthalmology* **65**: 25–32.
18. Leibowitz, H.M., Kreuger, D.E., Maunder, L.R. *et al.* (1980) The Framingham Eye Study monograph: an ophthalmological and epidemiological study of cataract, glaucoma, diabetic retinopathy, macular degeneration and visual acuity in a general population of 2831 adults. *Survey of Ophthalmology* **34** (Suppl.): 335–610.
19. Kornzweig, A.L. (1972) The prevention of blindness in the aged. *Journal of the American Geriatrics Society* **20**: 383–6.
20. Galin, M.A., Obstbaum, S.A., Boniuk, V. *et al.* (1977) Iris-supported lens implantation *v* simple cataract extraction. *Transactions of the Ophthalmological Society, UK* **97**: 74–7.
21. Jaffe, N.S., Eichenbaum, D.M., Clayman, H.M. and Lights, D.S. (1978) A comparison of 50 Binkhorst implants with 500 routine intracapsular cataract extractions. *American Journal of Ophthalomology* **85**: 24–7.
22. Binkhorst, C.D., Loones, L.H. and Nygaard, P. (1977) Biomicroscopical observations on a corneal endothelium in pseudophakia. *Transactions of the Ophthalmology Society, UK* **97**: 67–73.
23. Kaufman, H.E. (1980) The correction of aphakia. *American Journal of Ophthalomology* **89**: 1–10.
24. Glass, J.M.D. (1977) *Stereocopic Atlas of Macular Disease – Diagnosis and Treatment*, 2nd Edn. C.V. Mosby, St. Louis.
25. Talbot, J. and Bird, A. (1980) Krypton laser in the management of disciform macular degeneration. *Transactions of the Ophthalmological Society, UK* **100**: 423–4.
26. Hollows, F.C. and Graham, P.A. (1966) Intraocular pressure, glaucoma, and

glaucoma suspects in a defined population. *British Journal of Ophthalmology* **50**: 570–86.

27. Bankes, J.K.L., Perkins, E.S., Tsolakis, S. and Wright, J.E. (1968) Bedford glaucoma survey. *British Medical Journal* **1**: 791–6.

28. Editorial (1977) Screening for glaucoma. *Lancet* **2**: 437–8.

29. Armstrong, J.R., Daily, R.K., Dobson, H.L. and Girard, L. (1960) The incidence of glaucoma in diabetes mellitus. *American Journal of Ophthalmology* **50**: 55–68.

30. Becker, B. (1971) Diabetes mellitus and primary open angle glaucoma. *American Journal of Ophthalmology* **71**: 1–16.

31. Wilensky, J.Y., Podos, S.M. and Becker, B. (1974) Prognostic indicators in ocular hypertension. *Archives of Ophthalmology* **91**: 200–2.

32. Mapstone, R. and Clark, C.V. (1985) Prevalence of diabetes in glaucoma. *British Medical Journal* **291**: 93–5.

33. Brown, N. and Hungerford, J. (1982) The influence of the size of the lens in ocular disease. *Transactions of the Ophthalmology Society, UK* **102**: 359–63.

34. Spina, J. (1982) Fear of cataract extraction: mental health aspects of a geriatric health problem. *Clinical Gerontologist* **2**: 68–70.

35. Meyer, E. (1981) The blind and social deprivation. *International Journal of Rehabilitation Research* **4**: 353–64.

36. Milne, J.S. (1979) Longitudinal studies of vision in older people. *Age and Ageing* **8**: 160–6.

37. Maule, M.M., Milne, J.S. and Williamson, J. (1984) Mental illness and physical health of older people. *Age and Ageing* **13**: 349–56.

38. Josephson, E. (1968) *The Social Life of Blind People*. American Foundation for the Blind, New York.

39. Gray, P.G. and Todd, J.E. (1967) *Mobility and Reading Habits of the Blind: An Inquiry Made for the Minister of Health Covering Registered Blind of England and Wales in 1965*. Government Social Survey, London.

40. Abel, R.A. (1976) *An Investigation into Some Aspects of Visual Handicap*. Department of Health and Social Security Statistical and Research Report Series No. 14. HMSO, London.

41. Cullinan, T., Silver, J., Gould, E. and Irvine, D. (1979) Visual disability and home lighting. *Lancet* **1**: 642–44.

42. Dodds, A.G. (1983) The sonic pathfinder – an objective evaluation. *International Journal of Rehabilitation Research* **6**: 350–1.

43. Law, R. and Chalmers, C. (1976) Medicines and elderly people: a general practice survey. *British Medical Journal* **1**: 565–8.

15

Falls and balance disturbances

Incidence, morbidity and mortality

Balance disturbances, especially when associated with falling, are some of the commonest causes of admission and readmission to hospital [1]. As many as one-third to one-half of the elderly population have suffered one or more falls [2-9], and probably the true number is about twenty times that reported to the general practitioner [8]. The prevalence of falls increases markedly with advancing age [2, 3, 5, 7, 9-11], with an average annual rate of falls per 1000 population being about 670 for those 65 years and over; and 890 for those 85 years and over [12]. A study in the 1950s found that 37 per cent of those 65-70 years of age, and 45 per cent of those over 75, had fallen at some time [2]. For some reason the prevalence of falls is higher in women [2, 3, 5, 6, 9-14] – the female:male ratio being 2:1 – though this difference narrows in very advanced old age.

Falls not only cause distress to the patient and the family but are also associated with much long-term morbidity and some lethal complications [15-17]. For instance, in one study of residents of a nursing home, 65 per cent of those who had had six or more falls died within the first year [18]. This, however, does not take into account the relatively high mortality of elderly people who require nursing home care. A number of studies have shown that there is an excess morbidity and mortality in old people who have fallen at home compared with an age/sex matched controlled group [5, 8, 19, 20]. In one study, 89 per cent of 3200 people who died as a result of a fall at home were over the age of 85 [16], while another study found that three-quarters of fatal accidents in the home involved those over the age of 65 [21]. The prevalence of fatal falls per 100 000 of the population at risk increases from 14.6 for the 65-74 age group, through 76.1 for the 75-84 age group, to 268.4 for the 85 years and over group [17]. Non-fatal trauma is also common, with an injury rate from falls of between 1.4 and 1.9 per cent of those 60 years and over [5, 22].

Causes of falls

The causes of falls are complex and multifactorial. Although a large amount of knowledge is available about the aetiology of falls, this has had limited effect on the ability to treat the conditions. Basically the causes can be subdivided into those that are external to the individual, and those that are due to physical disorders within the individual.

External causes

These include slipping and tripping and are thought to be responsible for about one-third of all falls [21, 23]. They tend to occur in otherwise healthy younger elderly people [8, 24], and the prognosis is good, usually only requiring simple advice. Underfoot accidents occur when the foot slips, is arrested in its stride (caught, tripped, stumbled) or is twisted, or when the ankle is turned, or when there is unexpected movement of the surface (e.g. a slipping mat on a smooth floor) [25].

The majority of falls occur in the home [18], especially in the toilet or on the stairs [2, 5, 7, 12] . Slipping on stairs is relatively infrequent [26, 27], mostly being due to 'overstepping'. This is more likely to occur on the bottom step owing to thinking wrongly that the ground level has been reached, and so most falls occur when descending stairs [28]. Two-flight stairs and those that are U-shaped seem to cause fewer problems than do long, single-flight stairs.

The use of handrails is also important. They should be on both sides of the stairway, and it seems that the optimal height should be 36–38 inches (about 95 cm) above the tread [29], though this is higher than the 31–33 inches (about 82 cm) recommendation based on bio-mechanical and anthropometric measurements [30]. The higher levels are probably more appropriate for safety when descending the stairs. A handrail with a circular cross-section of 1.75 inches (44 mm) diameter seems to be the best for achieving a power grip [29], or a circumference of 4.4–5.2 inches (112–132 mm) [30].

It must be noted that falls are very common in long-term residential institutions [12] and tend to occur at night, especially when transferring to and from bed or chair, or on the way to the toilet [12, 31, 32]. Falls in institutions are, ironically, probably a sign that there is a positive approach to rehabilitation, low levels being indicative of little activity [22, 23]. This is important to recognize if inhibitive 'protective' nursing is to be avoided owing to a fear of accusation of negligence.

The fact that falls tend to occur indoors does not necessarily mean that they were due to the environment, but may merely indicate the greater amount of time spent indoors by frail, elderly people. In the classical study by Sheldon [34], as many as one-third of all falls were thought to be accidental, of which one-third occurred on stairs. He found that 11 per cent of falls were due to tripping. This was also the commonest cause of falls in the study by Exton-Smith [9], especially for women in the 65–74 age group – falls due to giddiness also increased with advancing age. However, in two studies of people who fell either at home or in hospital, trips or slips were very rare [35]. Isaacs [35] has pointed out that patients often comment 'I must have tripped' or 'I must have slipped' and that this probably means that they did *not* trip or slip – patients presuming this to be the cause because they cannot account for why they did fall.

Gabell *et al.* [36] found trips or slips to be responsible for three-quarters of all falls, although they also identified ten other personal factors which were likely to have contributed: disturbances of gait following a period of rest, an abnormal plantar response, failure to wear prescribed spectacles, anxiety or depression, foot problems, two or more perceived limitations of disability, a history of previously having worn high-heel shoes, a sustained drop in the pulse pressure five minutes after a rest period, restricted neck mobility, and the presence of an inverse Romberg ratio. The slip or trip is therefore associated with underlying physical disabilities.

There is no doubt that some falls are due to inappropriate footwear, such as slippers which are too loose, or are due to inadequate lighting. However, the environment is usually contributory rather than causative in falls in elderly people. Nevertheless there is always an indication for checking for preventable environmental factors.

Intrinsic causes

These are usually present for all falls other than the one-off trip or slip. A fall is an inability to maintain the centre of the antigravity force between the supporting base (i.e. the feet when standing), or to respond quickly enough to any displacement. In effect this means that damage has occurred somewhere along the tract from the *control* (neurological) system, through the *actuating* (muscular) system to the *framework* (skeletal) system. Balance depends on the integrity of visual, vestibular, proprioceptive and tactile input, as well as on sensory integration within the central nervous system, visiospatial perception, effective muscle tone which adapts rapidly to change, muscle strength and joint flexibility.

When a fall occurs in the absence of a chronic balance disturbance, the cause is likely to be a cardiovascular disorder producing transient cerebral ischaemia, or to epilepsy. Transient ischaemic attacks are relatively common in the elderly. Broe *et al.* [37], in a community study, found a prevalence of 87 per 1000 population 65 years and over but did not show any sex difference or increase in frequency with advancing age.

The difficulty of associating cardiac dysrhythmias with falls is that, although abnormalities of cardiac rhythm are commonly found in patients who fall [38], they are also common in elderly people who do not fall [39, 40]. Nevertheless sudden collapse has been associated with acute onset of cardiac dysrhythmias [41, 42]. Other causes of syncope include aortic stenosis, especially when severe [43], other cardiac valve disorders, vasovagal attacks and syncopes due to coughing, micturition or defaecation.

It is generally felt that many falls are associated with drug therapy, especially by antihypertensives [8, 44–46], barbiturates [47, 48], sedatives/tranquillizers [14, 31, 47], antidepressants [6–8, 49, 50] or alcohol [7]; although others have found that the use of antihypertensive agents [51–53], sedatives [6, 32] or alcohol [6] are no more common in those patients who fall than those who do not.

It is important to recognize the association of drugs such as sedatives and tranquillizers in the aetiology of falls since these drugs are often prescribed to treat patients with dizziness and balance problems. Certainly clinical experience shows that stopping drugs helps to decrease the number of falls.

Factors which must be taken into account when discussing balance disturbances are whether they are acute or chronic in onset, and whether the disturbance occurs when standing still (static balance) or only when walking or changing position (dynamic balance).

Sway

Much of the study of balance has concentrated on static sway. Sheldon [54] showed that sway whilst standing was high in the infant but decreased by the late teens, remaining relatively constant until middle age, after which it continued to increase with advancing age; and this has been confirmed by other workers [55–57]. It also seems that sway is greater in females than in males [3, 58, 59], though the reason for this is unknown.

Overstall *et al.* (60), using stepwise multiple linear regressional analysis, found that for an association with sway, age was the most important single variable, with being female and increasing number of falls also being statistically significant. They also found that, although postural hypotension had a positive correlation with sway, tripping had a negative effect (i.e. people who tripped had low levels of sway).

The fact that sway increases with age does not necessarily mean that it is associated with falling – falls usually occur when walking rather than when standing still. Although there is an association between sway and falling [57, 59], the correlation is not as high as might be expected [56]. Probably more relevant is the finding that sway is strongly associated with the velocity of walking and the number of faults occurring on an obstacle course [60]. It is also of note that speed of sway is greater for non-fallers in an institution than for those who are at home [56], and this fits in with the finding that disturbances of gait parameters were as common in hospitalized elderly patients without a history of falls as in those fallers not admitted to hospital [62]. Sway and gait abnormalities may therefore be an indication of general ill-health.

Sway is greater with the eyes closed than when visual clues are available [54, 63]. It seems that the peripheral component of vision is the most important for normal balance [64]. To some extent the role of vision is seen in very young children when, in the laboratory situation, the walls are moved but the floor remains steady, with the result that the child falls. In this situation adults do not fall, though they may sway [65]. It is also a common sensation for 'normal' people in a stationary car or train to experience a sense of self movement when the adjacent vehicle moves.

It has been suggested that vision plays a less important role than is generally thought [66]. This is probably because vision is only one part of a complex feedback mechanism. However, vision is particularly important when the movement is complex and requires a high level of precision or speed. With a decrease in visual clues the postural and proprioceptive feedback becomes increasingly important [58, 67, 68]; that is, there was no decrease in the accuracy of spatial perception with the eyes closed, but when the head or the body was tilted there were significant errors of judgement of verticality, even in normal subjects. This is particularly relevent since disturbances of verticality perception and falls have been linked [69–70]. In addition, perception of tactile pressure and vibratory sensation also decrease with advancing age [71]. The relevance of the latter is uncertain since, although proprioceptive feedback decreases in the elderly under low or minimal feedback conditions, there is no difference under stronger feedback [72].

The rehabilitation implications are that every effort should be made to ensure that vision is optimal. Simple measures such as ensuring that there is bright light, that the spectacles are clean and that the lenses are providing optimal refraction go a long way to improving vision. Many patients do not wear their spectacles and this is associated with trips and slips [36]. Probably just as important is the need to avoid moving quickly from a bright light into a dimly lit environment.

One possible cause of increased sway may be the fear of falling. The evidence for this is slim but neurotics do seem to sway more than normal controls [73, 74]. Once a fall has occurred it is not surprising that an individual is frightened and is reluctant to stand and walk. Much rehabilitation is therefore to instil confidence.

Locomotion

One of the reasons why sway is not directly related to falling is that falls are more likely to occur during locomotion, which depends on the rapid response of the body's coordinating system to changes in speed and direction over a variety of surfaces whilst manoeuvring around obstacles. There are two aspects to this: one is the need for a highly developed awareness of the unbalancing mechanism [75]; the other is the ability of the dynamic forces generated by muscles to counteract the unbalancing forces [76].

A number of receptor organs are involved in control of balance. The vestibular labyrinth provides information about changes in position and speed, while the joint and tendon receptors give information about the relationship of different parts of the body during standing and changes in position.

Many of the possible balance control mechanisms are often disturbed at the same time. For instance, in one study of patients with unsteadiness the commonest abnormalities found were a peripheral neuropathy (85 per cent), cervical spondyosis (71 per cent), vestibular abnormalities (64 per cent) and cataracts (35 per cent) [77].

Dizziness and giddiness

Many patients complain of dizziness or giddiness when turning the head. This may be due to vestibular dysfunction or vertebrobasilar ischaemia, but it may also be associated with other systems in the body [77].

One of the problems is knowing what the patient means by the terms 'dizziness', 'giddiness' or 'lightheadedness'. These can vary from a heavy sensation within the head to severe rotational sensations. The commonest sensations are (figures in per cent); a momentary equilibrium disturbance (46), blackout or spots before the eyes (41), turning sensation (35), staggering or loss of balance (19) and a feeling of falling (14), with other sensations such as heaviness or confusion in the head or fainting being much less common [78].

Dizziness is more common in women (21 per cent) than in men (9 per cent in the 65–69 age group, but similar (24 per cent) in those 75–79) years of age of both sexes [79]. A similar difference between the sexes has been shown for vertigo, although the levels are somewhat higher (about two-thirds of those in the 75–79 age group) [3, 80].

Vertigo

Agate [81] described vertigo as 'a disagreeable sensation of instability or disordered orientation in space' and patients describe it in terms of a sensation of movement either of themselves or the environment. Vertigo is usually due to vestibular dysfunction [82], although it may, especially in the elderly, be due to a degenerative neuropathy of the vestibular nerve [83]. Treatment depends on correcting the underlying causes, and rehabilitation programmes usually have little part to play. However, if the cause is postural hypotension, vertebrobasilar ischaemia [84, 85] or cervical spondylosis [86], then the physical methods described for treating these conditions are applicable.

Balance problems on changing position

Positional dizziness is associated with a large number of activities [78], the commonest being (figures in per cent): sudden changes in position of the head or body (63), walking (56), standing up (50), lying down (20), looking up (13) or down (9), or bending over (12). It is obvious from these figures that a combination of these positional causes for dizziness is common.

Lightheadedness on standing may be due to a number of causes, such as vestibular hypersensitivity, vertebrobasilar ischaemia or postural hypotension. Vertebrobasilar ischaemia theoretically occurs in a number of disorders occurring singly or in combination. The diagnosis of vertebrobasilar ischaemia is commonly made on clinical grounds without any firm proof, and it has been questioned whether it is as common a cause of falls as is often thought [8].

Falls on standing are associated with a failure of the pulse pressure to return to its 'activity' level within five minutes of resting [36]. This has practical implications in training the patient to take deep breaths or flexing and extending the limbs before standing.

Postural hypotension

This is, as its name implies, a drop in the systemic blood pressure on standing. It is traditionally defined as a drop of system systolic blood pressure or 20 mmHg from the supine level after standing for two minutes. The problem with this definition is that patients who have symptomatic postural hypotension cannot stand for two minutes – they fall owing to decreased cerebral blood flow.

Symptoms are probably more related to the ability of the cerebral circulation to respond to the changes in systemic blood pressure. Some patients with only a slight drop in systemic blood pressure feel dizzy or lightheaded, whilst for others the cerebral blood circulation responds quickly even to a marked drop in systemic blood pressure, so that symptoms are not produced. Stark and Wodak [87] described four patients who developed classical symptoms of postural hypotension, such as faintness or dizziness on standing, but who did not have systemic postural drop in the blood pressure – though ophthalmodynamometry indicated that there was a fall in the cerebral blood flow. All had arterial stenosis in either the carotid or vertebral artery systems and eventually developed neurological signs.

Postural hypotension is found in up to about one-quarter of the elderly population [88, 89] and may be found in people who do not fall [90]. The exact prevalence is unknown. A study of patients in an acute geriatric unit found that 17 per cent had a fall of systolic blood pressure of 20 mmHg while 5 per cent had a fall of more than 40 mmHg [90]. These are obviously highly selected and ill patients. However, in a community study similar levels were found in an apparantly normal elderly population [89].

Rehabilitation involves training the patient to transfer from bed or chair correctly. When getting out of bed the patient should sit up in bed for a few minutes, then sit with the feet over the side of the bed for a while, and then stand. He should pause for a few moments before starting to walk. A similar technique is used for getting out of a chair.

Retraining of the baroreceptor reflexes by frequently changing the position of the patient has been shown to improve orthostatic tolerance [90]. Other suggestions are to sleep with the head of the bed raised (so that there is already some pooling of blood in the legs) and to exercise the limbs and take deep breaths before attempting to rise. It has been suggested that exercises such as flexion and extension of the ankle to increase the venous return before getting out of bed helps to reduce the symptoms. This has, however, been shown to increase sway and make some patients with postural hypotension feel less steady [60].

Long elastic stockings (covering above the knee as well as the lower leg) are effective but very difficult for many elderly people to manage on their own. They should be kept on both day and night, especially if the patient rises during the night to go to the toilet, but many patients find this impractical.

Drug therapy is generally unsatisfactory. Fludrocortisone raises the blood pressure temporarily but there is a risk of inducing heart failure. It has been suggested that parenteral thiamine should be effective because of its effect on both neurological and vascular functioning

[91–93]. Sympathomimetic drugs have been used, usually in conjuction with plasma expanders. Drugs such as phenylephrine, midodrine, monoamine oxidases with tyramine, or amphetamine do improve postural hypotension temporarily but also result in hypertension [94, 95]. Other drugs such as dihydroergotamine [96, 97], prostaglandin inhibitors [99, 100] and beta-blockers [101, 102] have also been used, but these produce marked side effects such as heart failure or supine hypertension at a level that is usually unacceptable.

Drop attacks

The term 'drop attack' means different things to different people [13, 34, 103–105]. It is usually taken to mean a sudden giving way of the legs without warning. There is no associated loss of consciousness or incontinence. Usually the person is unable to rise independently but once assisted to his feet can stand and walk normally. Some people find that if they can get their feet against a firm surface such as a wall and press several times this helps the legs to feel stronger, and it has been suggested that this is assisting the re-establishment of the lost proprioceptive sensation.

It is generally assumed that drop attacks are due to vertebrobasilar ischaemia producing acute, but temporary, spinal shock, resulting in the fall from sudden loss of tone in the legs. This is doubtful since there are rarely other signs of brain stem dysfunction, such as cranial or visual nerve involvement, and sensation does not seem to be affected. However, Gordon [106] described one case of infarction of the reticular formation in a patient with 'drop attacks' and postulated that these had been due to ischaemia in the vertebrobasilar territory. Overstall [107] suggested that the attacks may be due to a misinterpretation of visual stimulation without correcting information from proprioceptive feedback.

Vertebrobasilar ischaemia

There are several potential causes for vertebrobasilar ischaemia:

1. Atheromatous changes result in ischaemia whenever there is a decrease in blood flow through the vertebral arteries, as might occur in postural hypotension or acute dysrhythmias.
2. Decrease in height of the vertebral bodies and hardening and narrowing of the intervertebral discs produces kinking of the vertebral arteries as they take a tortuous course through the transverse processes of the cervical vertebrae.
3. Osteophytes arising from the neurocentral and apophyseal joints in cervical spondylosis encroach on the vertebral artery as it travels

through the foramen transversarium of the cervical vertebra [105, 108–110]. Turning the head causes nipping of the vertebral arteries by the osteophytes.

It should not be assumed that dizziness caused by head turning in the presence of cervical spondylosis is due to vertebrobasilar ischaemia, since cervical spondylosis is present in the majority of asymptomatic elderly people [111, 112], and balance disturbance could be due to decreased feedback from the receptors in the apophyseal joints [113]. Cervical spondylosis may produce balance disturbances in other ways. For instance, in one study 16 per cent of patients referred for assessment of gait disturbances had a myelopathy as diagnosed by spasticity in the legs, proprioceptive deficit and myleography [114]. There is also a decrease in the sensitivity of the afferent system from the cervical joints with advancing age [115].

These considerations are important in the rehabilitation programme since the treatment for cervical spondylosis often includes a cervical collar, which will decrease further the feedback from the receptors in the neck. Injecting local anaesthetic into the facet joints of the cervical spine results in nystagmus and ataxia even in young normal people [116]. Cervical collars increase the sensation of unsteadiness in the dark where visual clues are absent [113]. Patients with dizziness and associated cervical symptoms may therefore benefit more from head and neck exercises than by immobilization. Animal experiments have shown that, following vestibular neurotomy, retraining by moving the head is associated with an increased rate of recovery [117].

Balance disturbances due to cervical spondylosis may be caused by osteophytes pressing on the spinal cord. Decreased vibration sensation was found in about 50 per cent of patients with cervical spine narrowing, but in none of those without radiological signs [111]. This cervical myelopathy may produce paraparesis with increased muscle tone which is particularly noticeable when trying to walk [118], or may produce proprioception abnormalities [119].

Functional assessment of balance

Sitting balance

An inability to maintain sitting balance means that standing balance is impossible. It is essential that the postural mechanisms do not adapt to an abnormal position. For instance, the patient who has been lying in bed or in a trip-back chair for long periods almost invariably develops a backward leaning posture on attempting to stand.

There are several approaches to maintaining sitting balance. For example, support can be provided, by pillows, and to prevent slipping forward on the chair the patient can either be placed in a low chair or the front part of the seat cushion can be raised. This tends to produce backward leaning or, if left too long, flexion contractures, but it is helpful during periods when the patient is sitting passively. A tip-back chair is contraindicated if the patient is to become mobile.

Bracing or posture controllers come in several forms. Specially formed casts, made by an orthotics department to fit to the exact shape of the patient's body, provide optimal support. Though these are very useful for the severely disabled, they passively maintain position and prevent movement. More satisfactory is a vacuum-pack posture controller (see Chapter 3). This oblong bag contains small polystyrene beads which can be formed around the patient and 'set' by extracting the air with a vacuum pump. The advantage of this is that the position of the patient can be changed at regular intervals simply by reinflating the pack, repositioning the patient and then 'resetting' the pack.

A full-length mirror or a video system may be used to provide visual feedback about sitting positions.

Balance on standing

Several forms of imbalance may be seen when patients stand from a chair. In one form the patient is unable to stand without clutching on to furniture or a frame. This, which may be due to muscle weakness, arthritis or a neurological deficit, can largely be overcome by ensuring that the chair is of the right height to allow easy transfer of the centre of force over the feet. This usually means that the seat is at a height which allows the knees to be at right-angles and the feet to touch the floor. The seat should be horizontal or only a slight slope backwards, the cushion firm, the back of the chair near vertical and the arms of the appropriate height to provide easy leverage.

A further trend is for patients to lean backwards on standing. They grip the arms of the chair and move their feet forwards, producing a backward lean. There is also a tendency to this backwards lean when walking, which may be due to maladjustment of the 'posturostat' or be associated with a fear of open space. One way to overcome this is to provide a low table or bed in front of the chair so that the patient can stand by first leaning forwards on to this support. This does seem to be effective for a number of patients, partly by ensuring that the centre of force is placed over the feet, partly by providing a supportive surface to push against, and partly by breaking up the open space in front of the patient.

Standing balance

Many patients, although standing safely, do so with the feet apart to extend the base area. With the feet together, or with the eyes closed, sway increases and the patient feels insecure. This probably indicates that compensation is taking place under normal conditions but that the patient cannot respond to abnormal situations. A search for sensory and vestibular dysfunction is essential, as well as ensuring that there is optimal use of vision. It is essential that the eyes are protected from further damage by checking for, and treating if necessary, eye disorders such as diabetic retinopathy and glaucoma.

Displacement response is assessed by lightly pushing on the sternum. Normally there is only a slight increase in sway but the patient feels stable. Some patients take a step backwards, indicating that there is a slowing down of the response mechanism but that compensation is enough to prevent falling. A more serious situation is indicated if the patient produces a startle reflex with the arms and fingers extending in an attempt to correct the balance; there is no stepping backwards and the patient may fall if not supported. These patients invariably walk with a staggering, small-step gait and are easily displaced, especially on turning. In spite of this they may cope at home because of easy access to hand holds on furniture. Management of these patients includes building up muscle strength in the legs, retraining balance (see below) and making the environment as safe as possible.

Management of patients with static balance problems is designed to improve proprioceptive information.

Increasing sensory feedback

The exercises suggested by Cooksey [120] and Cawthorne [121] forty years ago are still applicable. These exercises encourage a whole range of movements of the eyes, neck, shoulders and arms. A ball may be used, in both individual and group exercises, to improve reaction time as well as range of movement. For instance, a ball can be thrown from one hand to the other with the arms held above the head, or it can be passed backwards and forwards under the knees.

Another approach is to stand the patient in a standing frame so that he or she is supported in a three-point splint at the chest, buttocks and knees. Various exercises can be carried out, such as table activities, catching and throwing a ball or punching a balloon suspended from the ceiling – or any activity which involves changing the position of the centre of gravity of the patient.

One particularly useful modification of the standing frame is the Flexistand Major (Fig. 3.2 in Chapter 3) which allows not only three-point splinting but also controlled movement backwards and forwards and/or sideways. The amount of flexion can be controlled by a locking mechanism in the base of the stand.

Biofeedback

Newer approaches include providing biofeedback of sway which is translated from a balanced foot plate and displayed on a television set; or using light goniometry feedback [122]. These pieces of sophisticated equipment are becoming more readily available to general rehabilitation units.

A simpler method of providing feedback is to stand the patient in front of a mirror so that he observes his poor posture. This is of limited help in brain-damaged patients because the reversal of the image requires more concentration than the patient has available. An indirect method of providing feedback is to video-record the gait and balance disturbance and play the recording back so that the patient can see his mistakes [123].

It is important to observe the patient manoeuvring around objects or turning. Several abnormalities can occur, including an inability to initiate the turning as with the stammering gait or parkinsonism, a sudden loss of balance or a startle-type reflex. These are dealt with in Chapter 16.

Walking

Difficulty in initiating the movement

Apraxia, the inability to perform purposive movement on request in the presence of intact motor function, can be demonstrated by the observed action being carried out spontaneously on another occasion. This may present as a specific gait abnormality.

Wright [124] has graphically described the 'stammering gait' in which the patient stands with a broad base and the feet seem to stick to the ground, although when the patient is examined lying down leg function seems quite normal. There may be great difficulty in initiating the first steps, and then only a few stiff, shuffling steps are made before he stops again. Once the patient is walking the gait can sometimes be maintained until it is necessary to change direction or move on to a different surface. There are usually other signs of cerebral dysfunction, such as brisk reflexes, increase in muscle tone, speech disturbances and mental lethargy. In spite of these difficulties the patient often has little difficulty in climbing stairs. This had led to the technique of training the patient to start walking on the spot in exaggerated stepping fashion, as if climbing stairs, before starting to walk. Often if the attendant places her foot in front of the patient and tells him to step over it then walking can be initiated. This is a useful technique to teach relatives.

Wright has adapted the walking frame by attaching flexible strips low down on the rear legs of the frame: the patient then steps over the strip into the frame, thus initiating the walking pattern. One difficulty is that the frame itself prevents a smooth walking gait, and it is much better to use a frame which has wheels on the front legs to help maintain a smooth alternating gait.

Unfortunately these techniques do not have a carry-over effect and the condition rarely improves even after an intensive rehabilitation programme. Wright, however, does point out that if the stammering gait is associated with parkinsonism or cervical spondylosis then treatment of these may result in an improvement of the 'stammering' part of the gait.

Shuffling gait

Although the shuffling gait is classically seen in parkinsonism, it is not uncommonly found in cerebrovascular disease. Patients are generally unsteady and walk as though on ice, with short, low steps. Management should include exercises to strengthen muscles and increase step length, probably by the use of a treadmill or static bicycle.

Ataxic gait

Sensory ataxia occurs in a number of disorders. Diabetes mellitus is associated with a neuropathy and probably contributes to the high incidence of balance disorders in this condition. Pernicious anaemia may present with unsteadiness or dragging of the feet [125, 126], although the elderly do not necessarily present with either the anaemia or the paraesthesia. In fact it seems rare for subacute combined degeneration of the cord to be present when the pernicious anaemia is severe [127].

Ataxia is quite often very difficult to manage in the elderly. It is usually associated with motor weakness, and so it is logical to attempt to increase muscle strength by the appropriate exercises. The programme requires retraining of joint movement, initially passively, to increase proprioceptive input. Usually the patient eventually becomes dependent on a wheelchair for mobility. There have been reports of improvement in ataxic gait from fastening lead weights (about 60 g) around the ankles and on the thigh suspended by straps from a waistband [128]. In addition larger weights (about 120 g) were placed in slots on the waistband. The weights produced gait improvement in 11 of 14 patients, six being considered as good. The optimal position of the weights varied from patient to patient and it was not possible to correlate the position with the degree of apraxia. Frames are of limited value but some help can be achieved using a wheeled frame [129].

Similar success has been achieved on control of ataxic tremor of the hands by weighting the wrists [128, 130, 131].

Complications

The most obvious complication from falls is injury, especially serious injury such as fracture of the hip, wrist or skull. These are remarkably uncommon [12, 34, 132, 133] and are not directly associated with the number of falls. Indeed, it seem that fracture off the femur is more likely to occur on the first rather than later falls [134].

Rehabilitation approaches

General principles

The rehabilitation programme depends on the cause of the falls, and as can be seen from the foregoing discussion these are legion. It is necessary to assess which activities are most commonly associated. For instance, if the falls occur when getting out of bed or up from a chair, investigation of the environment may well show that the bed or chair is too low. Management is then to alter the environment rather than introduce specific techniques of patient treatment. Obviously in this situation further investigation for postural hypotension would also be necessary.

There are two types of faller, those who are frightened to stand and those who are careless, overconfident and dangerous. The first requires reassurance and careful support since a further fall under supervision tends to destroy confidence, making rehabilitation very difficult. The overconfident person is just as difficult and requires persuasion that he should seek assistance prior to walking. The problem then is to avoid inhibiting the determination so necessary to overcome balance disorders. Some of these patients show evidence of perceptual disorders and difficulty in recognizing their limitations even in the absence of more formal signs of a stroke.

It may first be necessary to help the patient to relax before starting the exercise programme. This helps to reduce unwanted increase in muscle tone and to gain the confidence of the patient. It is essential to recognize that walking is a frightening experience for someone who falls frequently or who is very unsteady.

The general principle is to start off with a stable, broad base and gradually increase exercises through a combination of increasing the instability, and decreasing the size, of the base.

Sitting balance

A natural progression for training of balance is from neck to trunk to sitting, and only then standing. If the patient is unable to control stability of the neck then all other balance will be disturbed.

To improve sitting balance the patient sits upright on a bed or plinth with the feet on the floor with a broad base, the hands providing additional support (Fig. 15.1a). In the early stages it may be necessary to provide visual feedback by placing a mirror in front of the patient. The next stage is to remove the support provided by the arms

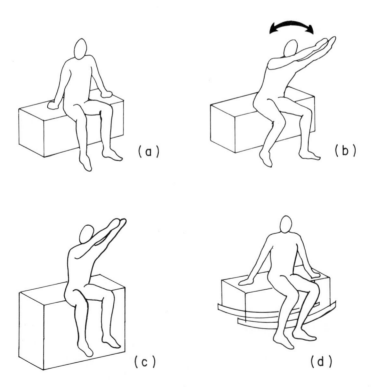

Fig. 15.1 Improving sitting balance: (a) stable surface, broad base; (b) stable surface, broad base but with movement; (c) stable surface, small base with movement; (d) unstable surface, broad base

(decreasing the base area) and gradually increase the amount of arm movement (increasing the instability) which shifts the centre of force and encourages corrective movements (Fig. 15.1b). The programme then progresses through raising the sitting base so that the feet are no longer supported on the floor (Fig. 15.1c), and further exercises to increase the displacing movements are carried out. These exercises follow the principle of decreasing the supporting base area whilst increasing movements which create instability. Once these activities can be carried out with the stable base then the exercises can be carried out using an unstable base. A satisfactory way of providing this is to use a rocking stool (Fig. 15.1d) – the rockers produce movement from side to side.

Standing up

Using a chair of the appropriate height, the patient slides forward to the front of the chair but keeps the heels below the front edge of the seat. By leaning forwards to bring the centre of gravity over the feet he then pushes up on the arms or seat of the chair. The habit of pulling up on the walking frame must be discouraged since this tends to topple over, causing a fall.

Sitting down

Many patients, especially those with parkinsonism, 'throw' themselves into chairs. The technique to overcome this is for the individual to stand with the back of the legs against the front of the chair, then to grasp the arms of the chair and lower himself down into it. If there are no arms on the chair then he should place the hands on the front edge of the seat or on his knees and lower himself into the sitting position in a controlled way.

Standing balance

A similar principle is used for training standing balance. If the patient is unable to stand still safely it is highly unlikely that he will be able to walk safely. The basic principles are for the patient to stand on a broad base (feet slightly apart) whilst standing at a table or a wall bar (Fig. 15.2a). If this is difficult to maintain then he may benefit from proprioceptive input by standing in a standing frame supported at the knees, buttocks and chest (see Chapter 3).

Dynamic standing balance is improved by providing exercises which allow the feet to remain in the same position but which encourage the amount of sway by means of table activities like playing card games or

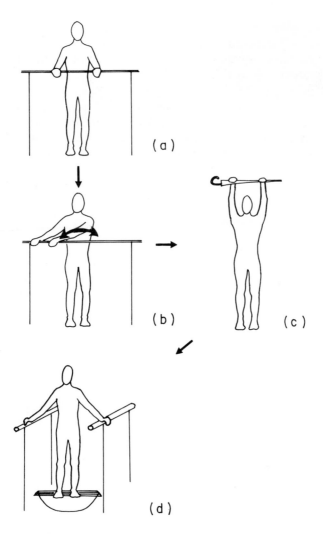

Fig. 15.2 Standing balance: (a) stable surface, broad base static; (b) stable surface, broad base with movement; (c) stable surface, small base with movement; (d) unstable surface, broad support

placing a plastic skittle into rings which are widely spaced on the able (Fig. 15.3). Other possible activities include playing games attached to the wall, such as solitaire (Fig. 15.4) or OXO. These allows later and stretching activities whilst adding interest and competition. Similar movement can be achieved by holding a stick or a towel above the head and moving the object from side to side (Fig. 15.2c). Some additional proprioceptive feedback can be provided using the Flexistand

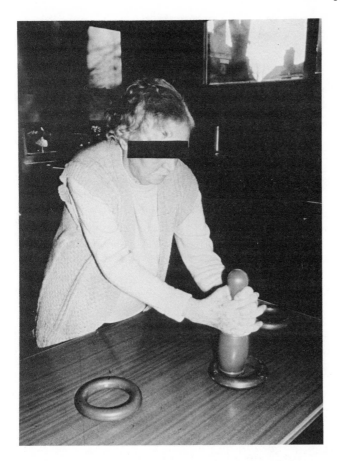

Fig. 15.3 Table activities to improve balance

standing frame (see Chapter 3); this provides support of the patient at the knees, buttocks and chest and can be moved in a lateral or antero-posterior direction.

When balance is good at this level then the base can be made unstable by standing on a rocking block or 'Wobble' board (Fig. 15.2d).

Backward leaners

A number of patients tend to lean backwards when standing, usually after long-term bed rest or a long time in tip-back chairs. This will be discussed further in Chapter 16. Early training includes standing the patient at the side of the bed leaning forwards on a number of pillows. This theoretically assists the 'posturostat' to realign in the erect

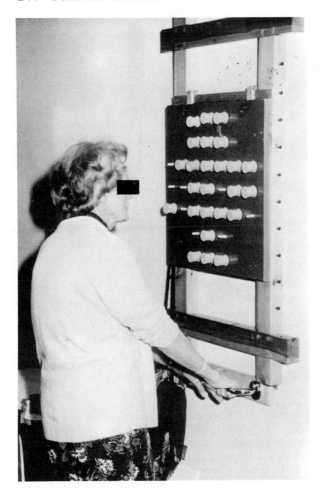

Fig. 15.4   Wall Solitaire to improve balance

position. There is no evidence that this is what happens, but in practice the technique does seem to be effective for some patients. Similarly the patient can be stood in the Flexistand frame, with the supporting frame set leaning forwards.

Falling and rising techniques

Patients should be taught to fall safely. In this they have first to be taught that if they are feeling dizzy they should reach for a stable support since, many injuries are caused by leaning on unstable furniture. If a fall is unavoidable, less damage is likely to be caused if the patient flexes like a parachutist on landing. This advice is rarely

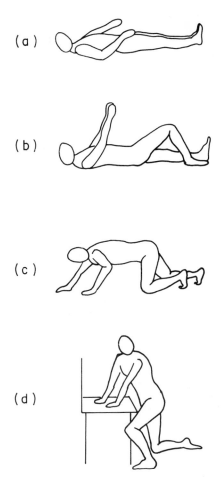

(a)

(b)

(c)

(d)

Fig. 15.5 Getting up from the floor after a fall

heeded since the fall produces a panic state, with resultant extension of arms, legs and neck. The patient should, however, be taught that once on the ground they should not panic but relax and plan how to get up.

Many patients find getting up from the floor very difficult. Part of this is due to difficulty in turning over or sitting up. If the patient is lying on his back then he can be taught to stretch out his arms in front of him, cross his legs, and rock the outstretched arms from side to side until he is able to roll over (Figs. 15.5a and b). Once he is prone the aim is to get on to the hands and knees and then crawl to a raised surface such as a chair, stool, sofa or bed (Fig. 15.5c). Using this sur- face as a lever he stands by supporting himself with the hands, bending one knee so that the foot is on the ground, and pushing himself up by pressing down with the arms and the leg (Fig. 15.5d).

If the patient is unable to get on to hands and knees he may be able to get into a sitting position and shuffle to a chair or sofa to pull himself up. An alternative is to move to the bottom of the stairs and sit on each step in turn until he is in a position to stand or pull on the hand rail. The patient must be strongly warned against trying to pull himself up on a frame, a low fragile table or an unstable chair since these easily topple over.

Where falls are frequent then a blanket and a pillow should be placed in a convenient place (e.g. under a chair) so that, if he does fall, he can keep warm until help arrives.

Attracting attention

There are a number of devices by which someone who has fallen can draw attention. These fall basically into two categories:

- Alarm systems (lights, which may or may not flash, or buzzers, sirens and bells). One system lights up a sign which says 'Help, please contact police'. These have the disadvanatage that they may attract the wrong form of attention and alert burglars to a vulnerable situation. For this reason it is more satisfactory if they are linked directly to a neighbour's house.
- Telephone links to either a relative or a 24-hour monitoring service. One social service department has instituted a system whereby radio-link home helps can be called to the home of a person who has fallen following the setting off of the alarm [135].

One of the problems is to ensure that the patient knows how to set off the alarm. There are a number of approaches to this. Some alarm systems require the patient to reach a switch or touch panel, which may not always be possible, and require a number of switches to be placed at strategic places around the home. Others set off an alarm if certain activities, such as going to the toilet or leaving the bedroom, are not carried out during a specified time period. This is achieved by fitting pressure mats at the appropriate doors.

There are also devices which the elderly person can wear around the neck as a pendant or on the wrist like a watch. These are radio-linked to a receiver which can, via the telephone, alert either specified supervisory services or relatives and friends. If there is no response from the first person contacted then the transmitter automatically contacts other telephone numbers until a reply is received.

It is essential that the patient be trained in the correct use of the alarm and that he is prepared to use it when required; and probably just as important, avoids using it unnecessarily.

Training the carer

Carers should be trained to assist the fallen patient correctly – to avoid damage to the patient and to avoid damage to the carer. One useful technique is for the carer to manipulate the patient into a sitting position and get him to clasp his hands together; the carer crouches behind him, puts her hands under his axillae and grips his forearms, and then stands, with back straight, bringing the patient to the upright position. This is protective for the attendant and is a safe method of standing. Another approach is to help the patient to get on to his hands and knees and then to lean on a chair and help him to push himself up.

Environmental control

Droller [2] pointed out that in addition to 'the liability to fall' there needs to be 'an opportunity to fall'. Therefore it is important to consider the environment in which the patient has to live. The common things to look for are loose rugs, worn and torn carpets (especially those with curled edges), draught bars across doorways, slippery surfaces and the absence of sufficient hand rails in passages and on stairs, or the presence of unstable supports used by the patient. The edges of steps should be clearly marked (for example by painting them white), especially when vision is poor.

Every opportunity should be provided for ease of movement. For instance, many patients have difficulty in getting out of a low chair and therefore have to 'throw' themselves out. This can be overcome by ensuring that the chair is at a height whereby the knees are at right-angles when sitting. This is just as applicable to bed and toilet seat height. The energy required to lift the body weight so that the buttocks rise above the level of the knees is quite large and this can be decreased by having chairs of the appropriate height. In addition, arms on the chair help with leverage. The use of spring-loaded seats should be discouraged for patients who are unable to rapidly correct changes in position. More useful are chairs which raise the height of the seat slowly and vertically rather than by tipping forwards.

Since many falls occur when stopping or bending, simple techniques are required to avoid these manoeuvres: for instance, a 'helping hand' extension grip to pick up objects; switches, plugs and heater switches raised to hip height; a cage on the letter box to collect the mail before it falls to the floor; and long-handled milk bottle containers to avoid bending. For dressing, stocking aids and long-handled shoe horns help to avoid the need to stoop. For those who fall frequently the telephone should be placed on a low table so that it can be reached from the floor in order to call for assistance.

It is easy to forget to examine the patient's footwear. Shoes or slippers should be well-fitting since loose slippers are a common cause of falls [28]. The soles should be smooth enough to allow easy walking without being too smooth to cause slipping. The latter is important since elderly people do seem to have a fear of slipping. This even applies to the type of surface on which they walk, since gait speed and step length are greater on carpeted floors than on a vinyl surface [136].

High-heeled shoes result in a smaller surface area in contact with the ground and also produce a less stable support. Flat shoes provide a firmer base, though some account should be taken of the patient's preference. It has been suggested that proprioceptive feedback adapts to the plantar flexion of the high-heeled position over the years and that reverting to flat shoes results in misinterpretation of feedback, with the effect that the brain interprets the flatter heel contact as implying that the patient is leaning backwards. This is a highly questionnable theory, but when balance depends on every bit of information available even a slight misinterpretation may be important.

Whilst considering footwear it is important to assess for unequal leg length. This more important when it has occurred recently, such as following fracture of the femur, rather than in chronic or congenital shortening. Whether the patient will benefit from a shoe raiser can easily be assessed by providing a temporary strap-on shoe raiser [137]. For very mild shortening, asking the patient to walk wearing a shoe on the affected side but not on the normal side can provide a quick assessment of the effect of a shoe raiser.

Confidence

It is not surprising that falls result in a loss of confidence. This further reduces the mobility of the patient, and a vicious circle is set up of inactivity, increasing weakness, more falls and a further loss of confidence. It is therefore important to break this circle. Admission to hospital may be necessary, but many patients can be managed in the day hospital or by domiciliary physiotherapy. The important point is to control as many factors leading to the falls as possible and to start strengthening and balance exercises. It is also important for the carers to recognize the importance of encouragement rather than 'protecting' the individual by discouraging activity.

References

1. Andrews, K. (1986) The relevance of readmission to hospital. *Journal of the American Geriatrics Society.* **34**: 5–11.

2. Droller, H. (1955) Falls among elderly people living at home. *Geriatrics* **10**: 239–44.
3. Sheldon, J.H. (1948) *The Social Medicine of Old Age.* Oxford University Press, London.
4. Rodstein, M. (1964) Accidents among the aged: incidence, causes and prevention. *Journal of Chronic Disease* **17**: 515–26.
5. Lucht, U. (1971) A prospective study of accidental falls and resulting injuries in the home among elderly people. *Acta Socio-Medica Scandinavica* **2**: 105–20.
6. Prudham, D. and Evans, J.G. (1981) Factors associated with falls in the elderly: a community study. *Age and Ageing* **10**: 141–6.
7. Waller, J.A. (1974) Injury in the aged: clinical and epidemiological implications. *New York State Journal of Medicine* **74**: 2200–8.
8. Wild, D., Nyak, U.S.L. and Isaacs, B. (1981) How dangerous are falls in old people? *British Medical Journal* **282**: 266–8.
9. Exton-Smith, A.N. (1977) Functional consequences of ageing: clinical manifestations. In: *Care of the Elderly: Meeting the Challenge of Dependency*, pp. 41–7 (Ed: Exton-Smith, A.N. and Evans, J.G.). Academic Press, London.
10. MacQueen, I.A. (1960) *Home Accidents in Aberdeen.* Churchill Livingstone, London.
11. Knowelden, J., Buhr, A.J. and Dunbar, O. (1964) Incidence of fractures in persons over 35 years of age. *British Journal of Preventive and Social Medicine* **18**: 130–41.
12. Gryfe, C.A., Amies, A. and Ashley, M.J. (1977) A longitudinal study of falls in an elderly population. I: Incidence and morbidity. *Age and Ageing* **6**: 201–10.
13. Stevens, D.L. and Matthews, W.B. (1973) Cryptogenic drop attacks: an affliction of women. *British Medical Journal* i: 439–42.
14. Brocklehurst, J.C., Exton-Smith, A.N., Lempert Barber, S.M. *et al.* (1978) Fracture of the femur in old age: a two centre study of associated clinical factors and the cause of fall. *Age and Ageing* **7**: 7–15.
15. Chapman, A.L. (1961) Accidents in the aged. In: *Accident Prevention* (Ed: Halsley, M.N.). MacGraw-Hill, New York.
16. Backett, E.M. (1965) *Domestic Accidents.* WHO, Geneva.
17. Berfenstam, R.D., Lagerberg, D. and Smedby, B. (1969) Victim characteristics of home accidents. *Acta Socio-Medica Scandinavica* **1**: 145–64.
18. Ashley, M.J., Gryfe, C.I. and Amies, A. (1977) A longitudinal study of falls in an elderly population. II: Some circumstances of falling. *Age and Ageing* **6**: 211–20.
19. Naylor, M.B. and Rosin, A.S. (1970) Falling as a cause of admission to a geriatric unit. *Practitioner* **205**: 327–30.
20. Evans, J.G., Prudham, D. and Wandless, I. (1979) A prospective study of fractured proximal femur. *Public Health* **93**: 235–41.
21. Agate, J. (1966) Accidents to old people in their homes. *British Medical Journal* ii: 785–8.
22. Waller, J.A. (1978) Falls among the elderly – human and environmental factors. *Accident Annual Review* **10**: 21–33.
23. Gray, B. (1966) *Home Accidents Among Older People.* Royal Society for the Prevention of Accidents, London.
24. Morfitt, J.M. (1983) Falls in old people at home: intrinsic versus environmental factors in causation. *Public Health (London)* **97**: 115–20.
25. Manning, D.P. (1983) Deaths and injuries caused by slipping, tripping and falling. *Ergonomics* **26**: 3–9.
26. Alessi, D., Brill, M. *et al.* (1978) *Home Safety Guidelines for Architects and Builders.* National Bureau of Standards NBS-GCR 78-156, Washington, DC.

27. Archea, J.C., Collins, B.L. and Stahl, F.I. (1979) *Guidelines for Stair Safety.* National Bureau of Standards NBS-BSS 120. Washington, DC.
28. Svanstrom, L. (1974) Falls on stairs: an epidemiological accident survey. *Scandinavian Journal of Social Medicine* 2: 113–20.
29. Maki, B. and Fernie, G.R. (1983) *Biomechanical Assessment of Handrail Parameters with Special Consideration for the Needs of Elderly Users.* Report prepared for National Research Council of Canada, Division of Electrical Engineering, Medical Engineering Section, Ottowa.
30. Armstrong, T., Chaffin, D.B., Miodonski, R., Stobbie, T. and Boydstuw, L. (1978) *An Ergonomic Basis for Recommendations Pertaining to Specific Sections of OSHA Standard 29CFR, Part 1910, Subpart D: Walking and Working Surfaces.* US Department of Labor, Occupational Safety & Health Administration, Washington, DC.
31. Manjam, N.V.B. and Mackinnon, H.H. (1973) Patient, bed and bathroom. *Nova Scotia Medical Bulletin* 52: 23–7.
32. Sehested, P. and Severin-Nielsen, T. (1977) Falls by hospitalized elderly patients: causes and prevention. *Geriatrics*, April: 101–8.
33. Morris, E.V. and Isaacs, B. (1980) The prevention of falls in a geriatric hospital. *Age and Ageing* 9: 181–5.
34. Sheldon, J.H. (1960) On the natural history of falls in old age. *British Medical Journal* ii: 1685–90.
35. Isaacs, B. (1978) Are falls a manifestation of brain failure? *Age and Ageing* 7 (Suppl): 97–105.
36. Gabell, A., Simons, M.A. and Nyak, U.S.L. (1985) Falls in the healthy elderly: predisposing causes. *Ergonomics* 28: 965–75.
37. Broe, G.A., Akhtar, A.J. Andrews, G.R. *et al.* (1976) Neurological disorders in the elderly at home. *Journal of Neurology, Neurosurgery and Psychiatry* 39: 362–6.
38. Liversey, B. and Atkinson, L. (1974) Repeated falls in the elderly. *Modern Geriatrics* i: 40–7.
39. Henderson, J.M. (1975) The place of the electrocardiograph in the study of cardiovascular problems in the elderly. *Journal of the Royal College of General Practioners* 25: 451–3.
40. Goldberg, A.D., Raftery, E.B. and Cashman, P.M.M. (1975) Ambulatory electrocardiographic methods in patients with transient syncopal attacks or palpitations. *British Medical Journal* 4: 569–71.
41. Brown, A.K. and Anderson, V. (1980) The contribution of 24-hour ambulatory ECG monitoring in a general medical unit. *Journal of the Royal College of Physicians of London* 14: 7–12.
42. Abdon, N.J. (1981) Frequency and distribution of long-term ECG-recorded cardiac arrhythmias in an elderly population. *Acta Medica Scandinavica* 208: 73–6.
43. Gann, D., Fernandes, H. and Samet, P.L. (1979) Syncope and aortic stenosis: significance of conduction abnormalities. *European Journal of Cardiology* 9: 405–13.
44. Jackson, G., Mahon, W., Pierscianowski, T.A. and Condon, J. (1976) Inappropriate antihypertensive therapy in the elderly. *Lancet* ii: 1317–18.
45. Stout, R.W. (1978) Falls and disorders of postural balance. *Age and Ageing* 7: 134–6.
46. Hale, W.E., Stewart, R.B. and Marks, R.G. (1984) Central nervous system symptoms of elderly subjects using antihypertensive drugs. *Journal of the American Geriatrics Society* 32: 5–10.
47. MacDonald, J.B. and MacDonald, E.T. (1977) Nocturnal femoral fractures

and continuing widespread use of barbiturate hypnotics. *British Medical Journal* ii: 483–5.

48. Sloan, J. and Holloway, G. (1981) Fracture of the femur: the cause of the fall? *Injury* 13: 230–2.

49. Glassman, A.H., Bigger, J.T., Giardina, E.V. *et al.* (1979) Clinical characteristics of imipramine induced orthostatic hypotension. *Lancet* i: 468–72.

50. Campbell, A.J., Reinken, J., Allen, B.C. and Martinez, G.S. (1981) Falls in old age: a study of frequency and related factors. *Age and Ageing* 10: 264–70.

51. Baker, M.R. (1980) *The Epidemiology and Aetiology of Femoral Neck Fracture.* MD thesis, University of Newcastle upon Tyne.

52. Stegman, M.R. (1983) Falls among elderly hypertensives – are they iatrogenic? *Gerontology* 29: 399–406.

53. Rashiq, S. and Logan, R.F.A. (1986) Role of drugs in fractures of the femoral neck. *British Medical Journal* 292: 861–3.

54. Sheldon, J.H. (1963) The effect of age on the control of sway. *Gerontologia Clinica* 5: 129–38.

55. Hasselkus, B.R. and Shambes, G.M. (1975) Ageing and postural sway in women. *Journal of Gerontolgy* 30: 661–7.

56. Fernie, G.R. and Holliday, P.J. (1979) Postural sway in amputees. *Journal of Bone and Joint Surgery* 60A: 895–8.

57. Murray, M.P., Seireg, A.A. and Sepic, S.B. (1975) Normal postural stability and steadiness: quantitative assessment. *Journal of Bone and Joint Surgery* 57A: 510–16.

58. Bannermeister, M. (1964) The effect of body tilt on apparent verticality: apparent body position and their relation. *Journal of Experimental Psychology* 67: 142–53.

59. Overstall, P.W., Exton-Smith, A.N., Imms, F.J. and Johnson, A.L. (1977) Falls in the elderly related to postural imbalance. *British Medical Journal* i: 261–4.

60. Overstall, P.W., Johnson, A.L. and Exton-Smith, A.N. (1978) Instability and falls in the elderly. *Age and Ageing 7 (Suppl.)*: 92–6.

61. Imms, F.J. and Edholm, O.G. (1981) Studies of gait and mobility in the elderly. *Age and Ageing* 10: 147–56.

62. Guimaraes, R.M. and Isaacs, B. (1980) Studies of gait and balance in normal old people and in people who have fallen. *International Rehabilitation Medicine* 2: 177–80.

63. Dornan, J., Fernie, G.R. and Holliday, P.J. (1978) Visual input: its importance in the control of postural sway. *Archives of Physical Medicine and Rehabilitation* 59: 586–91.

64. Begbie, G.H. (1967) Some problems of postural sway. In: *Myotic, Kinaesthetic and Vestibular Mechanisms* (Eds: de Reuck, A.V.S. and Knight, J.). Churchill Livingstone, London.

65. Lee, D. and Lishman, R. (1975) Vision in movement and balance. *New Scientist* 65: 59.

66. Brocklehurst, J.C., Robertson, D. and James-Groom, P. (1982) Clinical correlation of sway in old age – sensory modalities. *Age and Ageing* 11: 1–10.

67. Weintraub, D.J., O'Connell, D.C. and McHale, T.J. (1964) Apparent verticality: fundamental variable of sensori-tonic theory reinvestigated. *Journal of Experimental Psychology* 68: 550–4.

68. O'Connell, D.C., Weintraunb, D.J., Lathop, R.G. and McHale, T.J. (1967) Apparent verticality: psychophysical error *v* sensory tonic theory. *Journal of Experimental Psychology* 73: 347–53.

69. Hulicka, I.M. and Beckenstein, B.S. (1961) Perception of verticality by

hemiplegic patients. *Archives of Physical Medicine and Rehabilitation* **42**: 192–200.

70. Tobis, J.S., Nyak, L. and Hochler, F. (1981) Visual perception of verticality and horizontality among elderly fallers. *Archives of Physical Medicine and Rehabilitation* **62**: 619–22.

71. Corso, J.F. (1971) Sensory processes and age effects in normal adults. *Journal of Gerontology* **26**: 90–105.

72. Levin, H.S. and Benton, A.L. (1973) Age effects of proprioceptive feedback performance. *Gerontologia Clinica* **15**: 161–9.

73. Eyseck, H.J. (1952) *The Scientific Study of Personality.* Routledge and Kegan Paul, London.

74. Ingham, J.G. (1954) Body sway suggestibility and neurosis. *Journal of Mental Science* **100**: 247–53.

75. Rasch, P.J. and Burke, R.K. (1978) *Kinesiology and Applied Anatomy: The Source of Human Movement.* Lea and Febiger, Philadelphia.

76. Eberhardt, H.P. (1976) In: *Neural Control of Locomotion* (Ed: Herman, R.M. *et al*,. Plenum Press, New York.

77. Drachman, D.A. and Hart, C.W. (1972) An approach to the dizzy patient. *Neurology* **22**: 323–34.

78. Orma, E.J. and Koskenoja, M. (1957) Postural dizziness in the aged. *Geriatrics* **12**: 49–59.

79. Tanja, T.A., Hofman, A. and Valkenburg, H.A.C. (1979) Een epidemiologisch onderzoek onder bejaarden. II: Duizeligheid bij bejaarden, mogelijko oorzaken en gevolgen. *Nederlasndsch Tijdschrift voor Gerontologie* **10**: 195–201.

80. Droller, H. and Pemberton, J. (1953) Vertigo in a random sample of elderly people living at home. *Journal of Laryngology and Otology* **67**: 689–94.

81. Agate, J. (1983) *The Practice of Geriatrics.* Heinemann, London.

82. Dix, M.R. (1973) Vertigo. *The Practitioner* **211**: 295–303.

83. Schuknecht, H.F. and Kitamura, K. (1981) Vestibular neuritis. *Annals of Otology, Rhinology and Laryngology* **90** (Suppl. 78): 1–19.

84. Loeb, C. and Meyer, J.S. (1965) *Strokes Due to Vertebrobasilar Disease.* Thomas, Springfield, Illinois.

85. Fisher, C.M. (1970) Occlusion of the vertebral arteries causing transient basilar symptoms. *Archives of Neurology* **22**: 13–19.

86. Davis, D. (1953) A common type of vertigo relieved by traction of the cervical spine. *Annals of Internal Medicine* **38**: 778–86.

87. Stark, R.J. and Wodak, J. (1983) Primary orthostatic cerebral ischaemia. *Journal of Neurology, Neurosurgery and Psychiatry* **46**: 883–91.

88. Rodstein, M. and Zeldman, F.D. (1957) Postural blood pressure changes in the elderly. *Journal of Chronic Disease* **6**: 581–8.

89. Caird, F.I., Andrews, G.R. and Kennedy, R.D. (1973) Effect of posture on blood pressure in the elderly. *British Heart Journal* **35**: 527–30.

90. Johnson, R.H., Smith, A.C., Spalding, J.M.K. and Wollner, L. (1965) Effect of posture on blood pressure in elderly patients. *Lancet*: 731–3.

91. Barraclough, M.A. and Sharpley-Schafer, E.P. (1963) Hypotension from circulatory reflexes. *Lancet* i: 1121–6.

92. Birchfield, R.I. (1964) Postural hypotension in Wernicke's disease. *American Journal of Medicine* **36**: 404–14.

93. Paulley, J.W. (1965) Posture and blood pressure in the elderly. *Lancet* i: 1076–7.

94. Bannister, R., Ardill, L. and Fentem, P. (1969) An assessment of various methods of treatment of orthostatic hypotension. *Quarterly Journal of Medicine* **38**: 377–95.

95. Schirger, A., Sheps, S.G., Thomas, J.E. and Fealey, R.D. (1981) Midodrine: a

new agent in the management of orthostatic hypotension and Shy–Drager syndrome. *Mayo Clinic Proceedings* **56**: 429–33.

96. Fouad, F.M., Tarazi, R.C. and Bravo, E.L. (1981) Dihydroergotamine in idiopathic orthostatic hypotension: a short term intramuscular and long term oral therapy. *Clinical Pharamacology and Therapeutics* **30**: 782–9.

97. Bevegard, S., Castenfors, J. and Lindblad, L.E. (1974) Haemodynamic effects of dihydroergotamine in patients with postural hypotension. *Acta Medica Scandinavica* **196**: 473–7.

98. Jennings, G., Esler, M. and Holmes, R. (1979) Treatment of orthostatic hypotension with dihydroergotamine. *British Medical Journal* **2**: 307.

99. Abate, G., Polimeni, R.M., Cuccurullo, F. *et al.* (1979) Effects of indomethacin on postural hypotension in Parkinsonism. *British Medical Journal* **2**: 1466–8.

100. Watt, S.J., Troke, J.E., Perkins, C.M. and Lee, M.R. (1981) The treatment of idiopathic orthostatic hypotension: a combined fludrocortisone and flubiprofen regime. *Quarterly Journal of Medicine* **50**: 205–12.

101. Davies, I.B., Bannister, R. and Mathias, C. (1981) Pindolol in postural hypotension: a case for caution. *Lancet* **2**: 982–3.

102. Goldstraw, P. and Waller, D.G. (1981) Pindolol on orthostatic hypotension. *British Medical Journal* **283**: 310.

103. Kremer, M. (1958) Sitting, standing and walking. *British Medical Journal* **ii**: 63–8.

104. Lund, M. (1963) *Drop attacks in association in Parkinsonism and basilar artery sclerosis. Acta Neurological Scandinavica* **39 (Suppl. 4)**: 226–9.

105. Kubala, M.J. and Millikan, C.H. (1964) Diagnosis, pathogenesis and treatment of 'drop attacks'. *Archives of Neurology* **ii**: 107–13.

106. Gordon, M. (1978) Occult cardiac arrhythmias associated with falls and dizziness in the elderly: detection by Holter monitoring. *Journal of the American Geriatrics Society* **26**: 418–23.

107. Overstall, P.W. (1978) Falls in the elderly. In: *Recent Advances in Geriatric Medicine*, p. 65 (Ed: Isaacs, B). Churchill Livingstone, Edinburgh.

108. Sheehan, S., Bauber, R.B. and Meyer, J.S. (1960) Vertebral artery compression in cervical spondylosis: arteriographic demonstration during life of vertebral artery insufficiency due to rotation and extension of the neck. *Neurology* **10**: 968–86.

109. Williams, D. and Wilson, T.G. (1962) The diagnosis of major and minor syndrome of basilar insufficiency. *Brain* **85**: 741–74.

110. Kameyama, M. (1965) Vertigo and drop attacks: with special reference to cerebrovascular disorders and atherosclerosis of the vertebro-basilar system. *Geriatrics* **20**: 892–900.

111. Pallis, C.A., Jones, A.M. and Spillane, J.D. (1954) Cervical spondylosis. *Brain* **77**: 274–89.

112. Adams, K.R.H., Yung, M.W., Lye, M. and Whitehouse, G.H. (1986) Are cervical spine radiographs of value in elderly patients with verebrobasilar insufficiency? *Age and Ageing* **15**: 57–9.

113. Wyke, B.D. (1979) Cervical articular contributions to posture and gait: their relation to senile disequilibrium. *Age and Ageing* **8**: 251–8.

114. Sudarsky, L. and Ronthal, M. (1983) Gait disorders among elderly patients. *Archives of Neurology* **40**: 740–3.

115. Arnold, N. and Harriman, D.G. (1970) The incidence of abnormality in control of human peripheral nerves, studied by single axon dissection. *Journal of Neurology, Neurosurgery and Psychiatry* **33**: 55–61.

116. De Jong, P.T.V.M., De Jong, J.M.B.V., Cohen, B. and Jongkees, L.B.W. (1977) Ataxia and nystagmus induced by injection of local anaesthetics in the

neck. *Annals of Neurology* **1**: 240–6.

117. Lacour, M., Roll, J.R. and Appaix, M. (1976) Modifications and development of spinal reflexes in the alert baboon following an unilateral vestibular neurotomy. *Brain Research* **113**: 255–69.

118. Clarke, E. and Robinson, P.K. (1956) Cervical myelopathy: a complication of cervical spondylosis. *Brain* **79**: 483–510.

119. Yuhl, E.T., Hanna, D., Rasmussen, T. and Richter, R.B. (1955) Diagnosis and surgical therapy of chronic midline cervical disc protrusion. *Neurology* **5**: 494–509.

120. Cooksey, F.S. (1945) Rehabilitation of vestibular injuries. *Proceedings of the Royal Society of Medicine* **39**: 273–8.

121. Cawthorne, T.E. (1945) Vestibular injuries. *Proceedings of the Royal Society of Medicine* **39**: 270–3.

122. Mitchelson, D.L. (1978) Instrumented movement analysis as a means of motor function assessment and therapy. In: *Baclofen: Spasticity and Cerebral Pathology* (Ed: Jukes, A.M.). Cambridge Medical Publications, Northampton.

123. Van Gestel, A.P.M. (1971) Television and video-recorder in therapeutic exercise. *Scandinavian Journal of Rehabilitation Medicine* **3**: 79–85.

124. Wright, W.B. (1979) Stammering gait. *Age and Ageing* **8**: 8–12.

125. Cox-Klazinga, M. and Endtz, L.J. (1980) Peripheral nerve involvement in pernicious anaemia. *Journal of Neurological Sciences* **43**: 367–71.

126. Roach, E.S. and McLean, W.T. (1982) Neurological disorders of vitamin B_{12} deficiency. *American Family Physician* **25**: 111–15.

127. Matthews, D.M. and Wilson, J. (1971) Cobalamins and cyanide metabolism in neurological diseases. In: *Cobalamins and Cyanide Metabolism in Neurological Disease* (Ed: H.R.V. Arnstein, H.R.V. and Wrighton, R.J.). Churchill Livingstone, Edinburgh.

128. Morgan, M.H. (1975) Ataxia and weights. *Physiotherapy* **61**: 332–4.

129. Morgan, M.H. (1980) Ataxia – its causes, measurement, and management. *International Rehabilitation Medicine* **2**: 126–32.

130. Hewer, R.L., Cooper, R. and Morgan, M.H. (1972) An investigation into the value of treating intention tremor by weighting the affected limbs. *Brain* **95**: 579–90.

131. Morgan, M.H., Hewer, R.L. and Cooper, R. (1975) Application of an objective method of assessing intention tremor – a further study on the use of weights to reduce intention tremor. *Journal of Neurology, Neurosurgery and Pyschiatry* **38**: 259–64.

132. Iskrant, A.P. (1968) The aetiology of fractured hips in females. *American Journal of Public Health* **58**: 485–90.

133. Scott, C.J. (1976) Accidents in hospital with special reference to old people. *Health Bulletin* **18**: 330–5.

134. Evans, J.G., Prudham, D. and Wandless, I. (1979) A prospective study of fractured proximal femur: factors predisposing to survival. *Age and Ageing* **8**: 246–50.

135. Stockport Social Service Department (1979) *Mobile Alarm System for Home Emergencies.* Stockport SSD Cheshire, England.

136. Willmott, M. (1986) The effect of a vinyl floor surface and a carpeted floor surface upon walking in elderly hospital in-patients. *Age and Ageing* **15**: 119–20.

137. Squires, A. and Morris, M. (1984) Temporary shoe raise. *Physiotherapy* **70**: 466.

16

Parkinson's disease

Epidemiology and clinical features

The prevalence of Parkinson's disease increases with advancing age [1–6 and Table 16.1], although some have shown a decrease after the age of 80 years [7, 8]. Some of these studies were carried out in the 1960s, since when there has been a dramatic change in the survival of patients with the disease, especially for the very elderly [9].

It is important to recognize drug-induced parkinsonism in the elderly [10], especially that due to phenothiazines and butyrophones. The parkinsonian symptoms produced by these drugs may persist for up to two years, while others who initially improve when the drug is discontinued eventually develop Parkinson's disease [11], suggesting that the drugs were exacerbating the preclinical form of the disease.

The commonest symptoms of Parkinson's disease (12) are slowness in walking or dressing, getting out of a chair or turning over in bed [12]. Moderate to severe dysfunction, based on the Webster Scale [13] for rigidity, bradykinesia and gait disturbances, was found in about 50 per cent of patients.

Table 16.1 The prevalence of Parkinson's disease

Age range	USA: Kurland (1958) [1]	UK: Brewis (1966) [7]	Iceland: Gudmundson (1967) [8]	Australia: Jenkins (1966) [2]	Finland: Marttila (1976) [5]	Sweden: Broman (1963) [4]	UK: Mutch (1986) [6]
40–49	–	1.4	0.6	0.3	0.2	0.2	0.5
50–59	2.4	1.6	1.6	1.7	1.2	0.9	0.8
60–69	7.6	3.2	9.4	3.0	5.0	2.0	2.5
70–79	–	6.1	15.8	–	8.0	5.1	8.4
70	–	–	–	9.2	–	–	–
70–84	14.1	–	–	–	–	–	–
80–89	–	–	13.1	–	5.9	–	–
80	–	4.4	–	–	–	4.5	19.2
85	26.5	–	–	–	–	–	–
90–99	–	–	4.0	–	–	–	–

The value of rehabilitation

There is little scientific evidence as to the value of rehabilitation, partly owing to the difficulty in deciding how much of the effect is due to drug therapy and how much to the rehabilitation programme, as well as the difficulties of measuring improvement in a condition which varies in its rate of deterioration.

Most rehabilitation research into parkinsonism has studied small numbers of patients and has often tried to complete complex crossover studies or trials of two (or more) different approaches. Franklyn *et al.* [14] studied three groups of parkinsonian patients (5–8 in each group) who had a wide range of severity and compared group treatment twice weekly for ten weeks with individual treatment twice weekly for eight weeks; the latter group was also subdivided into physiotheraphy given at home or in hospital. Ten showed modest improvement, seven of whom retained the improvement for up to five weeks following the rehabilitation programme.

Another small study allocated 28 patients with Parkinson's disease into two study groups [15]. In one study the gait of 14 patients was assessed by polarized light goniometry. Seven of these patients were treated for three to eight weeks, the others acting as controls. Five of the treated group completed the study, three returned subjectively and objectively to a normal walking pattern, while there was no change in the control group. In the second part of the study seven patients, including three from the control subgroup of the first study, were treated by physiotherapy twice a week for three weeks and shown exercises to continue at home. Five of these patients developed a normal walking pattern.

In another study of patients randomly allocated in a crossover design study [16], six patients were given 'active' treatment (a neurophysiological rehabilitation programme), while 11 were included in the control group which received infra-red therapy to the thorax and diversional activities. Four of the controls were eventually transferred to the treatment group and two of the treated patients to the control group. There was no statistical difference in outcome between the two groups – both showing some improvement. This study has many difficulties. Apart from the small number of patients in each group, this was really a study of two different rehabilitation approaches rather than treatment versus non-treatment. Heat treatment helps to decrease the rigidity and any activity, diversional or otherwise, can be expected to have some effect on the general ability of the patient. It is also questionnable whether a crossover study design is feasible in a learning process such as rehabilitation.

Franklyn, and Stern [17] pointed out some of the difficulties with their own study, such as making allowances for the spontaneous fluctuations in motor performance and mental state which are common in parkinsonism. They also found it difficult to assess the influence of depression and motivation. Transport to the outpatient department proved to be tiring and many patients became rigid in anticipation of having to attend the hospital.

These studies emphasize the great difficulty of rehabilitation research and can only give pointers to understanding the role of physical therapy in the management of the parkinsonian patient.

Management

Rigidity

The rigidity of Parkinson's disease differs from the increased tone of spasticity in that it is not always associated with increased reflexes, clonus or pathological plantar response. However, in the elderly both rigidity and spasticity may occur in the same patient.

The early symptom of muscle stiffness may only affect fine finger movement but later progresses to involve the neck and trunk. The flexor muscles become more hypertonic than the extensors, producing the classical parkinsonian posture. Rigidity also affects the facial muscles, producing a staring appearance with a mask-like expression. The general increase in tone produces difficulty in rapid spontaneous changes and results in difficulty in carrying out activities such as turning over in bed. Even minor acts require a large amount of concentration and planning. Patients often feel tired and distraction limits the ability to carry out activities. Rigidity of the neck muscles results in headaches, while the increased tone in the chest muscles and the associated poor posture produce a decrease in lung function.

Bradykinesia

The functional problems due to bradykinesia are difficult to separate from those due to rigidity. Bradykinesia results in difficulty initiating new movements, in responding to changes in movement and in carrying out repetitive or simultaneous movements by different parts of the body.

Muscle tone and bradykinesia are generally increased by cold and by anxiety, which has implications for rehabilitation programmes and for general home activities.

Tremor

Tremor usually starts in the hands as a pill rolling action in which there is alternating flexion and extension at the metocarpophalyngeal joints whilst the fingers are held extended. One of the very early signs, before the tremor occurs, may be this flexion at the metocarpophalyngeal joints and extension of the fingers when the patient is asked to stretch out his hand.

Although tremor traditionally disappears during sleep and at rest, many patients also have an action tremor which is made worse by movement. This differs from the intention tremor of cerebellar disease in that it is worse in the early stages of movement and does not become worse as the movement progresses.

The resting tremor is worse during anxiety. Many patients try to hide the hand by putting it into a pocket. Other techniques which help to control the tremor include pressing the elbows into the side or holding a small lead weight in the hand. The latter, in effect, is producing an activity (i.e. gripping) which inhibits the resting component of the tremor probably by facilitating the distal muscle stabilizers.

Posture

Classically the parkinsonian patient has: neck flexion with an inability to maintain the head in a horizontal position when kneeling on all fours; kyphosis of the dorsal spine; elbow and/or wrist flexion; hip and knee flexion; ankle plantar flexion with the heels off the ground; weight bearing on the heads of the metatarsal bones and toes; and a tendency to lean to one side – usually to the contralateral side to the major signs [18] – which may be associated with a tilt of the head to one side.

These produce abnormalities of the normal standing posture. The base area is decreased to about one-third of normal. The synergistic actions of the flexors and dorsiflexors are lost since both groups of muscles are used to support the weight of the body. Since the knee is in flexion it cannot lock and therefore depends on continuous muscle activity to maintain standing: this is tiring and may result in the leg suddenly giving away. Management includes attaching a narrow strip of cork or wood to the shoes at the level of the metatarsal heads; this results in the knee being thrown into extension and spreads the body weight more evenly between the two feet [19].

Spinal kyphosis contributes to the difficulty of controlling the position of the centre of gravity, resulting in a tendency to fall forwards.

A number of simple techniques are available to alleviate these abnormalities in the early stages. For example, passive movement of the neck helps to release the increased tone, especially if the neck is warmed first. A cervical collar may help some patients, although this may be due to the heat produced, especially by the soft Plastozote type, as well as to the passive splinting. Some patients who lean to one side find that carrying something (a stick or a handbag, for example) in the contralateral hand helps to improve the posture.

Active repetitive resistive exercises may help [20]. Some examples are: raising and lowering the arms to shoulder level whilst lying prone; extending the neck to look as high as possible whilst lying prone; and raising the buttocks from the bed whilst lying supine with the hips and legs flexed.

In addition, the following are examples of possible stretching and extension exercises:

- The patient stands with his back to a wall with the heels as near to the wall as possible (Fig. 16.1a). The aim is to keep the shoulder blades and back of the head against the wall for 10 seconds and then relax for 10 seconds. This is repeated for five minutes several times a day.
- The patient stands facing the wall with the feet a few inches away from it (Fig. 16.1b). The outstretched hands are then placed on the wall and the patient tries to reach as high on the wall as possible. If he looks at the hands while doing so this encourages extension of the neck. This position is maintained for 5–10 seconds and then repeated after a short period of relaxation.
- A weight on a piece of string is hung from the patient's neck. He is instructed to bring the weight as close to this body as is possible. This helps to demonstrate when he is flexed too far forward.

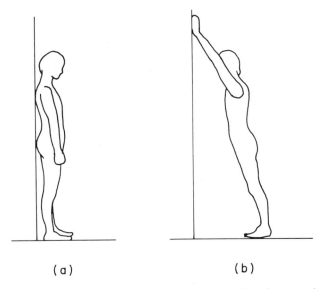

(a)   (b)

Fig. 16.1 Stretching and extension exercises (see text)

Visual feedback can be provided by a mirror or videotape to demonstrate the abnormalities.

Turning over in bed

Three-quarters of parkinsonian patients have difficulty turning over in bed [21]. This is usually due to the bradykinesia and rigidity making it difficult to initiate the movement.

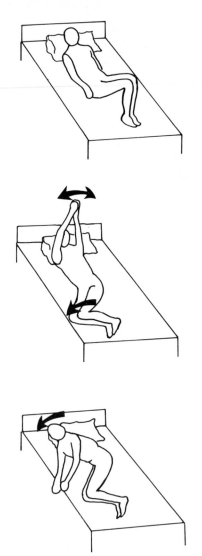

Fig. 16.2   Turning over in bed (see text)

A number of simple approaches may be of some help. First of all the bed should be firm since a soft bed makes turning over more difficult. On the other hand the patient who is unable to turn is at risk of pressure sores if the bed surface is too hard. Any resistance to turning should be avoided, and this includes heavy or tightly fastened bedclothes. It is usually not necessary to provide a bed cradle, but bed sheets should be loose and light – a duvet is ideal.

There are a few simple techniques to help the patient to turn over. Even if he is unable to use these techniques independently they will help the carer to turn him without excessive struggling.

The weight of the body can be used to advantage (Fig. 16.2). If the patient lies on his back with the legs bent and the feet flat on the bed, rocking the legs from side to side assists the legs to roll to the side on which he wants to lie. If at the same time the hands are clasped together and the arms extended, swinging them from side to side builds up momentum until the patient rolls over to the affected side. It is important for the patient to look and turn the head in the direction in which he wants to turn.

Where the patient is unable to turn by himself, the carer should stand so that she will be behind him when he has turned. The patient should then look in the direction in which he wants to turn and reach for that side of the bed whilst the carer places her hands under him at the shoulder and hip and gently pulls until he is in the correct position.

Getting out of bed

Many patients find it very difficult to get out of bed even when they have achieved the side-lying position. The difficulty seems to be in sitting up. There are several approaches to this problem:

1. Starting from the side-lying position (Fig. 16.3) the patient places the hand of the uppermost arm on the bed and moves the legs to the side of the bed until they begin to fall to the floor. He then pushes up against the bed while the weight of the legs helps to assist the action of sitting up.
2. For those starting from the position of back-lying (Fig. 16.4), the approach is to place the chin on the chest, ease up on to the elbows and lean forwards to sit up. The legs are then moved to the side of the bed, one leg at a time, until they are over the side. This is a difficult technique to carry out but may be helped if the head of the bed is raised.
3. A rope ladder attached to the bottom of the bed sometimes provides sufficient leverage to sit up.
4. A handrail attached to the side of the bed can also provide something to pull against.

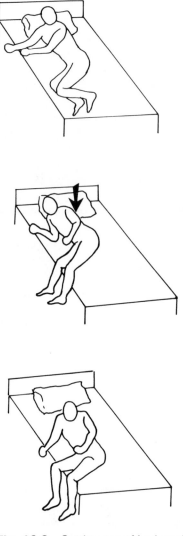

Fig. 16.3 Getting out of bed: technique 1 (see text)

Getting into bed

The technique involves sitting at the right spot on the side of the bed so that when the patient lies down the head automatically falls on to the pillow. The success of the technique depends on the patient using the mechanical action of the top half of the body falling on to the bed to assist lifting the legs on to the bed in one action.

Some patients find it easier to crawl on hands and knees on to the bed and then to roll over into the lying position.

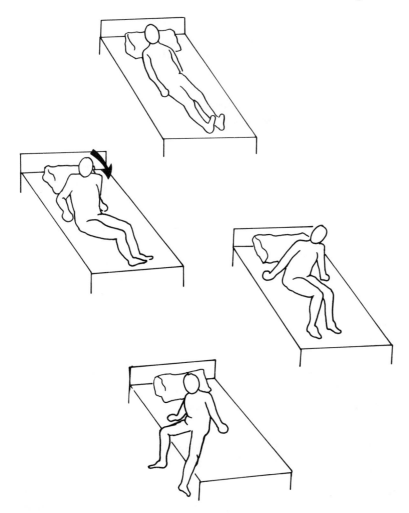

Fig. 16.4 Getting out of bed: technique 2 (see text)

Getting out of a chair

The difficulty in getting up from a chair is largely due to the rigidity of the back and the bradykinesia. The patient tends to try to stand with the legs extended and has difficulty getting the centre of gravity over his feet. There are several approaches to assist with this:

1. The chair should be of such a height that the ankles, knees and hips are at right-angles. This avoids the need to lift the body weight up to the level of the knees *before* beginning to stand. For this reason low chairs and those which are softly upholstered should be

avoided. Some patients find advantage in having a slight raise on the back legs of the chair to provide a slight forward tilt of the seat.

2. The patient brings his feet to the level of the front legs of the chair, moves his buttocks forwards to the edge of the chair to bring the centre of gravity over the feet, and then pushes up on the arms of the chair. When the chair does not have arms, pressing down on the front corners of the chair has the advantage of encouraging the patient to lean forward, but there may then be difficulty in straightening up.

3. This is as for (2) above, except that instead of pushing up on the arms of the chair the patient clasps his hands together and stretches them out in front of him to bring the centre of gravity forward over the feet. The essential ingredient is that the feet are placed far enough back to allow the centre of gravity to easily fall between them.

4. If the patient is sitting at a table, then he can lean forward on to the table (provided that it is stable) and push himself up.

5. For those patients who still find it difficult to stand because they do not seem to be able to release their grip on the arms of the chair, some can benefit by leaning forward and placing their hands on a stool, or other surface such as a bed, and then standing up. This is particularly helpful for the backward leaner.

6. Some patients find it easier to have a fixed and stable grabrail placed in front of the chair. The common practice of pulling on the walking frame should be discouraged since this can easily lead to an accident.

All these techniques may require a gentle rocking action to gain momentum to stand and may be supplemented by counting 'One, two, three, GO'.

Spring-loaded seats should be used with the greatest caution since parkinsonian patients usually have propulsion or retropulsion; if the spring loading is too powerful the patient may be catapulated on to the floor.

It must also be recognized that the patient will have the same difficulty in getting up from the toilet as from a chair. For this reason, depending on the height of the patient, it may be necessary to provide a raised seat on the toilet.

Sitting down

Sitting down is a hazardous procedure because the patient does not flex his back: he therefore falls backwards into the chair. One technique to overcome this is for the patient to place his hands on to his knees when sitting. This produces flexion of the trunk and allows the centre of gravity to move gently backwards, producing a more satisfactory sitting style.

Walking

One of the early signs of parkinsonism is the tendency to drag one leg. This eventually progresses into a gait that has shortening of the step length and a low step height, loss of rotation and arm swing, difficulty in initiating actions, and a tendency for activity to fade after a very short period. The rigidity of the neck affects some of the normal righting reflexes originating in the cervical muscles and apophyseal joints. The flexion of the trunk and limbs shifts the centre of gravity over the metatarsal heads, with a tendency for the patient to fall forwards when walking (propulsion).

Management involves reversing these abnormal gait patterns. Maintenance of a general level of exercise activity is preferred to sudden bursts of activity once or twice a week – though this is what usually happens with patients attending day hospitals. There is often a feeling of exhaustion after these bouts of unaccustomed exercise, and patients often express the view that the day hospital is making them worse. Those patients who maintain some exercise, either by walking or using an exercise bicycle or rowing machine at home, do not usually feel so tired after exercise.

Although many textbooks recommend swimming as an excellent exercise in parkinsonism, there is a tendency for parkinsonian patients to float head downwards with the buttocks rising. They should therefore never be in the swimming pool without an attendant, and they may need to swim with one hand on the side of the pool for stability.

Low step height and shuffling

The environment should be as free from obstructions as possible. This applies especially to rugs, torn carpets, curled lino and raised door sills. The soles of the shoes should be of leather or a hard composition and in good condition, the aim being to prevent a rough sole catching on the floor. Training the patient to walk with a high step can be helpful for short distances, but the tendency is for the step height to fade as the distances progresses.

Improving step rhythm

There have been several suggestions made on how to improve walking rhythm. For instance, the regular beat of a metronome, or an attendant saying 'left, right, left, right' whilst clapping her hands, can be used to indicate the rate of stepping. Some patients find it helpful to walk to a regular beat of music. Another approach has been to encourage the patient to listen to the sound of his own feet as they strike the ground – preferably when wearing leather-soled shoes or a metal heel bar to provide a louder noise. Deliberately striking the foot down hard increases the sound and provides sensory feedback.

Much of the problem of poor gait is due to the lack of arm swinging and trunk rotation. One technique to improve rotation is for the attendant to walk behind the patient and move his shoulders, or stand in front of him holding his hands and move the arms, in time to the walking.

The patient can be taught to swing the arms but this needs quite a lot of concentration and soon fades. Another approach is to concentrate on alternating patterns by having the patient pull on a piece of string passing from one hand, over a pulley, back to the other hand.

Exercise bicycles, pedalators or treadmills are used to provide alternating movement of the legs. Unfortunately in many of these exercises there is little transfer effect to normal walking. By far the best course is to encourage walking, and this needs persistence on the part of the patient, family and professional staff.

Improving step length

One technique is to place pieces of paper on the floor at suitable step length distances: the patient steps on these and the step length can gradually be increased. Another approach is to set a series of obstacles (such as books) at suitable distances on the floor for the patient to step over. This combines improving the length and height of the step.

Turning

Even when the patient is able to walk in a straight line, there is often difficulty changing direction or turning around. One solution is for the patient to walk in a semicircle rather than trying to turn around on the spot. This can be used as a training approach by first walking in a circle and then gradually narrowing this into an ellipse and eventually into a very narrow strip with a short turning point at each end.

Another approach is for the patient to stop when he wants to turn and then, by marching on the spot, turn with each step until facing in the direction in which he wishes to proceed.

Many patients lose the spontaneous act of turning the head to look in the direction in which they have to turn. If they can make a conscious effort to do so turning seems to be easier.

Propulsion and retropulsion

When walking with short steps the gait becomes increasingly fast, as though the patient is trying to catch up with his own centre of gravity. This will continue until he is saved by coming up against some object or until he falls. This may occur when going forwards (propulsion) or backwards (retropulsion).

Propulsion usually occurs when the patient walks with toe strike before heel strike, and so a training programme to increase heel strike should be attempted. Some patients benefit from a shoe raiser under the toe for propulsion or under the heel for retropulsion.

For those patients with a backward lean a walking frame is usually counterproductive. There are several reasons for this. First of all a walking frame inhibits a good alternating pattern of walking – the patient lifts the frame forward, steps into the frame, stops, lifts the frame forward, and so on. Secondly, the act of lifting the frame exacerbates the tendency to fall backwards. One way around this is to provide a wheeled frame which allows a more normal reciprocal walking gait without the frame having to be lifted.

When there is a very severe backward lean even the wheeled frame may be too light. In this case the patient should practise pushing a wheelchair with someone sitting in it, preferably a member of staff. The amusement of pushing the staff around distracts the patient from the fear of falling. In addition the force required to push a relatively heavy weight means that the patient must lean forward, thus overcoming the backward lean.

Freezing

Freezing is an inability to initiate an action and can be seen in all activities involving movement, such as turning over in bed, getting out of a chair or walking.

The flexed position of the trunk and legs results in the body weight being transferred over the metatarsal heads of the feet. It will be noted that many parkinsonian patients stand with the heel off the ground. Even normal people with no rigidity or bradykinesia find it difficult to start walking if they flex the trunk, bend their knees and stand forward on their toes.

A number of techniques are used to overcome freezing. They largely move the centre of gravity backwards from the metatarsal heads to encourage a more erect stance. The following ideas may help:

- Stand up straight, lift the head and place the heels on the floor.
- Take a step backwards (this puts the weight on to the heels) before making a step forward.

- Dorsiflex the toes.
- Start walking on the spot with exaggerated stepping. Swinging the arms also helps.
- Rock from side to side before starting to walk. Parkinsonian patients are usually stable on side-rocking [22] even when unstable on backward–forward rocking.
- Stepping over an object may help to initiate the first step. This can be the attendant's foot or a piece of paper dropped on the floor. One variation of the latter is to use a small object on a piece of string which allows retrieval for reuse and avoids littering the environment. For more difficult situations a flexible strip attached to the back legs of a walking frame [23] provides a suitable object to step over.
- Some patients find kicking their walking stick helps to initiate the movement.

Many of the hesitating or freezing actions, or those due to lack of initiation, are made worse by trying to force the activity. It is often better to overcome the problem by achieving spontaneous movement by stopping the action and starting again after a period of distraction. Some patients find that verbal commands, counting ('One, two, three, GO') or thinking angry or provocative thoughts helps them to 'unfreeze'. It has often been said that at the sound of the fire alarm the parkinsonian patients are usually the first people out of the room! However, when activity has been produced by a crisis situation there usually follows a worsening of the clinical features for a period.

Balance

Postural instability is common in Parkinson's disease, for several reasons. Vestibular activity is affected by basal ganglia lesions [24], while neck rigidity decreases feedback from the apophyseal joints and cervical muscles. It has also been shown that there is often a disturbance of perception of the vertical in Parkinson's disease, which increases the tendency to fall [25]. In addition, the peripheral mechanisms do not respond to change in posture because of the loss of automatic movement, rigidity and bradykinesia (i.e. the normal reaction of taking a corrective step and flinging out the arms does not occur).

Balance training uses the same techniques as described in Chapter 15.

Speech

Speech disturbances occur in 50 per cent of cases of parkinsonism [26,

27] and basically fall into five patterns: weakened volume and inaudibility;poor articulation and rhythm of speech with difficulty in sychronizing respiration with speaking; difficulty in verbal expression; poor initiation of speech; and a monotonous quality to the speech pattern owing to loss of prosody.

The main deficits in speech are in respiration, phonation, prosody and rate, with articulation being affected to a lesser extent [28].

Prosody is the emphasis that is put on different parts of a word or sentence to give it meaning. Thus we can say *re*habilitation or re*hab*ilitation or even rehabili*ta*tion. Prosody is essential for indicating the difference between 'it is me, Tom' (meaning Tom is speaking) from 'it is me, Tom' (meaning the person spoken to is Tom). This emphasis is often lost in parkinsonism, thereby influencing the intelligibility of speech [29]. This is one area which does respond to training by a speech therapist [30].

There has been a general nihilism about the use of speech therapy in the management of speech disturbances in parkinsonism [31], although there are strong claims [29] for benefits of therapy which can be maintained for up to three months after a two-week intensive speech therapy programme [28]. Some claim that the speech therapist is merely providing psychological support [32] and the will to communicate [33]. Even if this is all (!) that is achieved, the improvement in speech is greatly appreciated by the patient and the family.

The rigidity of the chest wall and the abnormal posture of the thoracic spine decreases the functional lung volume [34, 35], but the resulting low volume of speech is probably the most responsive to therapy [36]. Exercises can include lying on the back with a book on the chest, aiming to raise it as high as possible by taking deep breaths. It is also important to concentrate on expiration, such as blowing up a balloon or playing blow-football. Activities to improve posture also contribute to an improvement of speech volume.

During general exercises it is important for the patient to sit up straight, placing feet firmly on the floor (avoiding crossing the legs) whilst the hands are pressed on the arms of the chair to encourage 'boosting' of expiration.

Other approaches to improving the volume include forcing exercises [33] in which the patient practises laughing or coughing, attempts to pull apart clasped hands which are held at shoulder level, pushes the hands against a table whilst phonating on vowels, or uses exaggerated chewing activities whilst speaking.

Voice amplification has been used to increase the volume of speech [36], and there does seem to be a carry-over effect [37]. Relatives, especially those who are hard of hearing, may find amplification particularly beneficial, although it must be recognized that it will also amplify the other abnormalities of speech which may be irritating or unhelpful.

For the patient who is prepared to put a lot of work into improving his speech, the use of a tape recorder is sometimes helpful in providing feedback about the volume level. It has also been suggested that further visual feedback can be provided by watching the volume meter provided on many tape recorders [38].

The value of specific exercise techniques is uncertain, although there have been some quite dramatic effects shown using 'proprioceptive neuromuscular facilitation' in the management of volume and rate of speech [29]. The effects can continue for up to three months, though the technique is less effective for improving the rhythm, pitch or tone of speech.

Improving articulation requires the specialist skills of a speech therapist to provide the correct advice and management. In general the aim will be to train the patient in repetition of specific phrases and repeating words and sentences to improve the rhythm.

The use of machines which provide a delayed auditory feedback of 50 or so milliseconds has been shown to improve speech in at least two parkinsonian patients [39]. Another approach to visual feedback is the 'Visispeech' machine, which is normally used in the management of deaf people, allowing the therapist to demonstrate speech patterns on a television screen which the patient attempts to imitate.

The problem with any of these approaches is that they require determination and persistance on the part of the patient and his family. Unfortunately this is not always forthcoming in the elderly and can lead to a great deal of frustration within the family. Many patients develop a sign language to indicate their needs, and certainly if they have had a very close relationship with the carer much is 'known' without being said. This, of course, is not very helpful to the casual visitor. Unfortunately the non-verbal communication that we all use – such as smiling, raising an eyebrow and other facial expressions – is often lacking in parkinsonism. This is why many people with parkinsonism are regarded as being dull-witted and do not attract a friendly response. The fact that patients are unable to speak well should not mean that they are unable to communicate. Apart from gestures, simple aids include a communication board which may consist of a card on which the alphabet is printed in large letters along with selected words or even sentences; or a simple picture board may be of some help. Some patients find it easier to communicate with a typewriter or a Cannon communicator (a small portable printer with a keyboard). More sophisticated computerized equipment is available, including the SPLINK, a programmable board which allows the patient to create a vocabulary suitable to his own level of communication needs; messages are transmitted to a television screen for display. These more complicated aids are rarely used by the elderly, and it is usually more rewarding to train the patient and his family in communication by gesture to supplement the available speech, using a writing pad when words are not understood.

Swallowing difficulties

Swallowing difficulties are not uncommon in Parkinson's disease. Sometimes these result in a low calorie intake, although weight loss may be due to malabsorbtion of food secondary to damage to the autonomic nervous system.

A number of problems associated with feeding occur. There may be difficulty with chewing or with the swallowing reflex. Some patients experience nasal regurgitation of food, while others find that food accumulates in the cheeks. The rate of swallowing is decreased and food seems to be held up at the back of the mouth and in the cheeks. The embarrassment of drooling and feeding problems often causes the patient to withdraw from social occasions.

Simple advice is to find the type of food which is easiest to swallow. This varies from patient to patient, but frequently semi-solid food is found to cause less diffculty than solids or fluids. Sipping iced water sometimes helps to encourage swallowing reflexes. Swallowing is also assisted by a good sitting posture (sitting erect when eating).

As associated feature is the tendency to drool or dribble. This is exacerbated by the head hanging forward, and so the patient should be trained to sit erect. Lip exercises, such as sucking a spoon or a lollipop, helps to keep the mouth closed. Stroking with ice around the mouth helps to stimulate the mouth tone and resistive exercises for the tongue help with its mobility.

Perceptual disorders

It is generally regarded that Parkinson's disease primarily affects motor function, but there is evidence that visio-spatial perceptual difficulties also occur [40]. There may be difficulties, even in the absence of cognitive deficits, in obtaining non-visual clues to speech owing to the difficulty in interpreting facial expressions [41]. This possibly accounts for some communication difficulties since facial expression is important for interpreting the semantic and emotional part of communication. Fortunately this also seems to benefit from speech therapy retraining [30].

Activities of daily living

Eating

Some of the difficulties with eating are due to the inability to maintain a grip, the bradykinesia and the action tremor. Simple aids are helpful. A non-slip mat prevents the plate from sliding around the surface of the table. Heavy cutlery or weighted wristbands help to dampen down the modulations of the action tremor. The difficulty here is trying to balance the damping down of the tremor against the added weight on already weakened limbs. The patient should be taught to only partly fill a cup with fluid and to hold the cup with both hands. Supporting the elbows on the table or holding them against the chest wall can provide some stability. Thickening of the handles of cutlery improves grip.

There are a number of aids to assist carrying food. The patient will usually find it easier to carry even one object on a tray, especially those suspended from a handle.

When a normal person pours a cup of tea he starts by pouring slowly and then quickens as the tea flows. A parkinsonian patient pours slowly all the time. Since the patient can rarely hold the teapot for long this produces difficulties with spillage. If this occurs then a tilting teapot holder can be of assistance.

Because of the difficulties in feeding the patient may lose weight. It is therefore wise for him to eat a little at a time but often. To avoid food going cold insulated plates and cups can be used.

Dressing

It is important that the room is warm since rigidity and bradykinesia are made worse by cold. Sitting on a firm seat also assists dressing.

Selection of the type of clothes is important since dressing aids tend to be of little help. Where buttons and zips present real difficulties, fastening with elastic or Velcro should be considered. For lesser difficulty the use of larger buttons (and larger button holes) may make dressing much easier. Elastic shoe laces or slip-on shoes avoid the need for fastening laces. Clip-on ties may be more practical than the conventional type.

Psychological support

Parkinson's disease is a frustrating condition for both patient and family. The general appearances suggest a level of mental retardation and the patient is often treated as such, especially by strangers. The difficulties with speech emphasize this impression.

The experienced carer asks the patient to talk slowly, if necessary repeating what has been said to let the patient known how much has been understood. She or he will aim to encourage the patient to continue to communicate rather than inhibit the attempt.

There is a general decrease in what might be called motivation, although it is probably a biochemical effect – a bradykinesia of the spirit. This seems to respond to some extent to group therapy [42, 43], especially when the other members of the group also suffer from parkinsonism.

In general Parkinson's disease is a difficult condition to manage. This is largely due to progressive deterioration, but it is also partly due to the nature of the symptoms producing slowing of both physical and internal 'drive' mechanisms, making the carry-over effect of a formal rehabilitation programme difficult to achieve. Successful rehabilitation depends largely on the willingness and ability of the carer to encourage activity over the long term. Parkinson's disease is an example par excellence of the need to involve the carer in the rehabilitation programme.

References

1. Kurland, L.T. (1958) Epidemiology: incidence, geographical distribution and genetic considerations. In: *Pathogenesis and Treatment of Parkinsonism*, pp. 5–49 (Ed: Fields, W.S.). Charles C. Thomas, Springfield, Illinois.
2. Jenkins, A.C. (1966) Epidemiology of parkinsonism in Victoria. *Medical Journal of Australia* 2: 496–502.
3. Kessler, I.I. (1972) Epidemiological studies in Parkinson's disease. 3: A community based survey. *American Journal of Epidemiology* 96: 242–54.
4. Broman, T. (1963) Parkinson's syndrome: prevalence and incidence in Goteborg. *Acta Neurologica Scandinavica* 39 (**Suppl. 4**): 95–101.
5. Marttila, R.J. and Rinne, U.K. (1976) Epidemiology of Parkinson's disease in Finland. *Acta Neurologica Scandinavica* 53: 81–102.
6. Mutch, W.J., Dingwall-Fordyce, I., Downie, A.W. *et al.* (1986) Parkinson's disease in a Scottish city. *British Medical Journal* 292: 534–6.
7. Brewis, M., Poskanzer, D.C., Rolland, C. and Miller, H. (1966) Neurological disease in an English city. *Acta Neurologica Scandinavica* 42 (Suppl. 24): 31–6.
8. Gudmundsson, K.R. (1967) A clinical survey of parkinsonism in Iceland. *Acta Neurologica Scandinavica* 43 (Suppl. 33): 1–61.
9. Birkmayer, W., Ambrozi, L., Neumayer, E. and Riederer, P. (1974) Longevity in Parkinson's disease treated with L-dopa. *Clinical Neurology and Neurosurgery* 1: 15–19.
10. Stephen, P.J. and Williamson, J. (1984) Drug induced parkinsonism in the elderly. *Lancet* ii: 1082–3.
11. Wilson, J.A. and Primrose, W.R. (1986) Drug induced Parkinsonism. *British Medical Journal* 293: 957 (letter).
12. Mutch, W.J., Strudwick, A., Roy, S.K. and Downie, A.W. (1986) Parkinson's disease: disability, review and management. *British Medical Journal* 293: 675–7.
13. Webster, D.D. (1968) Cortical analysis of the disability in Parkinson's disease. *Modern Treatment* 5: 257–82.

14. Franklyn, S., Kohout, L.J., Stern, G.M., and Dunning, M. (1981) Physiotherapy in Parkinson's disease. In: *Research Progress in Parkinson's Disease* (Eds: Rose, F.C. and Capildeo, R.). Pitman Medical, London.

15. Flewitt, B., Capildeo, R., and Rose, F.C. (1981) Physiotheraphy and assessment in Parkinson's disease using the polarised light goniometer. In: *Research Progress in Parkinson's Disease* (Eds: Rose, F.C. and Capildeo, R.). Pitman Medical, London.

16. Gibbert, F.B., Page, N.G.R., Spencer, K.M. *et al.* (1981) Controlled trial of physiotheraphy and occupational therapy for Parkinson's disease. *British Medical Journal* 282: 1196–1197.

17. Franklyn, S. and Stern, G.M. (1981) Controlled trial of physiotherapy and occupational therapy for Parkinson's disease. *British Medical Journal* 282: 1969–70.

18. Duvoisin, R.C. and Marsden, C.D. (1975) Notes on the scoliosis of Parkinsonism. *Journal of Neurology, Neurosurgery and Psychiatry* 38: 787–93.

19. Cooper, I.S., Riklan, M., Stellar, S. *et al.* (1968) A multidisciplinary investigation of neurosurgical rehabilitation in bilateral parkinsonism. *Journal of the American Geriatrics Society* 16: 1177–306.

20. Partridge, M.J. (1962) Repetitive resistance exercise: a method of indirect muscle training. *Physical Therapy* 42: 405–6.

21. Martin, W.E., Loewenson, R.B., Resch, J.A. and Baker, A.B. (1973) Parkinsons disease: clinical analysis of 100 patients. *Neurology* 23: 783–90.

22. Martin, J.P., Hurwitz, L.J. and Finlayson, M.H. (1962) The negative symptoms of basal ganglia disease. *Lancet* ii: 1–6.

23. Wright, W.B. (1979) Stammering gait. *Age and Ageing* 8: 8–12.

24. Mettler, F.A. (1932) Connections of the auditory cortex of cat. *Comparative Neurology* 55: 139–83.

25. Proctor, F., Riklan, M., Cooper, I.S. and Teuber, H.L. (1963) Somatosensory status of parkinsonian patients before and after chemothalecomy. *Neurology* 13: 906–12.

26. Atarashi, J. and Uchida, E. (1959) A clinical study of Parkinsonism. *Recent Advances in Research in the Nervous System* 3: 871–2.

27. Selby, G. (1968) Parkinson's disease. In: *Handbook of Clinical Neurology*, Vol. 6 (Eds: Vinken, P.J. and Bruyn, G.W.). North Holland Publishing Co., Amsterdam.

28. Robertson, S.J. and Thomson, F. (1984) Speech therapy in Parkinson's disease: a study of the efficacy and long term effects of intensive treatment. *British Journal of Disorders of Communication* 19: 213–24.

29. Scott, S. and Caird, F.I. (1983) Speech therapy for patients with Parkinson's disease. *Journal of Neurology, Neurosurgery and Psychiatry* 46: 140–4.

30. Scott, S. and Caird, F.I. (1984) The respond of the apparent receptive speech disorder in Parkinson's disease to speech therapy. *Journal of Neurology, Neurosurgery and Psychiatry* 47: 302–4.

31. Allen, C.M. (1970) Treatment of non-fluent speech resulting from neurological disease – treatment of dysarthria. *British Journal of Disorders of Communication* 5: 1–4.

32. Sarno, M.T. (1968) Speech impairment in Parkinson's disease. *Archives of Physical Medicine and Rehabilitation* 49: 269–75.

33. Butfield, C. (1961) Dysarthria. *Speech Pathology and Therapy* 4: 74.

34. Kim, R. (1968) The chronic residual respiratory disorder in post-encephalitic Parkinsonism. *Journal of Neurology, Neurosurgery and Psychiatry* 31: 393–8.

35. Mueller, P.B. (1971) Parkinson's disease: motor speech behaviour in a selected group of patients. *Folia Phoniatrica* 23: 333–46.

36. Greene, M.L.C. and Watson, B.W. (1968) The value of speech amplification in Parkinson's disease patients. *Folia Phoniatrica* **20**: 250.
37. Green, M.L.C. (1980) *The Voice and its Disorders.* Pitman Medical, London.
38. Perry, A.R. and Das, P.K. (1981) Speech assessment of patients with Parkinson's disease. In: *Progress in Parkinson's Disease*, pp. 373–84 (Eds: Rose, F.C. and Capildeo, R.). Pitman Medical, London.
39. Downie, A.W., Low, J.M. and Lindsay, D.O. (1981) Speech disorders in Parkinsonism – usefulness of delayed auditory feedback in selected cases. *British Journal of Disorders of Communication* **16**: 135–9.
40. Villardita, C., Smirni, P., Le Pira, F. *et al.* (1966) Mental deterioration, visuoperceptive disabilities and constructional apraxia in Parkinson's disease. *Acta Neurologica Scandinavica* **1**: 114–20.
41. Scott, S., Caird, F.I. and Williams, B.O. (1984) Evidence for an apparent sensory speech disorder in Parkinson's disease. *Journal of Neurology, Neurosurgery and Psychiatry* **47**: 840–3.
42. Minnigh, E.C. (1971) The Northwestern University concept of rehabilitation through group physical therapy. *Rehabilitation Literature* **32**: 38–9.
43. Carroll, B. (1971) Fingers to toes. *American Journal of Nursing* **71**: 550–1.

17

Stroke

Stroke is the third major killer (after heart disease and cancer) in western society and the major cause of severe disability. The incidence of stroke has been decreasing over the last thirty years or so [1-9]. This is complicated by the various definitions of 'stroke' used by different researchers [10], as well as by changes in diagnostic fashion, coding practices, coverage of death certificates and the low accuracy of diagnosis. Most.studies are of mortality, but it is important to consider those who survive and to observe whether they are treated in hospital or at home [11]. These figures are much more difficult to obtain.

Table 17.1   The incidence of stroke by age group (per 100 000 population)

Age range	Matsumoto et al. (1973) [12]	Whisnant et al. (1971) [13]	Goldner et al. (1967) [14]	Wylie (1970) [15]	Gibson (1974) [16]	Oxford (1983) [19]
<35	4	2	} 65	1	–	} 54
35–44	35	34		29	41	
45–54	110	159		122	73	
55–64	364	369	412	346	275	305
65–74	791	1081	1072	830	831	645
75–84	} 2156	} 2494	2716	2242	} 1950	} 1546
85 +			5820	4858		

Age and stroke

The incidence of stroke increases with advancing age [12–18 and Table 17.1] There is, approximately, a doubling every decade after the age of 45, especially for males [12, 17, 19 and Table 17.2]. This is particularly relevant since the elderly population is increasing disproportionately in most western countries. Demographic trends in the United Kingdom suggest that there will be a 9 per cent increse in the number of stroke patients over the last quarter of the twentieth century. Within these figures there will be little change in the number of stroke victims

276

Table 17.2   Sex difference in incidence of stroke per 100 000 population

Age range	Matsumoto *et al.* (1973) [12]		Age range	Oxford (1983) [19]	
	M	F		M	F
<45	9	8	<55	17	16
45–64	313	157	55–64	318	292
65–74	1082	603	65–74	595	689
75 +	2504	1988	75 +	1782	1421

for those age groups under the age of 75 years, but an increase of 25–30 per cent in the number of those 75 years and over simply arising from demographic trends [Table 17.3]. Much will depend on which incidence figures are used, but they do give some idea of the future trends.

Table 17.3   Projected number of stroke patients in the United Kingdom 1975–2001

Year	Number of stoke patients 1975	Percentage increase from 1975		
		1981	1991	2001
Males				
<45	1660	<1	+ 5	+ 5
45–64	19720	– 3	– 3	+ 8
65–74	23800	0	0	– 9
75 +	22540	+ 11	+ 22	+ 33
All males	67720	+ 3	+ 7	+ 10
Females				
<45	1380	0	+ 4	+ 3
45–65	7850	– 4	– 6	+ 8
65–74	27740	– 2	– 9	– 15
75 +	37770	+ 11	+ 26	+ 26
All females	74740	+ 4	+ 10	+ 9
TOTAL	142460	+ 3	+ 8	+ 9

Recovery and age

Although some workers have found a close correlation between poor recovery and increasing age [20–28], others have not found so direct a relationship [29–34]. The elderly are more likely to start with a greater deficit [35], and the severity of the stroke influences the outcome. If survivors of stroke are examined at six months or one year following the onset, there is no statistically significant difference between those under 65 years, those 65–74 years or those 75 years and over for the level of recovery [35]. Indeed, the 75 + group showed a greater trend to reach better levels of recovery than the 65–74 year group. Of course, this only takes the survivors into account and the early mortality increases markedly with advancing age. Nevertheless it does give some optimism for rehabilitation of some elderly stroke patients.

Poor functional recovery is associated with the severity of the motor power loss [23, 29, 36, 37], sensory loss [36, 38], hemianopia [37], aphasia [24, 39] and incontinence of urine or faeces [23, 31, 34, 37]; but the major barriers are perceptual [23, 34, 37, 40] and cognitive dysfunction [23]. Poor functional capacity after the age of 70 is nearly always due to severe organic mental disorders [41], although it has been suggested [42] that the elderly face more demanding requirements than do younger patients. Multiple pathology might also be expected to limit the rehabilitation potential.

The rate of recovery

Most recovery takes place during the first six months following the stroke, but experience suggests that recovery can continue for up to about five years. This slow but important late recovery has not received the attention it deserves.

The literature suggests quite a wide time range for optimal recovery. For instance, little recovery is said to occur beyond three [43], four [44] or six months [45, 46], although others [21, 47–49] have reported recovery beyond six months. Little recovery is found in mobility and leg strength after the first two months [36], or in hand function after six months [50] following the stroke. Progress is likely to be poor if there is no apparent movement within three weeks or if motion in one segment of the limb is not followed by movement in another within one week [45], and there is little chance of recovery in walking or activities of daily living if severe neuromuscular disability is still present eight weeks following the onset of the stroke [51]. Maximum recovery has usually occurred within one month for activities of daily living [21]; while the ability to walk independently has variously been found to occur within two months [36], six months [51] or longer [49]; and muscle power within two months [36]. There are so many variables between the studies, including selection of patients, amount of rehabilitation and definition of recovery, that meaningful comparison is impossible.

Hurwitz and Adams [48] have expressed the view that it is seldom possible to confidently determine those with the potential for recovery earlier than three months following the stroke. Some of the late recovery may depend not so much on the brain damage as on overcoming negative emotions such as depression, fear, despair and lack of purpose [25].

It is obvious from the above that it is difficult to answer the question which is frequently asked: 'How long should we continue active rehabilitation for the stroke patient?'. It is logical to continue formal rehabilitation until there is no evidence of improvement in any of the parameters being assessed – usually functional – and then to transfer the management to a nursing rehabilitation model which is functionally orientated. This is not the same as discontinuing treatment but is changing the style of the rehabilitation programme. It is then worth continuing to monitor the process so that specific forms of therapy can be reintroduced as required.

The effectiveness of rehabilitation

The provision of therapy services for stroke varies widely, with one-third of stroke patients throughout the western world not receiving any [52]. In one study in England, 79 per cent of stroke patients received physiotherapy but only 26 per cent occupational therapy, and only one-quarter of those with communication problems received speech therapy [53]. These levels of provision depend more on the availability of therapist resources than on the specific needs of the patients.

Evidence for the effectiveness of rehabilitation in stroke is difficult to find. Several workers, in uncontrolled trials, report that rehabilitation was effective in improving functional recovery [32, 37, 54, 55]. Others have shown that those who start treatment early progress better than those who start late. These were not controlled trials and there is likely to be a reason why some patients received early rather than later treatment; this factor itself may influence the outcome, apart from the differences due to spontaneous recovery. Other studies have shown greater functional recovery in units with, than in those without, a specific interest in rehabilitation [54, 58, 59]. These were not controlled trials and it is likely that there were significant differences in the admission policies of the units. This is important when it is recognized that, in one city at least [60], the side of the stroke not only influenced whether an elderly patient was admitted to hospital but also to which type of unit – patients with a right hemiplegia were more likely to be admitted to hospital, and of the latter those with right hemiplegia were more likely to be admitted to general medical wards and those with left hemiplegia to geriatric wards. This probably relates to the perceived urgency, dysphasia being more obvious than the spatial problems of right hemisphere damage. Geriatricians are more likely to be contacted when recovery is slow or symptoms are 'bizarre'.

Another research approach has been to provide rehabilitation to a group of chronically severely disabled patients where spontaneous recovery could not be expected [61], with the encouraging result that about one-half showed some improvement which was maintained over six months. Here, again, factors other than the formal rehabilitation programme may have influenced the recovery. In studies of simple functional help versus formal rehabilitation [62, 63], there were no statistically significant differences in recovery, although functional help can be regarded as rehabilitation in its broadest sense.

The difficulty in carrying out controlled trials of rehabilitation is shown in the Northwick Park Hospital study [64]. Of 1094 stroke patients admitted to hospital 33 per cent died, 20 per cent recovered, 30 per cent were regarded as too frail or too ill to be considered for the study, and only 11 per cent fitted the criteria for a trial to assess the effect of different levels of rehabilitation. This is, nevertheless, an important study because many of the variables were controlled and a specified level of disability studied. The study assessed patients with moderate degrees of disability who could receive rehabilitation on an outpatient basis. The patients were allocated to one of three groups: 'intensive therapy' (rehabilitation for four full days a week), 'conventional therapy' (rehabilitation for three half days a week), or 'no treatment' (not attending for rehabilitation but visited by a health visitor at home and encouraged to carry out the exercises they had been shown whilst in hospital). Improvement was greatest among those receiving the most therapy and least in those receiving none. Deterioration occurred less often as the amount of treatment increased. From this study it does seem that recovery is associated with the amount of rehabilitation provided.

So far the discussion has been about rehabilitation in its broadest sense without an attempt to describe what the process consists of. There are, however, a large number of different neurophysiological approaches but there has been little attempt to assess the value of these concepts. In one randomly controlled study there was no statistically significant difference between one group of patients treated by a neurophysiological approach and another group treated by 'traditional' methods [65]. Another study of walking competence over a seven-year period, during which time different physiotherapy approaches had been tried, could not show any one technique to be superior [66]. These findings fit in with clinical experience that the techniques have to be adapted to the needs of the patient.

If the question of whether treatment is beneficial is difficult, then the decision of when to stop treatment is even more so. As was suggested above the evidence is that there is little recovery after six months following the onset of the stroke. However, this could have been due to treatment having been stopped before this stage was reached. There is evidence that, of those who were severely disabled at the onset of the stroke and showed evidence of improvement, 96 per cent had less than 105 days of physiotherapy; whereas 39 per cent of those who did not improve during the first year continued therapy for much longer periods. It would, therefore, seem reasonable, especially when therapy resources are scarce, to limit the period of treatment to less than six months provided that the patient is not showing evidence of further benefit from the rehabilitation programme. In many cases it will be obvious to discontinue treatment at a much earlier stage.

Home or hospital?

The appropriate place to treat a stroke patient has been much debated. The proportion of stroke patients admitted to hospital varies between and within countries, with figures between 30 and 60 per cent for those being treated at home [4, 44, 67, 68]. There is, of course, a wide variation for this throughout the world, with about one-quarter of those in European countries not being admitted to hospital [69].

Admission to hospital is not necessarily directly related to the severity of the stroke, with about one-half of mildly affected patients being admitted to hospital [68] and 13–23 per cent of severely disabled treated at home [68, 70]. Much of this is related to the local admission policy, the interest of the local physicians and the amount of social support locally available. For instance, Warren *et al.* [71] reported that, even where hospital treatment was requested, admission was obtained with difficulty in 35 per cent of cases and refused in 45 per cent. This was 20 years ago and it is hoped that a more enlightened view is taken in the 1980s.

Even when admission is obtained the quality of care often leaves much to be desired [72], probably because once the acute phase of stroke is over many doctors seem to lose interest [73]. Attempts to interest physicians in the problems of stroke have had limited effect. Waylonis [74] reported on the introduction of an educational programme directed at health professionals at all levels. Although some physicians became 'more aware of what could be done for stroke patients' it also 'become painfully apparent that the average physician was not significantly interested in stroke or other chronic diseases' and that within six weeks of the research grant discontinuing the nurses 'slid back into their former habit of playing Florence Nightingale to patients who needed independence rather than dependence'. This general disinterest in stroke is probably one of the strongest arguments for specialist stroke units.

Stroke units

There are two types of stroke unit: the intensive care unit which takes patients in the acute phase for investigation and medical treatment; and the rehabilitation stroke unit which takes patients once the acute medical emergency has settled.

Intensive care stroke units

These might be expected to save lives and prevent complications. There are mixed reports of their success in doing so. Pitner and Mance [58] compared 100 consecutive patients admitted to a stroke unit with 81 matched controls admitted to an adjacent neurological ward and concluded that the specialist stroke unit did not have an effect on mortality. This was not a randomly allocated controlled trial and there may have been differences in selection for each type of unit. In addition, there is probably not much difference in the management approach between a neurological unit and a stroke unit.

Reports of the effect of introducing intensive stroke units to a hospital suggest a decrease in mortality [75, 76], a reduction in complication-related deaths in younger and less impaired patients [77], or a decreased in complications, especially those involving the skin or urinary tract [78].

Rehabilitation stroke units

These have concentrated on patients who require an active rehabilitation programme in the post-acute stage. In Britain these have largely been associated with departments of geriatric medicine, although only 10 per cent of such departments had a stroke unit in 1983 [79]. In a study of 11 stroke units in the UK, eight were in departments of geriatric medicine, one was part of a regional rehabilitation unit, one of a sub-regional neurological rehabilitation unit and one part of a neurology ward – none was associated with a general medical ward [80]. The general provision was 0.5–1 beds per 10 000 total population.

The theoretical advantage of stroke units is that they provide greater emphasis on the total management of the stroke patient, with a better knowledge by all the staff in the prevention of complications such as spasticity and the painful hemiplegic shoulder. Probably the major advantage is not so much having therapists who have an interest in stroke, essential though this is, but that nurses, including night staff, are aware of the specialist techniques to employ (and avoid) throughout the whole 24-hour period. The specialization encourages improvement in rehabilitation techniques and offers greater opportunities for research and teaching. It has been argued that on economic grounds it makes sense to move stroke patients from a high-technology acute unit to a lower-cost area following investigation [81]. This is probably a misunderstanding of how costly a labour-intensive stroke rehabilitation unit has to be to be effective.

There are disadvantages to stroke units. They may increase the interest within the unit but reduce the training opportunities outside the department [82], thereby decreasing the expertise for those stroke patients not transferred to the stroke unit. Unless there is careful selection of patients for admission the unit gradually accumulates a large number of stroke patients who will require long-stay care. This has the effect of preventing those patients who would benefit from the skills of the unit from being admitted and has a demoralizing effect on staff who feel that they are not using their skills and expertise to the optimal level. This is a very real danger and implies that some guidelines and special arrangements have to be made to ensure that the unit is used effectively and efficiently. This usually means some arrangement with the original referring ward that they will accept patients back if the specialist skills of the stroke unit are no longer required but the patient cannot be discharged. In this case the stroke unit is acting like any highly specialized unit with limited resources, such as an intensive care or coronary care unit. The alternative is that high priority must be given to the stroke unit for places in long-stay care for those who do not reach discharge levels. These are problems which have to be solved at an early stage if efficient use of the unit is to be maintained and the best use of resources achieved.

The decision must then be made as to which patients to admit. Those with mild or moderate disability will probably make a good recovery wherever they are treated [49]. Evidence from stroke units suggests that it is the severely, as opposed to profoundly, disabled who benefit the most from specialist units [82, 83]. Rosenthal [84] suggested that rehabilitation should be reserved for those who did not recover quickly, and although he felt there were no absolute contra-indications to a rehabilitation programme he regarded receptive aphasia, bilateral involvement, balance difficulties and flexion contractions as major barriers to recovery. Anderson and Kottke [85] suggest that the criteria for acceptance for rehabilitation should be whether the patient can comprehend verbal or non-verbal directions, can follow two- or three-step instructions and can remember and apply today what he learnt yesterday.

These criteria are rather rigid and ignore the fact that the decision has to be made at an early stage before the potential for recovery can be assessed. It is important to decide the goals which are to be achieved for social coping. For instance, it may be reasonable to admit a confused patient to the stroke unit if the goal is to achieved transferring from bed to chair with the help of one person so that the family can cope. On the other hand, it may be less realistic to transfer a mentally alert patient who had difficulty coping alone prior to the stroke owing to severe arthritis if long-term care is inevitable. Sadly the decision often has to be made on the ground of the chances of being discharged from hospital rather than on giving the patient every opportunity. Each patient must be considered on his merits. This view is difficult for many relatives and staff to accept, but realistic goals have not only to be set but must be meaningful if achieved.

The effectiveness of stroke units is difficult to determine. The introduction of a rehabilitation stroke unit has been shown to increase the proportion of patients discharged home [86, 87] and to decrease the mean length of stay in hospital [88]. On the other hand, Waylonis [74] was unable to demonstrate any real functional benefit from the introduction of a stroke unit.

In a study of elderly hemiplegic patients randomly allocated to either a stroke unit or a general ward where the nurse in charge had rehabilitation exerience, no difference in outcome could be found between the two groups [89]. This may merely emphasize the importance of the nurses having a training in rehabilitation.

Other evidence from an uncontrolled study [81] is that, although patients admitted to one stroke unit were more disabled than those admitted to a general rehabilitation ward, they were more likely to achieve greater mobility and to be discharged home [81].

A different approach has been to compare the outcome of patients admitted either to a stroke unit or, when there was no bed available, to a general ward [83]. Although no difference could be found for those with moderate or profound stroke, those with a severe stroke reached better levels of ability, although they remained longer on the stroke unit and received more therapy than those on the general ward. There are obvious design problems and inevitably some degree of selection of patients is possible.

A significant contribution to the debate about stroke units comes from the Edinburgh study [90], where patients over the age of 60 who had had a stroke of moderate severity which had been present for more than six hours but less than three days, were randomly allocated to a stroke unit or a general medical ward. They found that a significantly higher proportion of patients on the stroke unit were independent at the time of discharge and had required less therapy time than those on the general ward. Although at the annual follow-up (91) there was no difference between the two groups owing to 'catching up' by the 'general medical' patients [91] it does suggest that the stroke unit was cost-effective in management of stroke.

Domiciliary rehabilitation

Domiciliary rehabilitation is discussed in Chapter 20, but there have been a number of studies of home rehabilitation specifically for stroke. Patients are much more likely to require admission to hospital if they have had a severe stroke or live alone [68, 70, 92], although these studies found that as many as one-quarter of the patients with severe stroke and 40 per cent who lived alone were treated at home. The main reasons general practitioners gave for admitting patients to hospital was for nursing care and social management rather than diagnosis or rehabilitation [68]. Similarly the reason for keeping patients at home was more related to the ability of the family to cope. This gives great scope for the setting up of domiciliary – based rehabilitation teams. However, an augmented domiciliary care team has not been shown to reduce the need for admission to hospital [93],

Community support

The importance of the size of the stroke problem lies in the increasing burden which is placed on the health and social services because of the requirements for long-term care [64].

Stroke affects the family as well as the patient, both physically and mentally [95]. The stroke family tends to become isolated as the intial phase of 'visiting the sick' declines and the patient and spouse become confined to the home. Even those patients who have gained mobility often remain housebound [96], partly due to lack of volition, partly to a sense of embarrassment and partly to dissatisfaction with the new lifestyle [97, 98].

Stroke clubs, which are usually run by voluntary bodies, have made a major contribution to these long-term problems. Clubs meet in a variety of places, including hospitals, social clubs, churches, factories and pubs. Some provide a small amount of therapy, whilst others are primarily social in nature. Although some clubs simply provide an entertaining evening out, others emphasize self-help, with workshops, outings to the cinema, theatre, restaurants, pubs or the countryside, or provide holidays. Outside speakers provide answers to a whole range of problems, often related to stroke and coping, including aids and appliances, welfare rights and clinical topics.

Probably the most important role of the stroke club is its self-help approach. Some clubs hold relatives' groups which allow frustrations to be vented and families to receive psychological support and practical tips from others who have been through the same diffi-culties. The psychological support of having the club often has a carry-over effect on the rest of the patient's life. Activities such as outings to pubs and restaurants are easier to cope with when in a group of people with the same disability. Many admit that they would not dare visit such places if they were not with the other stroke sufferers. These clubs, therefore, play a major part in the resettlement of the stroke family into the community.

Dysphasic patients do not always benefit from the stroke clubs because of the communication problems. For this reason some clubs have been specifically set up for the special needs of the dysphasic patient with the emphasis being placed on group activities. Most dysphasic clubs in Britain are associated with the Volunteer Dysphasic Scheme [99–101]. This originally started from the experience of Valerie Eaton Griffiths with the actress Patricia Neal, where it was found that untrained help could play a major part in the recovery from dysphasia. This was followed by a community study on 31 dysphasic stroke patients [99], and from this has grown a national scheme of volunteer groups. Each group is organized by a local manager and a number of volunteers are attached to a dysphasic family. These volunteers work in close cooperation with the local speech therapists and help the patients with their 'homework'. Relatives gain from the support of the volunteers who are not embarrassed by the communication problems and become family friends.

References

1. Garraway, W.M., Whisnant, J.P., Furlan, A.J. *et al.* (1979) The declining incidence of stroke. *New England Journal of Medicine* **300**: 409–52.
2. Levy, R.I. (1979) Stroke decline: implications and prospects. *New England Journal of Medicine* **300**: 480–91.
3. Haberman, S., Capildeo, R. and Rose, F.C. (1978) The changing mortality of cerebrovascular disease. *Quarterly Journal of Medicine* **47**: 71–88.
4. Baum, H.M. (1982) Stroke prevalence: an analysis of data from the 1977 National Health Interview Survey. *Public Health Reports* **97**: 24–30.
5. Bonita, R. and Beaglehole, R. (1982) Trends in cerebrovascular disease in New Zeland. *New Zealand Medical Journal* **95**: 411–14.
6. Haberman, S., Capildeo, R. and Rose, F.C. (1982) Diverging trends in cerebrovascular disease and ischaemic heart disease mortality. *Stroke* **13**: 582–9.
7. Dobson, A.J., Gibbert, R.W., Wheeler, D.J. and Leeder, S.R. (1981) Age specific trends in mortality from ischaemic heart disease and cerebrovascular disease in Australia. *American Journal of Epidemiology* **113**: 404–12.
8. Levy, R.I. and Moskowitz, J. (1982) Cardiovascular research: decade of progress, a decade of promise. *Science* **217**: 121–9.
9. Whisnant, J.P. (1984) The decline of stroke. *Stroke* **15**: 160–8.
10. Posner, J.D., Gorman, K.M. and Woldow, A. (1984) Stroke in the elderly. I: Epidemiology. *Journal of the American Geriatrics Society* **32**: 95–102.
11. Marquardsen, J. (1978) The epidemiology of cerebrovascular disease. *Acta Neurologica Scandinavica* **67 (Suppl)**: 57–75.
12. Matsumoto, N., Whisnant, J.P., Kurland, L.T. and Ikazaki, H. (1973) Natural history of stroke in Rochester, Minnesota, 1955 through 1969. *Stroke* **4**: 20–9.

13. Whisnant, J.P., Fitzgibbons, J.P., Kurland, L.T. and Sayre, G.P. (1971) Natural history of stroke in Rochester, Minnesota, 1945 through 1954. *Stroke* 2: 11–22.
14. Goldner, J.C., Payne, G.H., Watson, F.R. and Parrish, H.M. (1967) Prognosis for survival after stroke. *American Journal of Medical Science* 253: 129–33.
15. Wylie, C.M. (1970) The community medicine of cerebrovascular disease. *Stroke* 1: 385–96.
16. Gibson, C.J. (1974) Epidemiology and patterns of care of stroke patients. *Archives of Physical Medicine and Rehabilitation* 55: 398–403.
17. Robins, M. and Baum, H.M. (1981) The National Survey of Stroke: incidence. *Stroke* 12 (**Suppl. 1**): 1–58.
18. Abu-Zeid, H.A.H., Choi, N.W. and Nelson, N.A. (1975) Epidemiological features of cerebrovascular disease in Manitoba: incidence by age, sex and residence with etiological implications. *Canadian Medical Association Journal* 113: 379–82.
19. Oxfordshire Community Stroke Project (1983) Incidence of stroke in Oxfordshire: first years' experience of a community stroke register. *British Medical Journal* 287: 713–16.
20. Keeler, K.C. (1956) Appraisal of patient goals in a community rehabilitation centre. *Archives of Physical Medicine and Rehabilitation* 37: 293–6.
21. Carroll, D. (1962) The disability in hemiplegia caused by cerebrovascular disease: serial study of 98 cases. *Journal of Chronic Disease* 15: 179–89.
22. Wylie, C.M. (1968) Age and the rehabilitation of stroke. *Journal of the American Geriatric Society* 16: 428–35.
23. Marquardsen, J. (1969) The natural history of acute cerebrovascular disease. *Acta Neurologica Scandinavica* 35 (Suppl. 38).
24. Cain, L.S. (1969) Determining factors that affect rehabilitation. *Journal of the American Geriatrics Society* 17: 595–604.
25. di Benedetto, M. (1974) Optimal care of the severely involved stroke patient. *Rehabilitation* 91: 27–36.
26. Shafer, S.Q., Brunn, B. and Richter, R.W. (1974) Stroke: early portents of functional recovery in black patients. *Archives of Physical Medicine and Rehabilitation* 55: 264–8.
27. Haerer, A.F. and Woolsey, P.C. (1975) Prognosis and quality of survival in a hospitalised stroke population from the South. *Stroke* 6: 543–8.
28. Richter, R.W., Bengen, B., Brunn, B. *et al.* (1977) The Harlem regional stroke program. *Archives of Physical Medicine and Rehabilitation* 58: 224–9.
29. Boyle, R.W. and Scalzitti, P.D. (1963) A study of 480 consecutive cases of cerebrovascular disease. *Archives of Physical Medicine and Rehabilitation* 44: 19–28.
30. Litman, T.J. (1964) Influence of age on physical rehabilitation. *Geriatrics* 19: 202–7.
31. Bourestom, N.C. (1967) Predictors of long term recovery in cerebrovascular disease. *Archives of Physical Medicine and Rehabilitation* 48: 415–19.
32. Anderson, T.P., Bourstom, N.C., Greenberg, F.R. and Hilyard, V.C. (1974) Predictive factors in stroke rehabilitation. *Archives of Physical Medicine and Rehabilitation* 55: 545–53.
33. Feigenson, J.S., McCarthy, M.I., Messe, P.D. *et al.* (1977) Stroke rehabilitation: factors predicting outcome and length of stay – an overview. *New York State Journal of Medicine* 77: 1426–30.
34. Andrews, K., Brochklehurst, J.C., Richards, B. and Laycock, P.J. (1982) The recovery of the severely disabled stroke patient. *Rheumatology and Rehabilitation* 21: 225–30.

35. Andrews, K., Brocklehurst, J.C., Richards, B. and Laycock, P.J. (1984) The influence of age on the clinical presentation and outcome of stroke. *International Rehabilitation Medicine* 6: 49–53.
36. Stern, P.H., McDowell, F.M., Miller, J.M. and Robinson, M. (1971) Factors influencing rehabilitation. *Stroke* 2: 213–15.
37. Feigenson, J.S., McCarthy, M.L., Greenberg, S.D. and Feigenson, W.D. (1977) Factors influencing outcome and length of stay in a stroke rehabilitation unit. II: Comparison of 318 screened and 248 unscreened patients. *Stroke* 8: 657–62.
38. Steinberg, F.U. (1973) The stroke registry: a prospective method of studying stroke. *Archives of Physical Medicine and Rehabilitation* 54: 31–5.
39. Baker, R.N., Schwartz, W.S. and Ramseyer, J.C. (1968) Prognosis among survivors of ischaemic stroke. *Neurology* 18: 933–41.
40. Adams, G.F. and Hurwitz, L.J. (1963) Mental barriers to recovery from stroke. *Lancet* 2: 533–7.
41. Adler, E. and Tal, E. (1965) Relationship between physical disability and functional capacity in hemiplegic patients. *Archives of Physical Medicine and Rehabilitation* 46: 745–52.
42. Haber, L.D. (1973) Diabling effects of chronic disease and improvement. II: Functional capacity limitations. *Journal of Chronic Disease* 26: 127–51.
43. McDowel, F. and Louis, S. (1971) Improvement in motor performance in paretic and paralysed extremeties following non-embolic cerebral infarction. *Stroke* 2: 395–9.
44. Hewer, R.L. (1976) Stroke rehabilitation. In: *Stroke* (Eds: Gillingham, F., Mawdsley, C. and Williams, A.E.). Churchill Livingstone, London.
45. Bard, G. and Hirschberg, G.H.G. (1965) Recovery of voluntary motion in the upper extremity following hemiplegia. *Archives of Physical Medicine and Rehabilitation* 46: 567–72.
46. Miglietta, O., Chung, T–S and Rajeswaramma, V. (1976) Fate of stroke patients transferred to a long-term rehabilitation hospital. *Stroke* 7: 76–7.
47. Adams, C.F. and McComb, S.G. (1953) Assessment and prognosis in hemiplegia. *Lancet* 2: 266–9.
48. Hurwitz, L.J. and Adams, G.F. (1972) Rehabilitation of hemiplegia: indices, assessment and prognosis. *British Medical Journal* 1: 94–8.
49. Andrews, K., Brocklehurst, J.C., Richards, B. and Laycock, P.J. (1981) The rate and recovery from stroke and its measurement. *International Rehabilitation Medicine* 3: 151–61.
50. Moskowitz, E., Lightbody, F.E.H. and Freitag, N.S. (1972) Long term follow up of a post-stroke patient. *Archives of Physical Medicine and Rehabilitation* 53: 167–72.
51. Katz, S., Ford, A.B., Chinn, A.B. and Newill, V.A. (1966) Prognosis after stroke: long term follow up of 159 patients. *Medicine (Baltimore)* 45: 236–46.
52. Hatano, S. (1976) Experience from multicentre stroke register. *Bulletin of the World Organisation* 54: 541–53.
53. Brocklehurst, J.C., Andrews, K., Richards, B. and Laycock, P.J. (1978) How much physical therapy for patients with stroke? *British Medical Journal* 1: 1307–10.
54. Lowenthal, M., Tobis, J.S. and Howard, I.R. (1959) An analysis of rehabilitation needs and prognosis of 232 cases of cerebrovascular accident. *Archives of Physical Medicine and Rehabilitation* 40: 183–6.
55. Lehmann, J.F., Delateur, B., Fowler, R.S. *et al.* (1975) Does stroke rehabilitation affect outcome? *Archives of Physical Medicine and Rehabilitation* 56: 375–82.

56. Adams, G.F. and Merrett, J.D. (1961) Prognosis and survival in the aftermath of hemiplegia. *British Medical Journal* **1**: 309–14.
57. Geltner, L. and Lupo, G. (1964) Clinical problems of cerebrovascular accidents. *Israel Medical Journal* **23**: 241–8.
58. Pitner, S.E. and Mance, C.J. (1973) An evaluation of stroke intensive care: results in a municipal hospital. *Stroke* **4**: 737–41.
59. Anderson, T.P., Balbridge, M. and Ettinger, M.G. (1979) Quality of care for completed stroke without rehabilitation. *Archives of Physical Medicine and Rehabilitation* **60**: 103–7.
60. Andrews, K., Brocklehurst, J.C., Richards, B. and Laycock, P.J. (1982) Stroke: does side matter? *Rheumatology and Rehabilitation* **21**: 175–8.
61. Hoberman, M. and Springer, C.F. (1958) Rehabilitation of the 'permanently and totally disabled' patient. *Archives of Physical Medicine and Rehabilitation* **39**: 235–40.
62. Feldman, D., Lee, P.R., Unterecker, J. *et al.* (1962) A comparison of functionally orientated medical care and formal rehabilitation in the management of patients with hemiplegia due to cerebrovascular disease. *Journal of Chronic Disease* **15**: 297–310.
63. Waylonis, G.W., Keith, M.W. and Aseff, J.N. (1973) Stroke rehabilitation in a midwestern county. *Archives of Physical Medicine and Rehabilitation* **54**: 151–5.
64. Smith, D.S., Goldberg, E., Ashburn, A. *et al.* (1981) Remedial therapy after stroke: a randomised controlled trial. *British Medical Journal* **282**: 517–20.
65. Stern, P.H., McDowell, F.M., Miller, J.M. and Robinson, M. (1969) Effect of facilitation exercise technique in stroke rehabilitation. *Archives of Physical Medicine and Rehabilitation* **51**: 526–31.
66. Chin, P.L. (1982) Physical techniques in stroke rehabilitation. *Journal of the Royal College of Physicians of London* **16**: 165–9.
67. Cochrane, A. (1970) The burden of cerebrovascular disease. *British Medical Journal* **3**: 165.
68. Brocklehurst, J.C., Andrews, K., Richards, B. and Laycock, P.J. (1978) Why admit stroke patients to hospital? *Age and Ageing* **7**: 100–8.
69. Aho, K., Harmsen, P., Hatano, S. *et al.* (1980) Cerebrovascular disease in the community: results of a WHO collaboration study. *Bulletin of the World Health Organisation* **58**: 345–52.
70. Bamford, J., Sandercock, P., Warlow, C. and Gray, M. (1986) Why are patients with acute stroke admitted to hospital? *British Medical Journal* **292**: 1369–72.
71. Warren, M.D., Cooper, J. and Warren, J.L. (1967) Problems of emergency admission to London hospitals. *British Journal of Preventative Social Medicine* **21**: 141–9.
72. Wylie, C.M., Teich, K.W. and Slee, V.N. (1969) Evaluating the stroke effort in a regional medical program. *American Journal of Public Health* **59**: 974–81.
73. Sutherland, A. (1972) *A study of Long Stay Admissions in the Acute Medical Wards of the Aberdeen Hospitals.* Scottish Health Services Study No. 32, HMSO.
74. Waylonis, G.W. (1973) The community hospital in stroke care. *Archives of Physical Medicine and Rehabilitation* **54**: 151–5.
75. Truscott, B.L. (1972) Health care delivery in the community. *Journal of the American Medical Association* **221**: 289–91.
76. Taylor, R.R. (1970) Acute stroke demonstration project in a community hospital. *Journal of the South Carolina Medical Association* **66**: 225–7.
77. Drake, W.E., Hamilton, M.J., Carlsson, M. and Blumenkrantz, J. (1973)

Acute stroke management and patient outcome. *Stroke* **4**: 933-45.
78. Cooper, S.W., Olivet, J.A. and Woolsey, F.M. (1972) Establishment and operation of a combined intensive care unit. *New York State Journal of Medicine* **72**: 2215-20.
79. Andrews, K. and Brocklehurst, J.C. (1987) *Geriatric Medicine in the 1980s*. Kings Fund, London.
80. Stevens, R.S. and Isaacs, B. (1984) Stroke rehabilitation units in the United Kingdom. *Health Trends* **16**: 61-3.
81. Christie, D. (1976) Rationalisation of hospital services for stroke patients. *Australia and New Zealand Medical Journal* **6**: 407-10.
82. Blower, P. and Ali, S. (1979) A stroke unit in a general hospital: the Greenwich experience. *British Medical Journal* **2**: 644-6.
83. McCann, B.C. and Culbertson, R.A. (1976) Comparison of two systems of stroke rehabilitation in a general hospital. *Journal of the American Geriatrics Society* **24**: 211-16.
84. Rosenthal, H.A. (1961) Rehabilitation of the hemiplegic patient. *Pennsylvania Medical Journal* **64**: 56-9.
85. Anderson, T.P. and Kottke, F.J. (1978) Stroke rehabilitation: a reconsideration of some common attitudes. *Archives of Physical Medicine and Rehabilitation* **59**: 175-81.
86. Adams, G.F. (1974) In: *Cerebrovascular Disease in the Ageing Brain*. Churchill Livingstone, Edinburgh.
87. Dow, R.S., Dick, H.L. and Crowell, F.A. (1974) Failures and success in a stroke program. *Stroke* **5**: 40-7.
88. Schuman, J.E., Beattie, E.J., Steed, D.A. *et al.* (1980) Rehabilitation and geriatric teaching programs: clinical efficiency in a skilled nursing facility. *Archives of Physical Medicine and Rehabilitation* **61**: 310-15.
89. Gordon, E.E. and Kohn, K.H. (1966) Evaluation of rehabilitation in the hemiplegic patient. *Journal of Chronic Disease* **19**: 3-16.
90. Garraway, W.M., Akhtar, A.J., Prescott, R.J. and Hockey, L. (1980) Management of acute stroke in the elderly: preliminary results of a controlled trial. *British Medical Journal* **1**: 1040-3.
91. Garraway, W.M., Akhtar, A.J., Hockey, L. and Prescott, R.J. (1980) Management of acute stroke in the elderly: follow up study of a controlled trial. *British Medical Journal* **2**: 827-9.
92. Wade, D.T. and Hewer, R.L. (1985) Hospital admission for stroke: who, for how long, and to what effect? *Journal of Epidemiology and Community Health* **39**: 347-52.
93. Wade, D.T., Hewer, R.L., Skilbeck, C.E. *et al.* (1985) Control care of home-care services for stroke patients. *Lancet* **1**: 323-6.
94. Garraway, W.M. (1976) The size of the problem of stroke in Scotland. In: *Stroke* (Eds: Gillingham, F.J., Mawdsley, C. and Williams, A.E.). Churchill Livingstone, Edinburgh.
95. Brocklehurst, J.C., Morris, P., Andrews, K., Richards, B. and Laycock, P.J. (1981) Social effects of stroke. *Social Science and Medicine* **15A**: 35-9.
96. Labi, M.L.C., Phillips, T.F. and Gresham, G.E. (1980) Psychosocial disability in physically restored long-term stroke survivors. *Archives of Physical Medicine Rehabilitation* **61**: 561-5.
97. Hyman, M.D. (1975) Some psychological factors affecting disability among ambulatory patients. *Journal of Chronic Disease* **28**: 199-216.
98. Folstein, M.F., Maiberger, R. and McHugh, P.R. (1977) Mood disorders as a specific complication of stroke. *Journal of Neurology, Neurosurgery and Psychiatry* **40**: 1018-20.

99. Griffiths, V.E. (1975) Volunteer scheme for dysphasic patients. *British Medical Journal* **3**: 633–5.
100. Griffiths, V.E. (1980) Observation on patients dysphasic after a stroke. *British Medical Journal* **2**: 1608–9.
101. Griffiths, V.E. and Miller, C.L. (1980) Volunteer stroke scheme for dysphasic patients with stroke. *British Medical Journal* **2**: 1605–7.

18

Motor aspects of stroke

Introduction

A number of neurophysiological approaches to stroke rehabilitation have been developed and are described in specialist textbooks [1–7]. They all have in common a concentration on improving the function of the affected side, using a bilateral approach, emphasizing the importance of sensory input, utilizing reflex patterns and involving a large amount of therapist–patient contact.

The major contribution that can be made on any general ward is to avoid the complications which prevent optimization of spontaneous recovery, and this is the area to be dealt with in this chapter. The two major barriers to recovery are spasticity and the painful hemiplegic shoulder, and clinical experience shows that both of these are basically preventable by good nursing in the early days.

Spasticity

Spasticity occurs in the strongest muscle groups (i.e. those resisting the effect of gravity). The size of the muscles gives some clues; for example, the effect on latissimus dorsi results in the traditional hemiplegic posture of retraction of the shoulder and adduction of the arm, while that on glutimus maximus produces a retraction and outward rotation of the hip. In addition there is flexion of the elbow, wrist and fingers; and extension of the knee and plantar flexion at the ankle (Fig. 18.1). Tone may remain flaccid even after the acute phase and this has a poor prognosis.

Management of spasticity

Lying in bed

The nursing management is to control abnormal tonal patterns. Supine lying increases extensor tone and should be used only for short

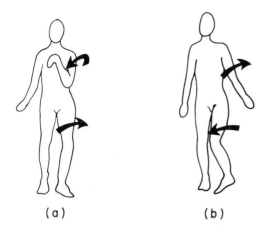

(a)   (b)

Fig. 18.1   (a) Dominant tonal pattern in stroke, and (b) corrective positioning

periods to relieve pressure. When lying supine the affected shoulder
should be supported (protracted) by a pillow and the arm held in
extension and outward rotation with the wrist and fingers extended
(Fig. 18.2a). Basically if the thumb is pointing away from the body the
arm is in a good position. It is important to support the arm on a
pillow to maintain the correct position of the shoulder.

Preventing the arm from returning to the dominant tonal pattern
can be difficult, though less of a problem in the early stages. One way
of overcoming this is to use an inflatable splint (Fig. 18.3) to keep the
arm in position. This probably also helps by retaining heat, which in
turn helps to lessen the spasticity. The other advantage of this splint is
that it is effective in keeping the fingers extended and abducted. To
control the tone in the leg the knee is semi-flexed supported by a pillow
and the leg internally rotated (Fig. 18.2a).

Since tonal pattern is influenced by the tonic neck reflexes, the head
should be kept in the neutral position or turned to the affected side.
The decerebrate pattern of tone is for the arm on the side to which the
head is turned to extend, with concomitant flexion in the contralateral
arm – the sword fencers pose. Flexion of the neck encourages flexion
of the body, extension encourages extensor tone. The head in stroke
tends to look away from the affected side and this helps to increase the
flexion of the affected arm. Turning the head towards the affected
side helps to control the tonal component caused by the tonic neck
reflexes.

Side-lying (Figs. 18.2 a and b) is a more neutral position, although
there are several points to observe:

1. It is important to ensure that there is good support for the back by

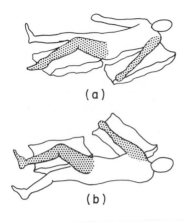

(a)

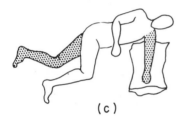

(b)

(c)

Fig. 18.2   Bed positioning for the hemiplegic patient: (a) lying on back; (b) lying on normal side; (c) lying on hemiplegic side

  pillows, otherwise there is a tendency to roll into the supine position, resulting in an increase in the dominant tonal pattern.
2. Whichever side the patient is lying on, it is important to aim for
  extension of the affected arm and semi-flexion of the leg.
3. When lying on the non-affected side the arm should be supported
  on several pillows to give good control at the shoulder (one pillow
  is rarely sufficient to maintain a neutral position) and the leg
  supported by a pillow allowing inward rotation (too many pillows
  will produce external rotation).
4. When lying on the affected side the shoulder should be held in a
  protracted position to avoid being trapped under the weight of the
  body.
5. The patient may find it more comfortable if the non-affected leg is
  supported on a pillow.

Bed activities

When sitting in bed a position as upright as possible should be maintained, assisted by placing a pillow under the knee and supporting the

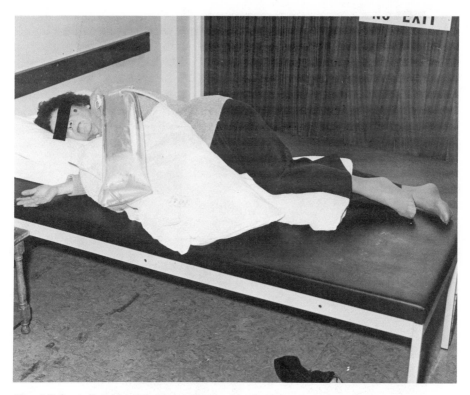

Fig. 18.3 Inflatable splint to assist positioning

arm in extension on several pillows.

To move across the bed the patient lifts the buttocks whilst pressing down on the bed with the good hand and with the foot in a bridging type movement. It may be necessary for the helper to hold the knees and feet in position with one arm whilst the other supports the affected scapular to assist the movement. This is more effective and less damaging (to both patient and helper) than being lifted).

One technique for rolling over in bed is for the patient to lie on his back, clasp the hands together and reach forwards (to protect the shoulder), cross the legs, look in the direction to which the movement is to be taken, turn the head in that direction and roll.

Sitting posture

Sitting posture is also important. The principle is to sit erect with the hips, knees and ankles at right angles. If the patient falls to the affected side, it is highly unlikely he will be able to stand until a good sitting balance has been achieved.

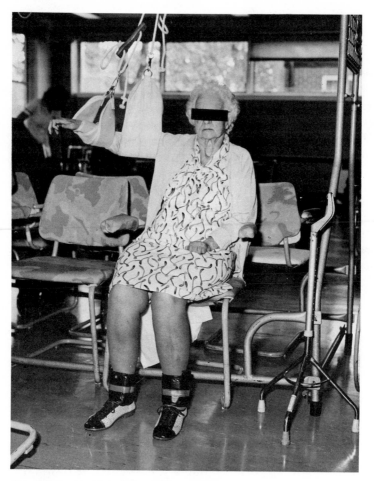

Fig. 18.4 Hemiplegic arm suspension

To maintain sitting balance a number of techniques have been used. For example, the patient may be supported by pillows to maintain the affected arm elevated, protracted and extended. Alternatively use can be made of a vacuum posture controller (see Chapter 3).

A number of other aids are available to maintain the arm in a good position. These include a gutter attachment to the arm of the chair; an inflatable splint; a sling supported by springs suspended from a bar (Fig. 18.4); a special table attached to the arm of the chair for support; or a padded cushion, attached to the arm of the chair, extending to the axilla [8].

A mirror or video tape can be used to provide visual feedback. There are, however, problems in using a mirror for visual feedback in stroke since many patients with balance problems also have unilateral visual neglect or spatial problems. Since the image in the mirror of the affected side falls into the blind field, the patient is often unable to appreciate his mistakes.

As static sitting balance improves the dynamic techniques described in Chapter 15 for the management of balance can be introduced; that is, starting from a broad, firm base and progressing by decreasing the size and stability of the sitting base.

Standing

Poor transferring technique is a common cause of the painful hemiplegic shoulder (see later). Standing the patient by dragging on the affected arm or lifting under the axilla disrupts the weak shoulder and must be avoided at all cost. The following are some appropriate standing techniques:

1. The attendant stands in front of the seated patient and supports his knees between hers (Fig. 18.5). The patient then puts his arm(s) around the helper, either at the level of the waist or neck according to their respective heights, and the helper supports the patient either at hip or scapula level. By the helper leaning backwards and the patient leaning forwards, the patient can stand without very much effort.
2. The patient places his feet under the front edge of the chair, leans forward to bring the centre of gravity over the feet, and stands by pressing down on the arm of the chair.
3. In another technique similar to (2) above, the hands are clasped

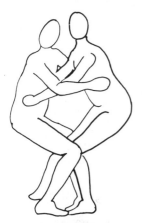

Fig. 18.5 Standing technique (patient on right, carer on left)

together and extended forwards before standing. This is a good use of the bilateral approach.
4. Another modification of this is to place the affected hand on the knee and press down on this with the good hand whilst standing.

Standing balance

It is normal practice for sitting balance to be achieved before standing is attempted, and for standing balance to be achieved before walking is attempted. There are slight difficulties with this approach since about 60 per cent of elderly stroke patients have had balance disturbances before they had the stroke and therefore may never gain good standing balance. Nevertheless attempts should be made to obtain a reasonable standing balance as described in Chapter 15.

Walking

Once a reasonable static balance has been achieved the patient can practice a few steps. There are numerous approaches to this. A few therapists with neurophysiological idealism insist that no walking aid should be used. For many elderly stroke patients a less dogmatic approach is required. The following are some possible techniques:

1. The patient stands facing the helper with his arms around her waist; she grips his forearms with the upper part of her arms whilst controlling pelvic movement with her hands.
2. The helper walks behind the patient controlling the pelvic movement whilst the patient walks with the hands clasped and extended out in front of him.
3. The helper walks beside the patient on his affected side and holds the affected hand in a handshake grip, keeping the patient's thumb uppermost and the arm externally rotated. The helper keeps the arm externally rotated and the shoulder protracted by passing her other hand behind the patient's elbow and placing the back of the hand on the patient's chest.
4. Many patients gain confidence to walk between parallel bars, though this does tend to cause a lean to the affected side.
5. Some patients feel more secure in walking in a tall frame which has gutters (a gutter frame) or a broad, flat surface at upper arm height (a pulpit frame). These have the advantage of allowing weight to be taken through both arms whilst the centre of gravity passes between the feet. An alternative frame is one with a central vertical bar for the patient to grip with both hands.
6. The use of sticks/canes or quadsticks/tripod have become unpopular with many physiotherapists because they result in the

centre of gravity falling between the good leg and the support, causing the affected hip to retract producing an abnormal stiff-legged hemiplegic gait. There is also the danger that the legs of the quadstick/tripod catch on furniture and carpets. Several patients treated by a full neurophysiological approach have commented that they not only feel safer but can walk quicker with a stick. These patients seem satisfied to sacrifice an aesthetically good gait for effective functional ambulation.

Some therapists compromise by allowing a tall walking stick with the handle pointing away from the patient, or a long pole, arguing that they are being used for balance rather than weight bearing. Observation suggests that this still results in the aid being used for weight bearing.

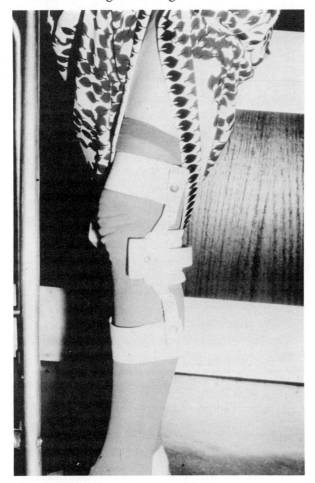

Fig. 18.6 Swedish knee cage

7. There are a few other approaches which, while not commonly used, may benefit a few patients. One is to use a stick held by both hands in front of the patient to encourage a bilateral approach and to ensure that the centre of gravity falls between the feet. This can be difficult for some patients but has had very impressive results with others. Another approach is to use a long stick on a wheeled base. This allows the patient to use the stick in the non-affected hand for balance without having to lift the stick. Some have used this in the affected hand to provide weight bearing through the hemiplegic side.

All of these approaches have advantages and disadvantages. The most appropriate technique is the one that the patient finds the most acceptable. Most elderly patients seem to prefer a safe technique even if the gait pattern leaves much to be desired aesthetically.

The knee that gives way

One problem occasionally encountered is the knee which suddenly gives way when the patient is walking, often at the end of the day when tired or distracted. There are a number of devices which might be of help:

- Long-leg rigid plastic splints certainly give rigidity to the knee but are cumbersome and unsightly. They prevent the knee from bending and create difficulties for transferring from a chair.
- The Swedish knee cage (Fig. 18.6) is light but has the disadvantages of limiting bending of the knee and being bulky. There is at least one report of a deep-vein thrombosis associated with wearing this orthosis.
- An elasticated knee support with hinged lateral supports (Fig. 18.7) is light, allows the knee to be flexed for sitting and the hinge can have a backstop to prevent hyperextension.

Footdrop

Theoretically, footdrop is preventable. A bed cradle for the foot region of the bed ensures that bedclothes do not exacerbate the foot drop. The patient should sit with the ankle maintained at right-angles. If it is impossible to stop the foot sliding forwards, then a wedged foot rest will keep the ankle at right-angles even when the leg is more extended. Sitting the patient in a high chair makes it less likely that the leg will extend.

Ankle–foot orthoses are available in a number of forms and help to improve walking gait [9–12]. They tend to change the dynamics of

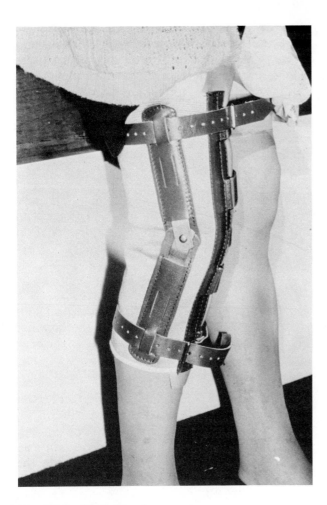

Fig. 18.7 Cinch knee brace

body positioning, produce unwanted changes in the contralateral limbs [13, 14] and may account for the early arthritic changes, discomfort and fatigue found in the unaffected leg [13]. These orthoses decreases the stride and step lengths and cause widening of the step width and foot angles in normal individuals [15], though whether this is relevant in practical stroke management is uncertain.

Calipers are still often used for foot drop but have several disadvantages. They are heavy, require the need for specially adapted shoes, emphasize the disability and, especially those with a toe spring, exacerbate the foot drop by putting stretch on the calf muscles.

Modern orthoses try to overcome these difficulties. The lightweight below-knee iron with an Exeter coil requires only slight modification

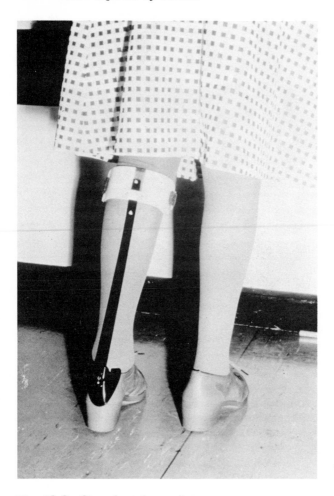

Fig. 18.8 Clasp foot drop splint

to the shoe but the spring loading of the coil increases the muscle spasm. The shoe clasp ankle-foot orthosis (Fig. 18.8) is a lightweight aid which straps around the upper calf and is attached by a bar to a clip attached to the back of the shoe. The shoes need to have a broad back and be of the lace-up type. The advantages are that it is light and does not require special shoe adaptation. The clasp does tend to wear the back of the shoe and is not very effective where there is marked spasm.

The polypropylene shoe-insert orthosis (Fig. 18.9) is a static splint which needs careful design for the individual patient, otherwise it is uncomfortable to wear. It has the advantages that it is light and can easily be hidden by trousers or more easily disguised by stockings than

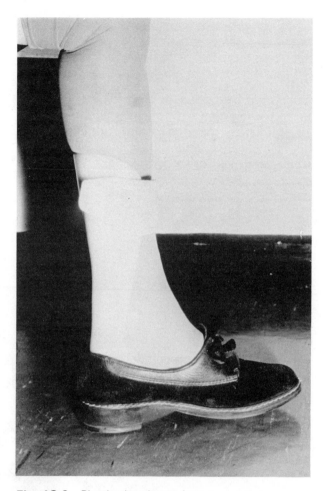

Fig. 18.9   Plastic shoe-insert foot drop splint

other forms of foot-drop splint. Some have a spiral component to inhibit inversion of the foot.

If a static shoe-insert orthosis is used it is important to angle the heel of the shoe to provide rolling on heel contact since the ankle is now in a fixed position.

Wheelchairs

The traditional one-arm-drive wheelchair provides control of the direction of turn by having two drive mechanisms on one side – push one rim and the chair goes left, push the other and it goes right, push both and it goes forward. Many patients do find this an effective mobility aid. There are several difficulties: the chair is heavy; many elderly people find it difficult to drive; the effort of pushing with the non-affected arm increases the tone in the affected limbs; and it encourages poor posture. Many patients still use the good foot to propel the chair, and so a lighter, foldable, more easily manoeuvrable, and cheaper, wheelchair would be more appropriate.

One very effective, though expensive, wheelchair suitable for the mentally alert stroke patient who needs good mobility is a lever-driven chair (Fig. 18.10). This uses a lever system as the drive mechanism as well as to guide the chair, and has forward, backward and neutral gears.

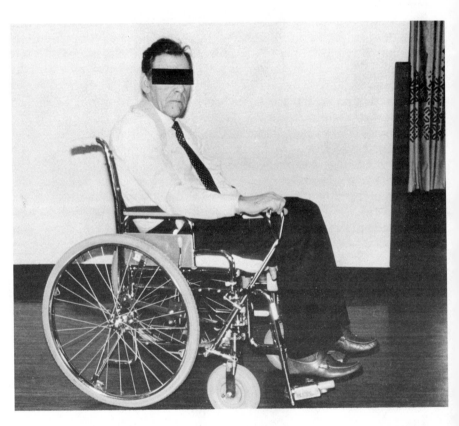

Fig. 18.10   Lever-driven one-arm-drive wheelchair

Controlling spasticity

Avoidance of exacerbating factors

Incorrect positioning, rapid or sudden changes in position, sudden loud noises, cold environments, anxiety or other forms of physical or emotional irritation should be avoided.

Heat

Heat helps to relieve pain, increase the blood supply, act as a non-specific relaxant and decrease spasticity [16]. It may be used in contractures to increase the extensibility of collagen [17].

Cooling

Ice locally decreases spasticity [18–20], probably by a neurological response from the skin afferents rather than by a direct response on the muscles [21]. Ice packs are the most convenient method of cooling the limb, or it can be immersed in iced water or sprayed with ethyl chloride. If ice packs are used it is important that crushed ice is used since ice cubes produce areas of local pressure. Chlorofluoromethane or 20% benzocaine sprays for 15 seconds [22], though ineffective for prolonged cooling, provide short-term relief to allow the physiotherapy techniques to be carried out.

Theoretically, the longer the limb is cooled the greater the effect on the spasticity. However, there is a danger, especially in the elderly, that prolonged cooling over a large area might produce ischaemia or hypothermia. In practice, muscle relaxation for up to three hours can be produced by cooling for half an hour. It is of note that those patients whose spasticity responds well to cooling also seem to be the group who respond to drug control of spasticity.

Ice can also be used to increase tone in the flaccid limb by stroking over the corresponding dermatome [23–26], while reflex relaxation of the spastic group can be produced by icing over the opposing muscle groups.

Vibration

Vibration over the dermatome opposing the dominant spastic pattern similarly produces muscle tone inhibition [27–30].

Splinting

The value of splinting of hemiplegic limbs has been debated for many years. For instance, the traditional concept has been to splint the hand

[31–33], although it has yet to be decided whether this should be on the palmar or dorsal surfaces [31, 34, 35]. Some have argued that a neuro-physiological approach is more appropriate to splinting [1, 36, 37], whereas others have combined splinting with a neurophysiological approach [34, 35, 38, 39].

The types of hand splinting vary: foam finger-spreaders [40], poly-propylene palmar splints, posterior dynamic splints [41] and inflat-able splints [3] are all used.

The advantages of splinting include the provision of appropriate joint positioning, inhibition of spasticity and contractures, and the relief of pain. Gentle, gradual stretching decreases spasticity [34, 35, 39], but misapplied splints are likely to cause deformities, stretch weak muscles and increase spasticity.

Passive splinting using weight-bearing plasters is particularly useful when severe spasticity progresses to contracture of the hand [42, 43] or the leg [44, 45]. This requires great skill since it is easy to produce abnormal tonal patterns if the splints are not correctly placed. The inflatable splint has the advantage that it is self-adjusting as the tone relaxes and the position of the limb can be observed through the clear plastic of the inflated sleeve.

The painful shoulder

Care of the shoulder is particularly important if there is to be a chance of good recovery in the arm. A painful shoulder following a stroke is unfortunately common, being found in 30–70 per cent of stroke patients [46–48]. The fact that there is such a wide range in the pre-valence suggests that a painful shoulder is preventable, and this fits in with clinical experience.

The need for a wide range of movement at the shoulder joint requires that the humeral head has very little area of contact with the glenoid fossa (Fig. 18.11). The humeral head is therefore vulnerable to subluxation in stroke since it is largely kept in place by muscle action.

To be free of pain and equal to the demands of normal living, mobility of the shoulder depends on maintenance of the joint plane between scapula and humerus, good control of the supraspinatus muscle, an intact rotator cuff ligament, and a mobile scapula. The two main causes of shoulder pain are related to abnormalities of muscle tone.

Flaccidity of the shoulder muscles results in sagging of the humerus within the lax shoulder girdle and stretching of the capsule, tendons and muscles. However, contrast arthrography of the painful shoulder has shown that in about one-third of patients there are actual tears in

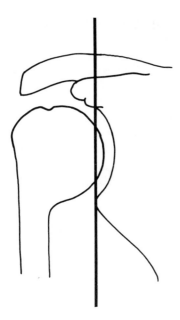

Fig. 18.11 Small area of head of humerus in glenoid fossa

the rotator cuff or the biceps tendon [49]. The flaccid shoulder tends to be painless until this damange has occurred. Once the tissues are torn then fibrosis results in a fixed shoulder.

For abduction of the glenohumeral joint to take place the scapular must rotate upwards and the humeral head be depressed and rotated externally. Spasticity in the muscles of the shoulder girdle prevents this free movements. Stretching the muscles by movement produces protective spasm, so exacerbating the spasticity and producing pain. For this reason it is the patient with spasticity who is more likely to complain of shoulder pain than the one with flaccidity [47, 50].

Management

Treatment of the condition is disappointing. Hazelman [51] could find little difference in the outcome between local steroid injections, physiotherapy or manipulation under anaesthetic, and McLaughlin [52] reported rotator cuff tears occurring commonly after manipulation under anaesthesia.

There is, however, some evidence that physiotherapy can reduce the recovery time [53]. The immediate treatment is to deal with the spasticity and make sure that further damage is prevented by corrective positioning. Analgesic drugs may be necessary, though these are very limited in their effectiveness. This can be supplemented by using ice packs or superficial heat to relieve the pain and spasm. Ultrasound [54–57], electromagnetic induction or shortwave diathermy have an effect on the deeper tissues. More persistent pain may require intra-articular injections of a local anaesthetic and a steroid. All of these require specialist management.

It is essential that good care is taken of the shoulder at all times. The patient should be trained in the care of his own shoulder. This includes training to keep the arm in the correct position throughout the day and when in bed. He should also be taught techniques to maintain mobility of the shoulder, including (Fig. 18.12) intertwining the fingers of the

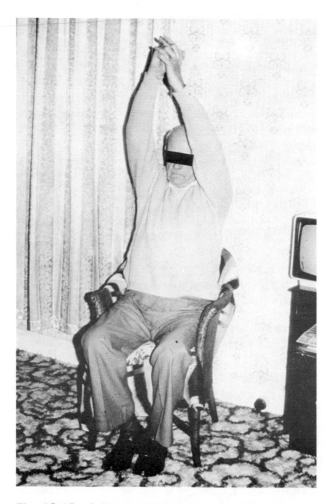

Fig. 18.12   Self care of the hemiplegic shoulder

normal hand between those of the affected hand (to help to release the spasticity in the rest of the arm); then extending the arms, pushing forwards with the arms (to relieve spasticity in the shoulder girdle muscles); followed by elevating the arms. The shoulder joint should not be abducted in the presence of spasticity since this will increase the spasticity when the scapular starts to rotate.

Slings

A common response to the painful shoulder has been to splint it, using slings, to support the subluxing shoulder and prevent stretching of the capsule. Slings, unfortunately, do not produce an improvement in the range of movement, the shoulder pain, the subluxation or the peripheral nerve damage [58]. The traditional triangular sling can, indeed, be counterproductive for the following reasons:

- The sling does not prevent subluxation since the elbow cannot be kept at right-angles with the forearm horizontal for very long – it tends to slip into the subluxed position.
- The arm is positioned in internal rotation and flexion, encouraging the dominant tonal pattern.
- The sling encourages spasticity of the shoulder and produces pressure on the neck.
- Balance is made difficult by encouraging an asymmetrical approach.
- The sling interferes with sensory input, disturbes the body image and discourages use of the arm.

Slings interfere with the distribution of body weight and inhibit redevelopment of the normal walking pattern, mainly because the sling positions the arm in front of the body [58–60]; although this is probably less relevant for gait characteristics over a normal walking distance [15].

If a sling is required then the simplest and most effective form is the figure-of-eight support. This is a soft foam support which passes over both shoulders and under the axillae in a continuous figure of eight. It supports the humeral head, encourages protraction of the shoulder whilst allowing the arm to move freely. Some therapists add a pad under the affected axilla to assist abduction of the arm. It is uncertain why this sling should be effective since it does not prevent subluxation according to radiological findings. It possibly creates its effect by alerting the carers to avoid damage to the shoulder.

Prevention

The fact that the painful shoulder is so difficult to treat emphasizes the importance of preventative measures and good shoulder care. All helpers must understand the dangers of suddenly moving the affected arm. The patient should not be helped to stand either by lifting under the axillae or by pulling on his arm. The correct technique for standing has been described earlier.

Since recovery takes place from proximal to distal, trunk and shoulder recovery should be considered early in the management. The techniques need to be carried out throughout the whole 24 hours if shoulder pain is to be prevented. The shoulder should not be allowed to rotate inwards. If the patient complains of pain during handling then this usually implies that the shoulder is wrongly rotated. One helpful clue to correct position is that with outward rotation of the arm and shoulder the thumb points away from the body. To assist good arm positioning when sitting, a coloured stripe can be placed down the centre of the table. If the affected hand strays across the stripe then the shoulder has turned into the unwanted pattern of inward rotation.

It is important to ensure that the elbow, too, is in a good position. Satisfactory control of the elbow will not be achieved unless there is good shoulder recovery. Similarly, hand recovery will be unsatisfactory until there is good elbow movement. The therapist will normally use techniques of elbow stabilization and weight bearing in the lying, sitting and crawling positions. This may be assisted by inflatable splints [3], with progressively shorter splints being used as the arm recovers. For example, a half-arm-length splint can be used to provide splinting of the wrist and fingers when the elbow is stable; and a hand splint can be used to maintain finger positioning while the wrist is mobilized.

It is essential that all those who come into contact with the stroke patient ensure that the above basic concepts are carried out. Excellent physiotheraphy and nursing care of the stroke patient is wasted if others, including relatives, damage the shoulder or encourage spasticity through lack of knowledge of simple correct procedures.

References

1. Bobath, B. (1978) *Adult Hemiplegia: Evaluation and Treatment* (2nd Edn.). William Heinneman, London.
2. Brunstrom, S. (1970) *Movement Therapy in Hemiplegia: a Neurophysiological Approach.* Harper and Row, New York.
3. Johnstone, M. (1983) In: *Restoration of Motor Function in the Stroke Patient* (2nd Edn.). Churchill Livingstone, Edinburgh.

4. O'Brien, M.T. and Pallett, P.J. (1978) *Total Care of the Stroke Patient.* Little, Brown and Co., Boston.
5. Eggers, O. (1983) *Occupational Therapy in the Treatment of Adult Hemiplegia.* William Heinneman, London.
6. Licht, S. (1975) *Stroke and Its Rehabilitation.* Waverly Press, Baltimore.
7. Mulley, G.P. (1986) *Practical Management of Stroke.* Croom Helm, London.
8. Steed, A. (1986) Using the Steed cushion in the treatment of flaccid hemiplegia. *Occupational Therapy*, February: 34–8.
9. Perry, J. (1969) The mechanics of walking in hemiplegia. *Clinical Orthopaedics* **63**: 23–31.
10. Perry, J. (1969) Lower extremity bracing. *Clinical Orthopaedics* **63**: 32–8.
11. Saunders, J.B., Inman, V.T. and Ebenhart, H.D. (1953) The major determinants in normal and pathological gait. *Journal of Bone and Joint Surgery* **35A**: 543–8.
12. Lehman, J.F.G. (1966) Lower limb orthotics. In: *Orthotics* (Ed: Licht, S.). Waverly Press, Baltimore.
13. Magora, A., Robin, G.C., Rozin, R. *et al.* (1973) Investigations of gait. 5: Effect of below knee brace on contralateral unbraced leg. *Electromyography and Clinical Nuerophysiology* **13**: 355–61.
14. Smidt, G.L. and Mommens, M.A. (1980) System of reporting and comparing influence of ambulation aids on gait. *Physical Therapy* **60**: 551–8.
15. Opara, C.U., Lavangie, P.K. and Nelson, D.L. (1985) Effects of selected assistive devices on normal distance gait characteristics. *Physical Therapy* **65**: 1188–91.
16. Lehmann, J.F., Warren, C.G. and Schain, S.M. (1974) Therapeutic heat and cold. *Clinical Orthopaedics* **99**: 207–47.
17. Lehmann, J.F., Masock, A.J. and Warren, C.G. (1970) Effects of therapeutic temperature on tendon extensibility. *Archives of Physical Medicine and Rehabilitation* **51**: 481–8.
18. Lee, J.M. and Warren, M.P. (1978) In: *Cold Therapy in Rehabilitation.* Bell and Hyman, London.
19. Hartviksen, K. (1962) Ice therapy in spasticity. *Acta Neurologica Scandinavica* **38** (Suppl. 3): 79–84.
20. Kelly, M. (1969) Effectiveness of cryotherapy technique on spasticity. *Physical Therapy* **49**: 349–53.
21. Miglietta, O. (1973) Action of cold on spasticity. *American Journal of Physical Medicine* **52**: 198–205.
22. Sabbahi, M.A. and Powers, W.R. (1981) Topical anaesthesia: a possible treatment method for spasticity. *Archives of Physical Medicine and Rehabilitation* **62**: 310–14.
23. Clarke, A.M. (1966) The effect of stimulation on certain skin areas on extensor motor neurones in the phasic reaction to stretch reflex in normal human subjects. *Electroencephalography and Clinical Neurophysiology* **21**: 185–93.
24. Eldred, E. and Hagbarth, K.E. (1954) Facilitation and inhibition of gamma efferents by stimulation of certain skin areas. *Journal of Neurophysiology* **17**: 59–65.
25. Clendenin, A. and Szumski, A.J. (1971) Influence of cutaneous ice application on single motor units in humans. *Physical Therapy* **51**: 166–75.
26. Spicer, S.D. and Matyas, T.A. (1980) Facilitation of tonic vibratory reflex by cutaneous stimulation. *American Journal of Physical Medicine* **59**: 223–31.
27. de Domenico, G. (1979) Tonic vibratory reflex: What is it? Can we use it? *Physiotherapy* **65**: 44–8.
28. Bishop, B. (1975) Vibratory stimulation. III: Possible applications of vibration

in the treatment of motor dysfunction. *Physical Therapy* **55**: 139–43.
29. Eklund, G. and Steen, M. (1969) Muscle vibration therapy in children with cerebral palsy. *Scandinavian Journal of Rehabilitation Medicine* **1**: 35–7.
30. Hagbarth, K.-E. and Eklund, G. (1969) The muscle vibrator – a useful tool in neurological therapeutic work. *Scandinavian Journal of Rehabilitation Medicine* **1**: 26–34.
31. Zislis, J.M. (1964) Splinting of the hand in the spastic hemiplegia patient. *Archives of Physical Medicine and Rehabilitation* **45**: 41–3.
32. Bearzy, H.J. (1954) Effective care of the hemiplegic. *Physical Therapy Review* **34**: 338–42.
33. Knapp, M.E. (1959) Problems in rehabilitation of the hemiplegic patient. *Journal of the American Medical Association* **169**: 224–9.
34. Kaplan, N. (1962) Effect of splinting on reflex inhibition and sensorimotor stimulation in the treatment of spasticity. *Archives of Physical Medicine and Rehabilitation* **43**: 565–9.
35. Charait, S.E. (1968) A comparison of volar and dorsal splinting of the hemiplegic hand. *American Journal of Occupational Therapy* **22**: 319–21.
36. Brunnstrom, S. (1956) Associated reactions of the upper extremity in adult patients with hemiplegia – an approach to training. *Physical Therapy Review* **36**: 225–36.
37. Rood, M. (1954) Nuerophysiological reactions as a basis for physical therapy. *Physical Therapy Review* **34**: 444–9.
38. Blashy, M.R. and Fuchs, R. (1959) Orthokinetics: a new receptor facilitation method. *American Journal of Occupational Therapy* **13**: 226.
39. Brennan, J. (1959) Response to stretch of hypertonic muscle groups in hemiplegia. *British Medical Journal* **1**: 1504–7.
40. Doubilet, L. and Polkow, L.S. (1977) Theory and design of a finger abduction splint for the spastic hand. *American Journal of Occupational Therapy* **31**: 320–2.
41. Fuchs, E.M. and Fuchs, R.L. (1954) Corrective bracing. *American Journal of Occupational Therapists* **8**: 88.
42. McPherson, J.J. (1981) Objective evaluation of a splint designed to reduce hypertonicity. *American Journal of Occupational Therapy* **35**: 189–94.
43. Neuhaus, B.E., Ascher, E.R. and Coullon, J. *et al.* (1981) A survey of rationales for and against hand splinting in hemiplegia. *American Journal of Occupational Therapy* **35**: 83–90.
44. Ada, L. and Scott, D. (1980) Use of inhibitory weight-bearing plasters to increase movement in the presence of spasticity. *Australian Journal of Physiotherapy* **26**: 57–61.
45. Hayes, N.K. and Burns, Y.R. (1970) Discussion on the use of weight-bearing plasters in the reduction of hypertonicity. *Australian Journal of Physiotherapy* **16**: 108–16.
46. Brocklehurst, J.C., Andrews, K., Richards, B. and Laycock, P.J. (1978) How much physical therapy for patients with stroke? *British Medical Journal* i: 1307–10.
47. Caldwell, C.B., Wilson, D.J. and Braun, R.M. (1969) Evaluation and treatment of the upper extremity in the hemiplegic stroke patient. *Clinical Orthopaedics* **63**: 69–93.
48. Najenson, T., Yacubovich, E. and Pikielini, S. (1971) Rotator cuff injury in shoulder joints of hemiplegic patients. *Scandinavian Journal of Rehabilitation Medicine* **3**: 131–7.
49. Nepomuceno, C.S. and Miller, J.M. (1974) Shoulder arthrography in hemiplegic patients. *Archives of Physical Medicine and Rehabilitation* **55**: 49–51.

50. Dardier, E. and Reid, C. (1972) Hemiplegia and painful shoulder. *Physical Therapy* **52**: 1208.
51. Hazelman, B.L. (1972) The painful stiff shoulder. *Rheumatology and Physical Medicine* **11**: 413–21.
52. McLaughlin, H. (1961) The frozen shoulder. *Clinical Orthopaedics* **20**: 126–30.
53. Sheldon, P.J.H. (1972) A retrospective survey of 102 cases of shoulder pain. *Rheumatology and Physical Medicine* **11**: 422–7.
54. Munting, E. (1978) Ultrasonic therapy for the painful shoulder. *Physiotherapy* **64**: 180–1.
55. Buchan, J.F. (1970) Use of ultrasonics in physical medicine. *The Practitioner* **205**: 319–26.
56. Echternach, M.S. (1965) Ultrasound in adjacent treatment for shoulder disabilities. *Physical Therapy* **4**: 865–9.
57. Goodman, C.R. (1971) Treatment of the shoulder hand syndrome. *New York State Journal of Medicine* **71**: 559–62.
58. Hurd, M.M., Farrell, K.H., Waylonis, G.W. (1974) Shoulder sling for hemiplegia: friend or foe? *Archives of Physical Medicine and Rehabilitation* **55**: 519–22.
59. Friedland, F. (1975) Physical therapy. In: *Stroke and Its Rehabilitation.* (Ed: Licht, S.). Williams and Wilkins, Baltimore.
60. Licht, S. (1975) Stroke rehabilitation program. In: *Stroke and Its Rehabilitation* (Ed: Licht, S.). Williams and Wilkins, Baltimore.

19

Sensory aspects of stroke

Sensory Loss

Epidemiology

Effective motor function depends on an intact sensory system. Although pure sensory strokes do occur [1], usually some motor deficit is present [2]. The incidence of hemisensory loss is between 23 and 38 per cent [2–4], although when thrombosis affected the cerebral cortex it was found in 80 per cent of cases. In the Framingham study [6] sensory deficits were found in 5 per cent of stroke survivors with no motor deficit and in 37 per cent of those with hemiplegia; there were only four patients with bilateral strokes and all of these had sensory loss. In one study, two-thirds of those with hemisensory loss had a left-sided hemiplegia [7].

Some studies have reported bilateral impairment of sensation in up to one-third of patients with unilateral cerebrovascular lesions [8–10]. These workers found no laterality difference for bilateral loss; but Vaughan and Costa [11] found it more common in left hemisphere lesions, whereas others [12, 13] have described it as being more common in right brain damage [12, 13].

Recovery and prognosis

Little information is available about the recovery of sensory loss. Two-point discrimination has been shown [14] to return to normal in 50 per cent of patients in about six weeks, whereas sensation improved in only one-quarter of those with impaired pain or vibratory sense – pain in an average of two months and vibration in an average of eighteen weeks.

Sensory loss is associated with poor functional improvement [7, 15, 16], probably because sensory loss was nearly always associated with perceptual or cognitive dysfunction which are major barriers to recovery. Similarly sensory loss is associated with a high mortality [16,

17], though Steinberg [15] did not find this. It is possible that it is not the loss of sensation itself which results in the poor recovery but the extent of the brain damage resulting in the sensory loss.

Sensory abnormalities

Sensory abnormalities are major barriers to recovery and are generally poorly understood, probably because the neuropsychological terminology (such as anosognosia, asomatognosia, atopographagnosia or prosopagnosia) has implied an unnecessary degree of complexity. Some oversimplification is warranted to understand the background to perceptual disorders.

To understand sensory dysfunction it is necessary to appreciate a few basic concepts:

1. Sensation from one side of the body is interpreted mainly by the contralateral side of the brain. This is only partly true since there is some bilateral innervation.
2. The front of the brain is primarily responsible for motor function and the posterior brain for sensory interpretation.
3. There are two *functional* systems: (a) the nerve *fibres* which carry information from the sensory organs on one side of the body, crossing over at some level in the spinal cord, to the contralateral cortex, and (b) the nerve *cells* which interpret the relevance of the sensory input. It must be stressed that we are considering *functional* rather than *anatomical* structures.
4. There is a hierarchical system of specialization within the brain. The more basic the sensation (e.g. touch, pain or temperature discrimination) the more likely that it has localized representation in one cortex. For the higher mental functions one hemisphere takes responsibility for detailed analysis of the different levels of sensation from both sides of the body – this applies, for instance, with speech and spatial relationships.

   Each hemisphere, therefore, has two levels of function. At one level it is responsible for interpreting primary sensations from the opposite side of the body; and at the other level it specializes in analysing complex degrees of sensory input.

Basically, information about the state of the body or its immediate environment is picked up by nerve endings, transmitted along a series of sensory nerves to the spinal cord where, at some point, it crosses over to the other side on its way to the contralateral cortex via the thalamus. Anaesthesia occurs when the nerve fibres, rather than the cortical nerve cells, are damaged. The ability to recognize that sensation is lost is dependent on intact cortical interpretation.

Thalamic sensation

The thalamus is the major sensory relay station on the way to the cerebral cortex. All sensory information, apart from smell, passes through the thalamus. It is at this level that the first awareness of sensation takes place. Infarction of the thalamus or its connections produces sensory loss, usually without motor involvement [1]. On the other hand, if it is irritated it may produce the very distressing 'thalamic syndrome' where there is sensory loss affecting all or many modalities, associated with excessive and extremely unpleasant sensation of pain when the sensory threshold is reached. This is a very difficult condition to treat. Only occasionally do patients benefit from drugs such as diphenylhydantoin or carbamazepine, and surgery has not been particularly helpful. A few patients have also been reported to benefit from levodapa treatment [18, 19].

The intractable severe pain is a major barrier to recovery since the patient will avoid any exercise or activity which is likely to bring on the pain. The advice that can be given is that the patient be kept warm, but not hot, that he avoid sudden movement, and that attendants be aware of the problem so as to avoid unnecessary stimulation of the affected side.

Primary sensory cortex

The first level of *interpretation* of sensation takes place in the primary sensory cortex. This is a narrow strip of brain tissue posterior to the central sulcus which has localized areas representing the various parts of the opposite side of the body; with the legs at the top tipping over on to the medial surface of the hemisphere and the head at the lower part of the lateral side. Some parts of the body, such as the hands and lips, have a greater area of representation in keeping with their greater sensory function. Electrical stimulation of this part of the brain results in the patient perceiving sensations of paraesthesia, touch or pressure but not pain. Ablation of this postcentral gyrus does not produces total loss of sensation but a difficulty in interpreting the difference between the modalities; that is, an inability to tell the difference between sharp and blunt, rough and smooth, hot and cold or soft and hard.

Testing for primary sensory damage is relatively simple. The difference between sharp and blunt is tested with a pin and a piece of cotton wool. It is essential to only lightly touch the skin with both pin and cotton wool since touch and not pressure is being tested. It is also important to avoid stroking the skin with the cotton wool since this gives a larger area of contact and may stimulate pain fibres by moving the hairs on the tested part. Heaviness is tested by giving the patient two small boxes each containing different weights. Differentation of degrees of roughness is tested by asking the patient to feel sandpaper of different textures. It is important to avoid visual clues: the patient should have his eyes closed, or the objects should be kept in a bag into which the patient puts his hand.

Association/secondary sensory cortex

Information from the primary cortex is further analysed in the secondary association cortex of the parietal lobes. The parietal cortex collects various types of information from different parts of the brain and builds up a picture of the opposite side of the body. There is no localized anatomical representation of the different parts of the body, but this part of the brain interprets the *existence* of the contralateral body.

The 'phantom limb' of the amputee is thought to be due to a parietal lobe misinterpretating sensation from the cut nerve fibres as though they were from the non-existent limb. In parietal brain damage the opposite applies: although the leg is present there is lack of awareness of its existence.

In the mildest form there is an inability to interpret sensation in the presence of competition from other sensations – inattention. This can be tested simply by touching both hands separately, in which case both stimuli are detected. Then both hands are touched simultaneously, in which case only the stimulus on the normal side will be felt. Other tests include asking the patient to identify familiar objects placed in his hand (with the eyes closed) or to detect by touch alone a number drawn on to the skin. Even minor difficulties such as these can have major implications for rehabilitation. Schwartz *et al.* [20] have shown that, although inattention occurs with damage to either hemipshere, it is more common when the right side of the brain is damaged. To complicate the matter further, they also found that left frontal lesions were more likely to produce extinction than right frontal lesions – but the inattention was almost always present on the left side of the body.

Patients with *tactile inattention* seem to be able to carry out activities when formally tested, since this is usually done unilaterally, yet become clumsy or have difficulty in carrying out bilateral activities such as dressing or eating because the affected limb is 'forgotten'.

In more severe forms there is complete unilateral tactile neglect (hemisomatoagnosia). This is often seen as the patient sitting with the limb in, what would seem to be, a most uncomfortable position, usually hanging by the side compressed against the chair. Tone is usually flaccid and there is often severe paralysis. However, occasionally the patient may seem to have good power when attention is

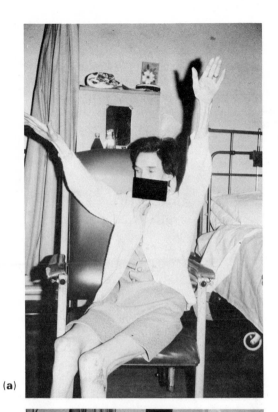

(a)

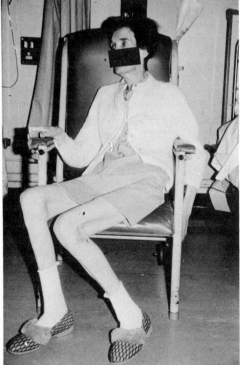

(b)

Fig. 19.1 Unilateral
inattention: (a) good power
when attention is drawn to
the affected side; (b) ignores
left side when attention is
distracted

drawn to the affected side (Fig. 19.1a) but soon 'forgets' the limb and it returns to the appearance of a flaccid dense hemiplegia (Fig. 19.1b). Some patients have bizarre associated symptoms: they may deny that the limb belongs to them, claiming that it was left there by the therapist, or refer to it as an inanimate object; others deny that there is anything wrong with the body at all (anosognosia). It is important to recognize that as far as the patient is concerned the limb or side of the body does *not* exist. Even if he responds to being reminded about the affected side this is usually temporary, and awareness rapidly decreases in the absence of stimulation.

Management

Attempts should be made to encourage the patient to take notice of the affected side. In the first instance this requires all staff and relatives being aware of the problem so that they can stimulate the affected side at every opportunity by stroking, tapping, using ice packs, vibrators or pneumatic intermittent compression. Other techniques include using vision or the sense of the ridiculous to draw attention to the affected side (for example, wrapping the limb in a brightly coloured sleeve or an inflatable splint). One patient responded remarkably well to having bells attached to the affected leg, not so much because they rang to remind her of the leg, but because she was so embarrassed that she became obsessed about having them removed. Whatever is used, the dual aim is to draw the patient's attention to the affected side as well as reminding the carers of the problem.

Position sense

Position sense loss may occur with or without the foregoing problems. Unless formally tested, position sense loss is easily missed, especially when mild. It is a difficult sign to demonstrate satisfactorily in stroke when there is concomitant arthritis, lack of concentration or difficulty in understanding detailed commands.

One approach is to ask the patient to grasp the affected thumb with his good hand whilst the eyes are open. If he has understood the command then he will grasp the thumb successfully – unless there are bilateral neurological problems (see below). The eyes are then covered, the affected arm moved to a different position and the patient requested to get hold of the thumb again. Several patterns of response are possible:

1. The patient has no difficulty in locating the affected thumb, suggesting that there is no gross loss of proprioceptive or perceptual abnormality.

2. The patient reaches for the upper part of the arm and follows it down to the thumb, implying that there is position sense loss but an appreciation of body image.
3. The patient reaches for where the thumb was before the eyes were closed but makes no attempt to use other techniques to find the thumb. This also implies position sense loss but indicates that the patient may well have difficulties in overcoming the problems.
4. The patient attempts to grasp the thumb by reaching out in front without aiming for the original position. This implies unilateral tactile neglect.
5. The patient makes no attempt to reach for the thumb. This implies that he has not understood the instruction, is dysphasic, deaf, confused, depressed or lacks insight or motivation. Some 'feeling' for which of these is the major factor can often be had by watching the patient, and this can be important in further management.

Bilateral incoordination

One further problem occasionally found is the inability to use both hands at the same time in a coordinated fashion. Each hand functions well when tested separately, but when the two hands attempt bilateral activities the actions become disjointed. Unfortunately most activities require bilateral control and coordination.

It is important to recognize these difficulties, otherwise the patient may be accused of not trying, being difficult, being clumsy or seeking attention. This attitude in the helper is not surprising when the function is good in each limb on separate testing.

Treatment of this problem is much more difficult. The patient should be encouraged in symmetrical bilateral exercises such as clapping hands or using a rolling pin before progressing to bilateral non-symmetrical activities. It is usually most productive to use activities which are relevant to the patient, such as washing the hands, picking up a knife and fork and simple dressing activities.

In summary, the tactile sensory brain is concerned with the immediate environment of the patient – what is happening within and in contact with the body. Many of the problems are made worse by the fact that the patient does not recognize the loss of the sensation and so is not in a position to complain about his difficulties. Although there are many sophisticated neuropsychological tests available, most problems can be detected by the aforementioned simple tests which can be carried out in the clinic and at the bedside.

Vision

Whereas tactile sensation is important for an appreciation of the immediate environment in touch with the body, vision is important for evaluation of distant activities.

Vision is affected in many ways in stroke. For instance, obstruction of the internal carotid artery below the level of the ophthalmic branch produces unilateral blindness on the ipsilateral side (Fig. 19.2b). Other symptoms relate to damage to the optic tracts or the occipital cortex, resulting in various degrees of homonymous quadrantanopia or hemianopia through to the visual agnosias.

For the purposes of this discussion the functional (as opposed to anatomical) approach will be used. Information from the left side of visual space passes to the right side of each eye and then on to the right occipital cortex. In effect, each occipital lobe interprets the information coming from the contralateral visual field but, because of the interchange of information across the corpus callosum, in practice both sides of the brain work together to produce a composite picture.

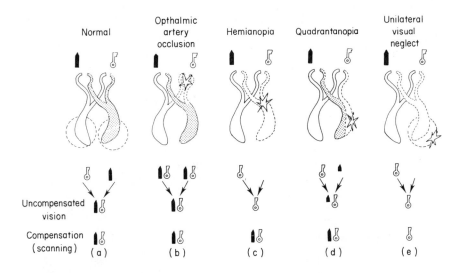

Fig. 19.2   Types of visual disorders in stroke (see text)

Hemianopia

The nerve fibres in the optic tracts and radiation travel over a very large area as they fan out through the temporal and parietal lobes, providing ample opportunity for damage.

Quadrantanopia is produced if only a part of the fibre tract is damaged (Fig. 19.2d). Lesions in the temporal lobe produce deficits in the upper visual field and those in the parietal lobes a lower quadrantic hemianopia.

In homonymous hemianopia (Fig. 19.2c) there is a loss in the contralateral visual field, affecting both eyes. The patient is aware of the deficit and although he may bump into objects in the blind field he is capable of compensating for the blindness.

Visual fields are classically tested by confrontation in which the examiner tests the patient's visual fields separately by comparing with his own visual field.

Since many stroke patients are confused, lack comprehension or cannot concentrate, accurate determination of visual fields is not always possible. In this case, assessment may have to be made by moving fingers at different points at the periphery of the visual fields to see if there is any reaction from the patient. This can only provide a crude assessment but it can usually detect homonymous hemianopia.

A more informative test is to hold up a pen in the patient's left visual field and a key in the right visual field. In a patient with normal visual fields both objects are 'seen', but with homonymous hemianopia the object in the blind field is not seen. The patient can compensate by turning his head or eyes; that is, if the patient is looking straight ahead he may at first only see the key, but if the examiner exchanges the postions of the two objects in front of the patient there will be recognition that there was a pen in the blind field and he will begin to compensate by moving his eyes to view that side of space. Similarly, if given a newspaper he will turn his head or eyes to see all the columns of print.

Some degree of hemianopia occurs in 20–40 per cent of stroke patients with unilateral lesions [6, 17] and three-quarters of those with bilateral lesions [6]. Visual field problems are associated with a high mortality [17, 21] and morbidity [23].

Unilateral visual neglect

In normal visual function there is a subcortical area responsible for alerting the cortex that some visual image is coming through. This is important since some patients who seem to be blind turn towards a light or an object and are therefore accused of not really being blind.

The first level of interpretation takes place at the tip of the occipital lobe in the primary visual cortex. This interprets angles and intensity of light, as well as providing some awareness of colour. Stimulation of this area produces flashes of light, usually in the form of blobs of colour especially at the red-orange end of the spectrum. More complex interpretation of shape takes place in the occipito-parietal area, adjacent to and overlapping that of the tactile association cortex. Electrical stimulation in this area produces formed visual hallucinations. Damage at this level produces blindness for the contralateral visual field. The difference from hemianopia, however, is that the patient is unaware that he is blind since the part of the brain which tells him whether he can, or cannot, see is not functioning. In effect one side of space does not exist and there is no reason for the opposite cortex to compensate. In the pen and key test (see above) the object in the blind field will not be seen even with encouragement. In other words, even if the pen and key are exchanged in, what should be, the full vision of the patient, he will continue to see only the object in the normal visual field. The patient does not seem to be surprised by the disappearance of the object and if asked where it has gone he will often accuse the examiner of playing a trick on him.

This unilateral visual neglect can produce some interesting clinical features, such as only half a column of newprint being read, even though it now no longer makes sense; food on only one side of the plate is eaten – the patient is often regarded as being off his food, disinterested or plain difficult; the time can be recognized only when the pointers are on the side of the clock falling in the normal visual field; the bedside container does not exist; or the patient ignores all activities going on in the affected visual field.

It is very difficult to understand why the patient should not be aware that a plate is round and therefore there must be another half. An explanation comes from studies of people who have had the corpus collusum divided [23]. In these patients the two sides of the brain are in effect working independently. If an individual with this 'split brain' is asked to look at a screen on to which a half square (the open end of the square on the right – Fig. 19.3) is flashed quickly before the eyes have had time to move, and is then asked to draw with the right hand what

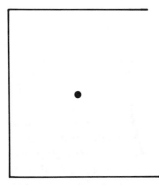

Fig. 19.3   Half square used in 'split brain' test

he saw, then he draws two parallel lines (i.e. the pattern received by the left hemisphere). If he is now asked to draw with his left hand what he saw he draws not a half square as might be expected, but a full square. Presumably there was some form of assumption that the other side of the brain must have been 'seeing' something similar. It therefore appears that the brain fills in gaps and sees what it expects to 'see', only modifying this in the presence of information to the contrary from the other hemisphere. This should not be surprising since the amount of visual stimulation reaching the brain is so vast that it must assume much from expectations based on past experience. This does help to explain the clinical picture of only one half of a plate of food being eaten or one half of a column of newsprint being read. Probably what happens is that at a subcortical level there is an awareness that there is an object in the visual fields. The normal visual cortex interprets the information coming from its visual field and, in the absence of information to the contrary from the opposite cortex, completes the picture. In the case of the plate of food, once the food on the side of the plate in the intact visual field has been eaten the plate is empty because the brain has completed the picture of the empty side of the plate. It is still puzzling why the patient should not be aware of the remaining food by turning his head or eyes slightly to the blind side. There are probably two reasons for this. The first is that patients with unilateral neglect do not look towards the affected side. The second is that there is probably a subcortical awareness of a whole object and each hemisphere concentrates on half of that object. This will still apply when the visual cortex is damaged except that only one cortex is concentrating on the work in hand – whilst assuming that the other side must be doing the same.

Implications of unilateral visual neglect

It is important to recognize that in unilateral neglect one side of the visual space does not exist, since many well-intentioned carers produce a very restricted environment for patients. Although it is an important part of the rehabilitation programme to encourage recognition of the neglected side this can only happen when there is 'active', as opposed to the 'passive', stimulation. This has major implications for positioning the patient in a room. For instance, if the healthy visual field is facing the wall, then the whole environment consists of a bank wall. Even if interesting activities are occurring on the blind side, this side of space does not exist and there is no reason to turn towards it. Similarly, putting the bedside container on the blind side to encourage him to look for his drink, or other object, is likely to fail.

Relatives should understand these problems since they may become distressed when they speak to the patient to find that he looks away from them when they approach from the affected side, interpreting this as the patient not wanting to speak to them, being awkward or as an insult. It is also important for carers to recognize that when food on only one side of the plate is eaten that this does not mean that the patient is not hungry but that he is unaware that there is still food on the plate. Similarly they should be aware that only half of anything which is placed in front of the patient is likely to be seen. When this is explained to relatives they are often relieved to find that the symptoms are due to the stroke and that the patient is not 'going mad'. They often ask about other observations they have made about the patient's activities and query whether they are related to the visual neglect.

Tests for unilateral visual neglect

When gross, unilateral visual neglect is usually so obvious that formal testing is unlikely to add much to the practical management. However, milder forms may be missed and therefore some simple bedside tests can be helpful.

It is important for all of these tests that the patient wears spectacles if applicable (i.e. spectacles for close vision). This might seem obvious but it is one of the most common mistakes made when testing.

Picture drawing test

The simplest test is to give the patient a piece of paper and a pen (preferably a large felt-tipped pen) and ask him to copy a simple picture of a house [24]. The patient should sit in a comfortable position in a good light and the paper should be supported on a firm surface – testing the ability to draw a picture whilst the patient is lying on his back and the paper supported on a soft pad cannot be expected to give optimal results.

Pictures drawn by patients with unilateral visual neglect vary widely. It is not uncommon for the patient to draw the outline of the house but to complete only half of the roof or other detail, such as the windows (Fig. 19.4a).

The copy test requires the patient to see, interpret and respond. It requires little long-term visual memory since the patient is presented with the picture to copy. A progression is to ask the patient to draw a picture, from memory, of a man, flower or a clock (Fig. 19.4c). This requires a higher degree of visual memory skill. In practice this rarely adds much to the information obtained from the copy test.

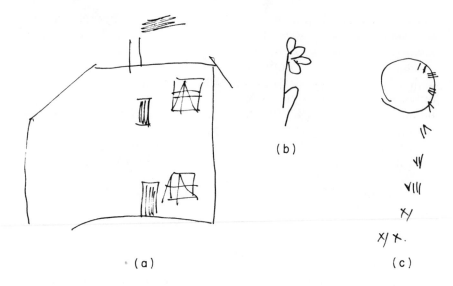

Fig. 19.4   Picture drawings in unilateral visual neglect

Pen–key test

Another test which can be carried out anywhere requires only simple objects, such as a pen and a key, which are readily available. One object (the pen, say) is held in the examiner's right hand (the patient's left visual field) and the other object (the key) in the left hand. These objects are held about 30 cm away from the patient's eyes and about 30 cm apart. The patient is asked what he can see. If he indicates only the object on the non-paralysed side then it is worth removing that object and asking the question again. If the patient then sees the object in the affected visual field this implies that there is visual inattention; that is, objects in the affected field will only be seen provided there is no distraction from the non-affected side. This is important to recognize since some clinicians test visual fields by holding up one hand or an object in each visual field separately, and so inattention will be missed.

Assuming that the patient has only seen the object in the normal visual field when two objects have been held up, this could mean that he has hemianopia and has not recognized that something is in the blind field, or that he has unilateral visual neglect and is unaware that there is another visual field. To differentiate between these two the patient is asked if anything else is being held up that he might have missed and he is invited to look around. Patients with hemianopia will then turn their eyes or the head and see the object in the blind field. If there is no attempt to look to the blind side then the two objects are exchanged within, what should be, the field of vision of the patient. In hemianopia there is recognition that there are two objects and compensation takes place by moving the head or the eyes. The patient with unilateral visual neglect will continue only to see the object in the normal visual field.

This test has some limitations if the patient is dysphasic or confused, but some clue can be obtained by simply watching the patient's reaction to moving objects. If, for example, he turns his eyes or head to follow an object moving from one visual field to the other, then it is unlikely that unilateral neglect is present.

Headline test

This test is based on the idea that only half of any object placed in front of the patient will be seen. If the patient is presented with a newspaper and asked to read the headline he will only read the words in the normal half of visual space. Thus

PERCEPTUAL DISORDERS ARE A MAJOR BARRIER

becomes

.... ARE A MAJOR BARRIER

This again is a simple test using an easily available newspaper or book. It has limitations if the patient is confused, dysphasic or cannot read.

Cloth man test

This uses the ability of the patient to construct a simple picture jig-saw puzzle (made of felt, cardboard or pieces of wood) shaped to represent the arms, legs, trunk and head of a man. In unilateral neglect the limbs on only one side of the trunk section will be added. A modification of this is to use a puzzle consisting of a face, the eyes, ears, nose, mouth and hair-piece. Abnormalities are also seen in the apraxias as well as the agnosias in this test.

Pegboard test

This consists of a wooden board into which a number of holes have been drilled in the shape of a square or a circle [26]. The patient is provided with a set of wooden pegs and asked to put them into the holes. In unilateral visual neglect only the holes on one side of the board will be filled. This is a close analogy to the problem of only one half of a plate of food being eaten. If this test is abnormal it is worth making a special effort to check on the patient's eating technique.

Deletion test

In this the patient is presented with a piece of paper on which a series of random letters have been typed and is asked to underline, or cross out, all of the A's or some other specified letter. In unilateral neglect only those on the non-affected side will be underlined; for example:

```
D   F   G   E   A   S   A   T   U   F   A   L   A   U   T   A   P   T   H   A   R
A   D   P   A   T   J   E   A   M   T   W   A   G   J   R   H   K   T   A   T   J
F   E   R   W   A   R   A   Y   E   D   L   W   A   R   E   A   R   A   V   R   A
```

Albert's test

This is a series of 41 lines about 2 cm long drawn on a sheet of paper at random [26, 27 and Fig. 19.5]. The patient is asked to cross out all the lines he can see. In unilateral visual neglect those lines in the blind field are left uncrossed (Fig. 19.5b). The advantage of this test is that it gives some standardization of the assessment and can provide evidence of improvement by counting the number of lines crossed on subsequent testing.

Quite a number of other tests are available, but these few should cover most clinical situations. It is not necessary to carry out all the tests on each patient since once unilateral neglect has been demonstrated there is nothing to be gained from persisting with tests which only confirm what is already known. Obviously some of the tests are more applicable for one patient than another. For instance, the headline test is inappropriate for dysphasic patients, and those tests requiring hand manipulation, especially when it is the non-dominant hand, will be of limited value in the presence of severe arthritis. One of the above tests

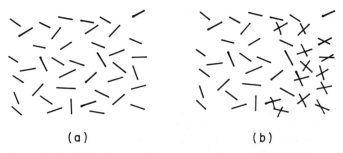

(a)   (b)

Fig. 19.5   Albert's test: (a) picture prior to testing; (b) response to a request to cross out the lines in left-sided unilateral visual neglect

should be of use in all but the comatosed or severely demented individual.

Treatment of unilateral visual neglect

There are three approaches to the rehabilitation of perceptual disorders which can be used separately or in combination. The first is to use the tests described above and train the patient to recognize what he is doing wrong. It is hoped by this approach that the ability to recognize the neglected side of space in the test material will carry over into other activities. This has the advantage that the information used is simple and consistent. There is a danger in trying to get the patient to recognize too much information in one go.

The second approach is a function one. Effort is put into recognizing specific problems of carrying out activities of daily living. The advantage of this is that it is of relevance to the patient and is dealing with real problems. There is a danger that too much will be attempted at once so it is worthwhile setting a definite programme of activities. This will require each stage of an acitivity to be established before progressing to the next stage. The problem with this approach is that it might disrupt the smooth sequential flow of events in carrying out the activity. It is impossible to define what the programme should be since this will vary from patient to patient. In general it is wise to find an activity about which the patient is enthusiastic, provided that it is not too complicated to be achieved at that stage. Simple goals will include learning to feed and recognize the part of the plate in the neglected visual field. This requires the attendant to constantly remind and persuade the patient to turn the head to, or to feel for, the affected side.

The third approach is to find techniques to encourage awareness of the neglected field. These again will vary from patient to patient and the scheme requires some ingenuity. For the following examples it will be assumed that the patient has left-sided visual neglect.

1. For reading place a brightly coloured band down the left-hand side of the page and instruct the patient to look for the band before reading.
2. A similar technique can be used for eating. A bright marker is placed on the edge of the neglected side of the plate.
3. Spread out a series of consecutively numbered cards starting with number 1 on the right and progressing to number 9 on the left. Instruct the patient to start counting and pointing to the cards in turn. He will probably stick at number 4 or 5, which will be in the midline, and should then be encouraged to continue counting.
4. A similar approach can be taken with a series of flashing lights on a

board. As the lights flash in series from right to left it is hoped that the patient will gradually become aware of the neglected field.

5. Start off with any activity (blowing a whistle, say) whilst standing on the right-hand side of the patient, and gradually move towards the left. This has the advantage that it uses a different modality – in this case hearing.

6. Other modalities can be used, such as putting a brightly coloured inflatable splint on the affected arm; this acts partly by tactile stimulation and partly by the absurdity of the situation.

These are only a few suggestions and they can obviously be adapted to the needs of the patient. For instance, instead of the numbered cards there could be letters of the alphabet in order; or the names of towns in the neighbourhood used as a game in which he has to pick up as many as possible; or coins of different denominations placed out in order starting with the lowest denomination in the right field, so that the patient has to collect as much money as is possible. The game element has the advantage that competition encourages more interest.

Visual memory problems

Unilateral visual neglect is an obvious visual problem, but there are others which can often be picked up when using the tests already described. One common problem is seen when the patient is asked to

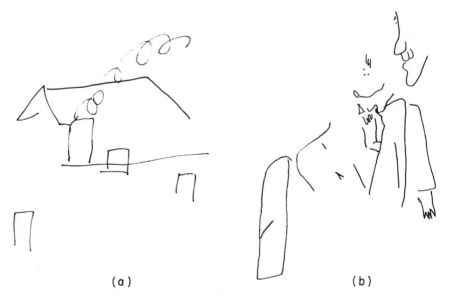

(a)   (b)

Fig. 19.6 Picture drawings in visual memory defects: (a) a house; (b) a man

draw a picture and he draws a house, or a man, similar to that seen in Fig. 19.6. The difficulty he seems to be having is one of visual memory. When we look at any object we rapidly focus on different parts of it to construct a visual image of the whole object. If the position of one part of the object is forgotten as soon as attention is moved to another part, then it is impossible to understand the role of the object or at least to use it productively. What seems to have happened in the figure is that, after drawing the head, the patient has difficulty in remembering the spatial relationships of the head to the body to the arms, and so each has been drawn separately without any true relationships. A similar pattern is seen when constructing the cloth man, the parts of the body being placed in inappropriate positions. Some therapists believe that this is due to a disruption of the patient's image of his own body, but it could also be a problem of visual memory of spatial relationships. The relevance of this for day-to-day activities is that we need to understand the relationship of at least two objects, or parts of objects, for every action that we take. For instance, to put on a jumper we need to know where the neck is in relation to the left sleeve in relation to the right sleeve and so on. For feeding we need to know the relationship of the knife to the fork to the food to the plate, etc.

Treatment of this condition is very difficult. It is probably best approached by giving the patient very simple tasks to carry out which involve connecting only two objects, such as putting a spoon into a cup, and then progressing to more complex tasks. It may, for instance, be possible to train the patient to put his hand into a bag and then progress to putting the arm into a disconnected sleeve, and thus progressing to putting on a full jumper. Since the more parts the object has the more difficulty the patient is likely to have, it is logical to make the environment as simple as possible. For instance, a sleeveless jumper is going to be easier to manage than one with sleeves. Similarly, it will be easier to learn to eat if only the fork is used and only one type of food is on the plate – or to learn to eat soup with a spoon before progressing on to more complex feeding programmes.

An alternative approach for complex activities, such as dressing, is to use 'guides'. For example, to help to put on a shirt coloured tapes can be attached to various parts of the garment – yellow at the bottom, red at the neck, blue at the sleeve. The patient can then feel along the tapes in sequence from one colour to the next in the order required for dressing.

Some patients benefit from training in sequence by numbers. By this is meant that an activity is broken down to individual actions, each of which is given a number, and the activity built up in a series of sequential steps. Thus filling a kettle with water would be: (1) turn on tap; (2) pick up kettle; (3) place kettle under tap; (4) watch for water reaching a specified level; (5) turn off tap; (6) put on kettle lid; and so on. The reason for this approach is that, as will be seen later, the right side of the brain requires information to be presented sequentially to be effective and this approach attempts to utilize this concept.

Other problems

Several other patterns are seen when asking patient is asked to draw a picture. One common pattern, usually in right hemiplegia, is perseveration: the patient starts by drawing a line or a word and repeats this over and over. It seems that once an idea has been started it gets into a perpetual loop into or out of which it is difficult to break. This obviously has implications for any activity that the patient wants to perform.

There are two other common picture types seen. In on the patient overcopies whatever has been drawn, and in the other he draws, totally unrelated and usually meaningless scrawls. Both of these patterns have a very bad prognosis because they indicate severe brain damage and are associated with a high early mortality rate.

Prognosis

Some form of abnormality of structure of the picture drawings which could not be accounted for by poor artistry or drawing with the non-dominant hand was found in about one-half of the stroke patients who survived the first two weeks following a stroke [28]. Although 42 per cent of those with picture drawing abnormalities had a mild loss of motor power, only 6 per cent had a mild loss of ADL function, indicating the importance of perceptual and cognitive dysfunction on functional ability. Picture drawing abnormalities were also associated with other evidence of cortical dysfunction, such as incontinence of urine or faeces, depression and confusion. Mortality was very much higher in those with picture abnormalities – only 56 per cent being alive at one year following the stroke compared with 83 per cent of those who drew normal pictures. Functional recovery was poorer in those with abnormal pictures even when only those who started with severe loss of function were studied – 79 per cent of those with severe ADL loss at two weeks who drew normal pictures improved, whereas only 38 per cent of those with abnormal pictures improved (and this was to a lower functional level than those who drew normal pictures).

It would, therefore, seem that even simple tests may be of some help in detecting the problems the patient has and give some indication as to the likely prognosis. There are many other tests and a clinical psychologist will be able to give a more detailed breakdown of the patient's problems. These simple tests can, however, be very helpful when a psychologist is not available and can be carried out in the clinic or the patient's home without the need for complicated equipment.

Hemisphere specialization

The features described so far occur when either hemisphere is damaged. The greater the complexity of information, the more likely it is that one hemisphere will take responsibility for analysis [29, 30]. Although the left side of the brain is generally regarded as being the dominant hemisphere, it is now recognized that the right hemisphere has an equally major role to play in its recognition of spatial relationships.

The left brain seems to take information in parallel, juggle it around and come up with a 'logical' answer, making it efficient for analysing logic, mathematics and language. The right brain, on the other hand, is more effective when taking information in series and making a spot diagnosis. It is, therefore, more efficient at recognizing pictures and spatial relationships. The left hemisphere, being more efficient for analysing speech, will predominantly be responsible for communication. However, if the 'speech centre' in a young child is damaged, speech may still develop as the right hemisphere can take over this function. The serial function of speech can sometimes be seen in a dysphasic patient who, when asked how many cigarettes he smokes, although unable to say the number immediately, will start at 'one' and count up to the appropriate number. Similarly, the dysphasic patient may be able to recite a nursery rhyme (e.g. 'Jack and Jill went up the hill to fetch a pail of water'); if the patient is stopped at the word 'hill' and then asked to continue he will have to go back to the start again. This applies to a large extent in normal people, showing the need to have information in a set order before it is analysed or utilized. The effectiveness of the right brain in serial learning possibly explains why some dysphasic patients can sing songs, recite poems or mathematical tables learnt in childhood. The problem in stroke is that there is less plasticity of the brain, and after 50, 60 or 70 years of hemisphere specialization it is more difficult for the other hemisphere to take over a function.

As discussed earlier, much of the evidence for the differing functions of each hemisphere comes from split-brain studies (that is, of people who have had division of the callosum which joins the two halves of the brain). In tests which required each hand to respond to different forms of visual stimuli, the left hand showed superiority in responding to three-dimensional forms [31]. Levy concluded that the right hand was more efficient when the pictures were easily described but were visually difficult to analyse, while the reverse was the case for the left hand.

The right brain is efficient at analysing pictures from very little information. It is also effective in analysing clues as to the distance between two objects. This is important for very simple activities such as putting milk into a cup of tea or sugar on to cereal, or picking up a comb. Where this difficulty is not recognized the patient is regarded as clumsy, difficult, not trying, confused, lacking in cooperation or having poor motivation [25]. All carers must be aware of this if they are to be constructive in their handling of the patient and to avoid frustration.

Just as judging distances of near objects can be a problem, so can judging the relationship of more distant objects. This makes it difficult to find the way around even familiar places (atopographagnosia). This has implications for treatment in hospital since, if the patient is having difficulty within the immediate environment, it does not make sense to move his bed to different positions on the ward from time to time. Similarly, patients who are beginning to adapt to a very limited environment around the bed become disorientated in space when taken to the physiotherapy or occupational therapy departments, and so these people will benefit more from ward rehabilitation. Indeed, they may become disorientated even when moved to sit in the day room of a ward. Similar principles apply to management at home.

The patient who is unable to judge distances feels that he is falling or will bump into furniture because he thinks it is more widely spaced than it is. These patients panic when faced with an open space and have a very real fear of falling.

The foregoing are all problems which are poorly recognized but are very real to the patient. Specific tests are not very helpful in picking up these problems, and it is only by an awareness that they may exist that they will be identified.

One further common feature seen in right brain damage is denial of illness (anosognosia). An extension of being unaware of the affected side of the body is a denial that there is anything wrong. It can be extremely difficult to manage a patient with a dense hemiplegia who, because he cannot recognize that he is disabled, insists that he will manage at home all alone.

Speech

The left hemisphere is particularly effective in dealing with verbal and language concepts. There are, however, a number of speech disorders found in stroke which, thought they are not all related to left brain damage, result in communication problems.

Deafness is the first barrier to communication and should certainly be ruled out before more complex speech disorders are diagnosed. The next step is for the brain to be primed that a sound is coming in and there does seem to be a subcortical awareness of sound before cortical function begins to analyse the sound. Thus, even very dysphasic patients may turn towards a sound but be unable to analyse its meaning. This is very similar to the thalamic function for tactile sensation and the superior colliculus for vision.

Dysphasia

Damage to the communication centres of the brain produces symptoms varying from complete inability to understand the spoken or written word with failure to express thoughts in speech and writing, to mild word-forming difficulties, slowing down in word formulation of sentences, slight spelling difficulties and slowing down of reading [33]. There have been many classifications of dysphasia based either on functional difficulties [34–36] or on anatomical localization [36, 37].

Investigation

There is a large battery of tests for dysphasia, though these are not practicable for people not trained in speech therapy. The detailed analysis of speech problems requires the expertise of a speech therapist, but some clue as to the difficulties can be provided by a few simple tests. The main aim is to determine the level of the patient's comprehension since functional recovery will largely depend on his ability to understand and learn.

The simple tests used by clinicians (like asking the patient to name common objects) can only detect crude communication problems; complete comprehension requires a greater understanding of a large amount of language more sophisticated than simple nouns. More complex instructions like 'put your left hand into your pocket' are misleading and can be difficult to interpret. Many of the comprehension difficulties will be picked up by careful observation of the problems the patient has in understanding what he has been requested to do in his general activities. A more satisfactory method is the Frenchay aphasic screening test [38], which is a standardized short assessment using picture cards and which can be used by those who are not speech therapists. The test covers areas of comprehension, expression, reading and writing in dyphasia. It is not designed for the assessment of dysarthria or speech dyspraxia (see later).

It is important not to miss comprehension difficulties since other ways of improving communication will be required. On the other hand it is unfortunate to assume that there are no communication difficulties just because the patient has been able to carry out a few basic communication tests.

Treatment

The value of speech therapy is debatable. Vignolo [39] compared 69 aphasic patients who received speech therapy with 27 untreated controls and concluded that speech therapy did not have a specific effect on recovery; while Lenneberg [40] felt that speech returns because the nerve cells in the brain recover and not because of a retraining programme.

Unfortunately many of the studies of speech therapy have not included control groups. As early as 1946 Butfield and Zangwill [41] investigated the recovery of 70 dysphasic patients and concluded that treatment had been effective. One of the first adequately controlled trials of speech therapy was that of Sarno *et al.* [42] who concluded that speech therapy did not modify the verbal behaviour in a group of severely dysphasic patients. This study has been criticized for including only grossly aphasic patients who had a very poor prognosis and for inadequate matching of the groups [43]; to this might be added that the numbers in each group were too small if slight changes were to be detected. Research findings are, therefore, not particularly optimistic about the benefit of speech therapy. This is probably because the amount of therapy provided is so limited that recovery could not be expected. There is evidence that 18 hours a week of speech therapy is effective at improving dysphasia [44], but lower levels were no better than none [45]. This is the danger of spreading scarce resources over all patients rather than selecting those most likely to improve.

Since lay volunteers are probably as effective as speech therapists in gaining some improvement in speech [46], certainly in the amounts of treatment time generally available, it is useful to use volunteers to assist the speech therapist in continuing the long-term support.

It is beyond the scope of this book to give detailed speech therapy techniques. There are, however, simple approaches to use such as games and activities with a language base, which can go a long way to providing the right type of encouragement to the dysphasic patient [47]. The following basic advice can be given to all those who come into contact with the dysphasic patient:

1. Do not treat the dysphasic patient as a child. This is easier said than

done. The published experiences of a dysphasic person expressed only too well his frustration as carers talked over him as though he did not exist [48].

2. Do not ask other people what the patient will want ('Does he take milk?'). The patient should be encouraged to take part in the decision making about his own needs and environment.
3. Try to avoid completing the sentence for the patient. This simply removes the need to speak and is demoralizing: it is rather like putting the patient into a wheelchair every time he tries to walk. Our embarrassment at watching the patient's difficulties makes us want to help but it is in fact hindering recovery.
4. Try to find a task that the patient is interested in. It is always easier to find words about a subject we know something about than one in which we hve no involvement.
5. Be patient. Frustration by the attendant at the slow rate of communication inhibits the patient and makes the situation worse.

Prognosis

Speech disorders due to head injuries are generally regarded as having a better prognosis than those due to stroke [41, 49–51]. Some workers have found an association between poor recovery of aphasia and the age of the patient [39, 52, 53], although others could not find such an association [54, 55].

Dysphasia results in learning defects [56–58] and so it is not surprising that it is associated with poor functional recovery. On the other hand, some workers [16, 59] did not find such a strong association with poor recovery, probably because they included both motor and sensory forms. Peszcynski [60] found that receptive, and sometimes global, aphasia did not interfere basically with the hemiplegic patient's ability to learn to walk, dress or feed himself. However, dysphasia, especially when severe or mixed, is associated with a high mortality rate [17, 61], probably because of the amount of brain that is damaged.

There is also disagreement about the time it takes to reach maximal recovery of speech. Culton [62] found that recovery was limited to the first month, while others have found the greatest improvement in the first three months [42, 52, 54], six months [39, 41, 63], or even continuing for several years [64].

If dysphasia is going to recover there is nearly always evidence of improvement within the first 40 days [65]. The final level of recovery is generally related to the severity of the dysphasia at onset [65, 66].

This uncertainty about the outcome and effectiveness of speech therapy does make it difficult to know what is best for the patient. It is probably appropriate to regard the benefit of speech therapy as unproven but to be optimistic as far as the patient is concerned. For this reason it is important that all members of the rehabilitation team and the family make efforts to involve the dysphasic patient in communication at all levels.

In spite of this lack of research support for the value of speech therapy, speech problems require the expertise of a speech therapist since the whole rehabilitation team, including the family, need her help and advice. Speech therapists are able to define and explain the problems that the patient is having and this is important in helping the team to develop the most appropriate ways of working with the patient. In addition they can provide prognostic guidelines and give advice to carers on how to cope with the communication handicap [67].

Other speech problems

It is important to differentiate dysphasia from other speech disorders such as dysarthria, dyspraxia and dysphonia.

Dysarthria

Dysfunction of coordination of the tongue and lips produces dysarthria, whereby speech is slurred but understanding of the spoken word and the ideas expressed are normal. It must be noted that, since dysarthria is mainly a disorder of transmission of information from the brain to the muscles of speech, it can be found with strokes on either side. However, it usually implies bilateral damage.

Dyspraxia

Dyspraxia (or apraxia) of speech describes the situation when there is no apparent weakness of the muscles of speech but there seems to be a block between the formulation of words and the organization of the muscles to act in the correct order. It therefore falls between motor dysphasia and dysarthria. It is an impairment of the programming of articulation. Dyspraxic patients have increasing difficulty with multi-syllabic words [68], and speeding the speech may increase the intelligibility and decrease the errors made [69].

Aphonia

Aphonia, and its milder form dysphonia, implies a difficulty in producing sufficient sound in the larynx to produce speech. The voice is hoarse and low volume. Spasticity in the laryngeal muscles produces a strangled type of voice. Since the muscles of the throat are bilaterally innervated the presence of dysphonia implies bilateral strokes or a brain stem lesion.

Laterality

Since each hemisphere has specific functions it might be expected that damage to one side of the brain would have an outcome different from damage on the other side. The adverse effects of dysphasia on functional recovery have been described above. However, a poor functional recovery is also associated with right hemisphere features such as prosopagnosia [70–73], anosognosia [74], emotional disturbances [75] and spatial agnosia [76]. A number of studies have shown that both hemispheres are equally affected [7, 16, 77, 78], and there does not seem to be a correlation between the dominant handedness of the patient and the side of the stroke.

In multiple strokes attacks occurred on the same side in three-quarters of cases [7]; while Marquardsen [2] found that, although recurrent lesions seemed slightly more common on the previously affected side, fatal attacks more often occurred on the contralateral side. The implication of this is not clear.

The side of the stroke does not seem to be related to the severity of dysfunction [16, 79]. Although Carroll [78] did find that functional disability was greater in patients with left hemisphere lesions, this was complicated by communiction problems being included in the scoring system.

No difference has been found between the hemispheres for survival [17, 80], physical recovery [16, 59, 80] or response to a rehabilitation programme [82], or for whether the patient was able to be discharged home [80]. In a study of elderly stroke patients, no difference was found between the two sides for survival, though 43 per cent of patients with a left hemiplegia compared with only 31 per cent of those with right-sided weakness eventually required long-stay care [83]. This could have been due to differential admission of left-sided stroke patients to geriatric units [16].

At least one group of workers found that patients with a left hemiplegia gained greater ambulatory improvement than did those with a right-sided weakness, although this did not influence the length of stay in hospital [84]. Most other studies which identify laterality differences have reported poorer functional recovery in patients with a left hemiplegia [2, 85, 86]. Di Benedetto [87] found that greater functional recovery for patients with a right-sided hemiplegia was only applicable to those less severely involved and that the outcome for the more severely affected patient was poor irrespective of the side of the lesion.

One of the problems with most of these studies is that they were nearly all carried out after selection of patients, either for specialist units or by admission to hospital. The relevance of this can be seen from the finding that for patients not admitted to hospital those with a right hemiplegia started with a better functional level than did those with left hemiplegia [88]. How much of this was related to the influence of the side of the lesion on admission to hospital is uncertain. In one study of elderly stroke patients it was found that those with a right hemiplegia were more likely to be admitted to hospital [16]. It is also of interest that, in the same study, of those who were admitted to hospital 66 per cent of patients with a right hemiplegia were admitted to general (internal) medical units whereas 69 per cent of those with a left hemiplegia were admitted to geriatric units. This differential referral pattern according to the laterality of the lesion must be taken into account when considering the findings of research from specialist units.

Probably the most logical conclusion about the influence of the side of the stroke and outcome comes from Isaacs and Marks [89]. They suggested that it is not so much the side of the stroke that matters but whether there are complicating perceptual or communication problems present. This at least provides the emphasis on the conditions which can be influenced.

References

1. Fisher, C.M. (1965) Pure sensory stroke involving the face, arm and leg. *Neurology* **15**: 76–80.
2. Marquardsen, J. (1969) The natural history of acute cerebrovascular disease. *Acta Neurologica Scandinavica* **45** (Suppl. 38).
3. Anderson, E.K. (1971) Sensory impairment in hemiplegia. *Practical Otorhinolaryngology* **33**: 293–7.
4. Brocklehurst, J.C., Andrews, K., Richards, B. and Laycock, P.J. (1978) How much physical therapy for patients with stroke? *British Medical Journal* **1**: 1307–10.
5. Lascelles, R.G. and Burrows, E.H. (1965) Occlusion of the middle cerebral artery. *Brain* **88**: 185–96.
6. Gresham, G.E., Fitzpatrick, T.E., Wolf, P.A. *et al.* (1975) Residual disability in survivors of stroke: the Framingham study. *New England Medical Journal* **293**: 954–56.
7. Moskowitz, E., Lightbody, F.E.H. and Freitag, N.S. (1972) Long term follow up of the post stroke patient. *Archives of Physical Medicine and Rehabilitation* **53**: 167–72.
8. Carmon, A. (1971) Disturbances of tactile sensitivity in patients with unilateral cerebral lesions. *Cortex* **7**: 83–97.
9. Corkin, S., Milner, B. and Taylor, L. (1973) Bilateral sensory loss after unilateral

cerebral lesions in man. *Transactions of the American Neurological Society* **98**: 118–22.

10. Essing, J.P., Gersten, J.W. and Yarnaell, P. (1980) Light touch thresholds in normal persons and cerebrovascular disease patients: bilateral deficits after unilateral lesions. *Stroke* **11**: 528–33.
11. Vaughan, H.G. and Costa, L.D. (1962) Performance of patients with lateralised cerebral lesions. II: Sensory and motor tests. *Journal of Nervous and Mental Diseases* **134**: 237–43.
12. Fontentot, D.J. and Benton, A.L. (1971) Tactile perception of duration in relationship to the hemisphere locus of lesion. *Neuropsychologia* **9**: 83–8.
13. Boll, T.J. (1974) Right and left cerebral hemisphere damage and tactile perception performance of the ipsilateral and contraleteral side of the body. *Neuropsychologia* **12**: 235–8.
14. van Buskirk, C. and Webster, D. (1955) Prognostic value of sensory deficits in rehabilitation of hemiplegia. *Neurology* **5**: 407–11.
15. Steinberg, F.U. (1973) The stroke registry: a prospective method of studying stroke. *Archives of Physical Medicine and Rehabilitation* **54**: 31–5.
16. Andrews, K., Brocklehurst, J.C., Richards, B. and Laycock, P.J. (1982) The recovery of the severely disabled stroke patient. *Rheumatology and Rehabilitation* **21**: 225–30.
17. Waylonis, G.W., Keith, M.W. and Aseff, J.N. (1973) Stroke rehabilitation in a Midwestern County. *Archives of Physical Medicine and Rehabilitation* **54**: 151–5.
18. Plasencia, R.J., Gilroy, J. and Cullis, P. (1984) Treatment of thalamic pain syndrome with levodopa. *Neurology* **34** (Suppl. 1): 137.
19. Grant, R. and Behan, P.O. (1984) Resistant thalamic pain treated by levodopa. *British Medical Journal* **289**: 1272.
20. Schwartz, A.S., Marchock, P.L., Kreinick, C.J. and Flynn, R.E. (1979) The asymmetric lateralisation of tactile extinction in patients with unilateral cerebral dysfunction. *Brain* **102**: 669–84.
21. Brust, J.C., Shafer, S.C., Richter, R.W. and Brunn, B. (1976) Aphasia in acute stroke. *Stroke* **7**: 167–74.
22. Miller, L.S. (1973) The significance of homonymous hemianopia in stroke. *Archives of Physical Medicine and Rehabilitation* **54**: 592–3.
23. Trevarthen, C. (1974) Analysis of cerebral activities that generate and regulate consciousness in commissurotomy patients. In: *Hemisphere Function in the Human Brain* (Eds: Dimond, S.J. and Beaumont, J.G.). Elk Science, London.
24. Adams, G.F. (1974) *Cerebrovascular Disability and the Ageing Brain*. Churchill Livingstone, Edinburgh.
25. Adams, G.F. and Hurwitz, L.J. (1963) Mental barriers to recovery from stroke. *Lancet* **ii**: 533–7.
26. Albert, M. (1973) A simple test of visual neglect. *Neurology* **23**: 658–64.
27. Fullerton, K.J., McSherry, D. and Stout, R.W. (1986) Albert's test: a neglected test of perceptual neglect. *Lancet* **i**: 430–432.
28. Andrews, K., Brocklehurst, J.C., Richards, B. and Laycock, P.J. (1980) The prognostic value of picture drawings by stroke patients. *Rheumatology and Rehabilitation* **19**: 180–8.
29. Wexler, B.E. (1980) Cerebral laterality and psychiatry. *American Journal of Psychiatry* **137**: 279–91.
30. Butler, S.R. (1971) Organisation of the cerebral cortex for perception. *British Medical Journal* **4**: 544–7.
31. Levy, J. and Sperry, R.W. (1968) Differential perceptual capacities in major and

minor hemispheres. *Proceedings of the US National Academy of Science* **61**: 1151.

32. Levy, J. (1974) Psychobiological implications of bilateral asymmetry. In: *Hemisphere Function in the Human Brain* (Eds: Dimond, S.J. and Beaumont, J.G.). Elk Science, London.
33. Butfield, E. (1966) Treatment of aquired speech and language disorders associated with hemiplegia. *Physiotherapy* **53**: 350-6.
34. Hurwitz, L.J. (1971) The word: a neurologists view on aphasia. *Gerontologia Clinica* **13**: 307-19.
35. Schuell, H., Jenkins, J.J. and Jimenez-Pabon, E. (1964) In: *Aphasia in Adults.* Harper and Row, New York.
36. Butler, R.B. and Benson, D.F. (1974) Aphasia: a clinical – anatomical correlation. *British Journal of Hospital Medicine* **12**: 211-17.
37. Geschwind, N. (1972) Language and the brain. *Scientific American* **226**: 76-83.
38. Enderby, P.M., Wood, V.A., Wade, D.T. and Hewer, R.L. (1987) The Frenchay aphasic screening test. (in press).
39. Vignolo, L.A. (1964) Evolution of aphasia and language rehabilitation: a retrospective exploratory study. *Cortex* **1**: 344-67.
40. Lenneberg, E.H. (1967) *Biological Foundations of Language.* John Wiley, New York.
41. Butfield, E. and Zangwill, O.L. (1946) Re-education in aphasia. *Journal of Neurology, Neurosurgery and Psychiatry* **9**: 7-9.
42. Sarno, M.T., Silverman, M. and Sands, E. (1970) Speech therapy and language recovery in severe aphasia. *Journal of Speech and Hearing Research* **13**: 607-23.
43. Hopkins, A. (1975) The need for speech therapy for dysphasia following a stroke. *Health Trends* **7**: 58-60.
44. Hagen, C. (1973) Communiction abilities in hemiplegia: effect of speech therapy. *Archives of Physical Medicine and Rehabilitation* **54**: 454-63.
45. Lincoln, N.B., McGuirk, E., Mulley, G.P. *et al.* (1984) Effectiveness of speech therapy for aphasia in stroke patients: a randomised controlled trial. *Lancet* **i**: 1197-200.
46. David, R.M., Enderby, P.M. and Bainton, D. (1982) Treatment of acquired aphasia: speech therapy and volunteers compared. *Journal of Neurology, Neurosurgery and Pyschiatry* **45**: 957-61.
47. Griffiths, V.E., Oetliker, P. and Oswin, P. (1983) *A Time to Speak.* Chest, Heart and Stroke Association, Tavistock House North, Tavistock Square, London.
48. Ritchie, D. (1960) *Stroke: A Diary of Recovery.* Faber and Faber, London.
49. Marks, M.M., Taylor, M.L. and Rusk, L.A. (1957) Rehabilitation of the aphasic patient. *Neurology* **7**: 837-43.
50. Luria, A.R. (1970) *Traumatic Aphasia.* Mouton, Thittague.
51. Alekoumbides, A. (1975) Hemisphere dominance for language. *Acta Neurologica Scandinavica* **57**: 97-140.
52. Kertesz, A. and McCabe, P. (1977) Recovery patterns and prognosis in aphasia. *Brain* **100**: 1-18.
53. Wepman, J.M. (1951) *Recovery from Aphasia.* Ronald Press, New York.
54. Sarno, M.T. and Levita, E. (1971) Natural course of recovery in severe aphasia. *Archives of Physical Medicine and Rehabilitation* **52**: 175-8.
55. Sarno, J.E., Sarno, M.T. and Levita, E. (1971) Evaluating language improvement after completed stroke. *Archives of Physical Medicine and Rehabilitation* **52**: 73-8.
56. Katz, L. (1958) Learning in aphasic patients. *Journal of Consultative Psychology* **22**: 143-6.
57. Tifosky, R.S. and Reynolds, G. (1962) Preliminary study: non-verbal learning in aphasia. *Journal of Speech and Hearing Research* **7**: 295-8.

58. Rosenberg, B. and Edwards, A. (1964) The performance of aphasia in three automated perceptual discrimination programmes. *Journal of Speech Hearing Research* **7**: 295–8.
59. Cain, L.S. (1966) Determining factors that affect rehabilitation. *Journal of the American Geriatrics Society* **17**: 295–8.
60. Peszcynski, M. (1961) Prognosis for rehabilitation of the older adult and in aged hemiplegic patients. *American Journal of Cardiology* **7**: 365–9.
61. Baker, R.N., Schwartz, W.S. and Ramseyer, J.C. (1968) Prognosis among survivors of ischaemic stroke. *Neurology* **18**: 933–41.
62. Culton, G.L. (1969) Spontaneous recovery from aphasia. *Journal of Speech Hearing Research* **12**: 825–32.
63. Douglass, E. (1953) Diagnostic classification and re-education in aphasia. *Canadian Medical Association Journal* **69**: 376–81.
64. Sands, E., Sarno, M.T. and Shanlweiler, D. (1969) Long term assessment of language function in aphasia due to stroke. *Archives of Physical Medicine and rehabilitation* **50**: 202–7.
65. Lendrum, W. and Lincoln, N.B. (1985) Spontaneous recovery of language in patients with aphasia between 4 and 34 weeks after stroke. *Journal of Neurology, Neurosurgery and Psychiatry* **48**: 743–8.
66. Wade, D.T., Hewer, R.L., David, R.M. and Enderby, P.M. (1986) Aphasia after stroke: natural history and associated deficits. *Journal of Neurology, Neurosurgery and Psychiatry* **49**: 11–16.
67. Wade, D.T. (1983) Can aphasic patients with stroke do without speech therapy? *British Medical Journal* **286**: 50.
68. Deal, J.L. and Darley, F.L. (1972) The influence of linguistic and situational variables of phonemic accuracy in apraxia of speech. *Journal of Speech and Hearing Research* **15**: 639–53.
69. Johns, D.F. and Darley, F.L. (1970) Phonemic variability in apraxia of speech. *Journal of Speech and Hearing Research* **13**: 556–683.
70. De Renzi, E. and Spinnler, H. (1966) Facial recognition in brain damaged patients. *Neurology* **6**: 145–52.
71. Warrington, E.K. and James, M. (1967) An experimental investigation of facial recognition in patients with unilateral cerebral lesions. *Cortex* **3**: 317–26.
72. Meadows, J.C. (1974) The anatomical basis of prosopagnosia. *Journal of Neurology, Neurosurgery and Psychiatry* **37**: 489–501.
73. Hacaen, H. and Angelergues, R. (1962) Agnosia for faces. *Archives of Neurology* **7**: 92–100.
74. Nathanson, M., Bergman, P.S. and Gordon, G.G. (1952) Denial of illness. *Archives of Physical Medicine and Rehabilitation* **68**: 380–7.
75. Gainotti, G. (1972) Emotional behaviour and hemiplegic side of stroke. *Cortex* **8**: 41–5.
76. Battersby, W.S., Bender, M.B., Pollak, M. and Kahn, R.L. (1956) Unilateral spatial agnosia. *Brain* **2**: 139–49.
77. Lowenthal, M., Tobis, J.S. and Howard, I.R. (1959) An analysis of rehabilitation needs and prognosis of 232 cases of cerebrovascular accident. *Archives of Physical Medicine and Rehabilitation* **40**: 183–6.
78. Carroll, d. (1962) The disability in hemiplegia caused by cerebrovascular disease: serial study of 98 cases. *Journal of Chronic Disease* **15**: 179–89.
79. Feldman, D.J., Lee, R.R. and Unterecker, J. (1962) A comparison of functionally orientated medical care and formal rehabilitation in the management of rehabilitation of hemiplegia. *Journal of Chronic Disease* **15**: 297–310.
80. Granger, C.V., Greer, D.S., Liset, E., Coulcombe, J. and O'Brien, E. (1975)

Measurement of outcome of care for stroke patients. *Stroke* 6: 34–41.

81. Bourstom, N. (1967) Predictors of long term recovery in cerebrovascular disease. *Archives of Physical Medicine and Rehabilitation* 48: 415–19.

82. Lorenze, E.J., Simon, H.B. and Linden, J.L. (1959) Urological problems in rehabilitation of hemiplegic patients. *Journal of the American Medical Association* 169: 1042–6.

83. Droller, H. (1960) Survival after apoplexy – a five year follow up. *Gerontologia Clinica* 2: 120–8.

84. Anderson, A.L., Hanvik, L.J. and Brown, J.R. (1950) A statistical analysis of rehabilitation in hemiplegia. *Journal of the American Medical Association* 169: 1042–6.

85. Lehmann, J.F., Delateur, B. and Fowler, R.S. (1975) Stroke rehabilitation: outcome and prediction. *Archives of Physical Medicine and Rehabilitation* 56: 383–9.

86. Cassvan, A., Ross, A.L., Dyer, P.R. and Zane, L. (1976) Lateralisation in stroke syndrome: a factor in ambulation. *Archives of Physical Medicine and Rehabilitation* 57: 583–7.

87. Di Benedetto, M. (1974) Optimal care of the severely involved stroke patient. *Rehabilitation* 91: 27–36.

88. Rogoff, J.B., Cooney, D.V. and Kutner, B. (1964) Hemiplegia: a study of home rehabilitation. *Journal of Chronic Disease* 17: 539–50.

89. Isaacs, B. and Marks, R. (1973) Determinants of outcome of stroke rehabilitation. *Age and Ageing* 2: 139–49.

20

Organization of rehabilitation services

There are three main ways of providing rehabilitation for an elderly person: as an inpatient, in a day hospital or at home. Each of these has advantages and disadvantages.

Admission to hospital

The advantage of admitting an elderly person to hospital for rehabilitation is that the setting provides support at a time when disability may be so marked that it is difficult to cope at home. It provides the opportunity for a full team assessment over the whole day and allows access to expensive investigational and treatment resources.

The disadvantage is that the environment is artificial. The patient functions in a stimulating and encouraging environment; chairs and beds are usually of an ideal height; there is plenty of space to manoeuvre frames; and the floor is usually free of obstacles such as unsuitable carpeting. In purpose-built units there are suitable handrails and wide doors which allow easy access to a toilet of the correct height.

Assessment flats

The hospital can be made like home by having wards carpeted and by using the type of bed that will be used at home. This is rarely achieved except in an assessment flat: a separate room or suite of rooms set out like a home in which the patient can live for several days. If necessary a relative, too, can stay in the flat and both be trained for the return home. One advantage of the assessment flat is that it allows observation of what the patient *will do* when left alone as well as what he *can do* when encouraged. It has another advantage that the patient can be allowed to manage his own medication, which is rarely possible on an open ward.

Even with the best intentions the flat is not the same as home. Many patients who do not manage in the flat still insist that they will manage when they return home, and this may or may not be the case. Similarly, even if the patient has coped in the flat this does not necessarily mean that he will manage at home.

Home assessment visits

In many cases it will be necessary to carry out a home visit with the patient prior to discharge. There has been some debate as to when this should take place. There is a point of view which states that a detailed knowledge of the patient's home is necessary from the time of admission so that the whole programme can be based on this information. This is rarely an appropriate use of scarce staff resources. In general it is satisfactory to take the patient home when he is at a level of ability where discharge is being planned – usually a week to ten days before discharge. This allows the opportunity to pick up the problems that the patient is likely to have, and also allows time for minor modifications to the home – such as nailing down carpets, raising the height of the bed or chairs and advising about reorganization of the furniture in the house. It also allows time to arrange for the provision of aids, such as chemical toilets, and to organize the necessary social service support.

For some patients several home visits are required until the team is satisfied that optimal conditions in both patient and environment have been achieved.

Some patients benefit from being taken home in a morning and brought back to hospital in the evening, which allows an assessment of how they are likely to cope in their own home without support. This may then progress to them being allowed to stay overnight and then for a few days with regular checking by members of the rehabilitation team. This gradual withdrawal of support is especially important both for the patient who has little confidence in his own abilities and for those who are overconfident. In both cases the visits help them to adjust to the realities of returning home safely. The other use for the planned short-term discharge is to help the carer gain confidence in their ability to cope with the disabled elderly person.

Day hospitals

Day hospitals originated from the need to provide hospital-based management without the need for hotel-type accommodation. They differ from the conventional outpatient rehabilitation service by providing an integrated service rather than the separate physiotherapy, occupational therapy and medical services otherwise provided [1, 2].

The philosophy of day hospitals has probably changed over the last 20 years. In the early 1960s they were used for elderly people who lived alone and needed care, who were lonely and had some physical or personality defect, and those who were pleasantly confused [3]. Pathy [4] described four categories of day hospital patients:

- those needing hospital services but not acutely ill and not requiring 24-hour nursing, especially for physically disabling conditions;
- those requiring detailed special procedures and investigations;
- those discharged from hospital and requiring continuing physical, therapeutic or nursing supervision;
- As a half-way house between being an inpatient and being totally at home, especially those who were worried about returning home.

By the late 1970s the functions of the day hospitals in rank order were rehabilitation, physical maintenance, nursing procedures, relief for relatives and medical procedures [5]. This swing towards the rehabilitation and medical components and away from social support has largely been made possible by the number of alternative support systems, such as Social Service and charitable day centres for those requiring social support, and the growing speciality of psychogeriatric medicine with its own day hospitals for the demented patient.

This change in role has seen the number of attendances per patient decrease to about twenty [6] spread over, on average, three months [4, 5, 7, 8]. There is some evidence, from a very large study of 2711 elderly people discharged from acute hospitals, that most of those who are attending the day hospital at three months are still attending at the end of the first year [9].

The effectiveness and efficiency of day hospitals is difficult to assess. It is obvious that at the time of their introduction day hospitals played a major role in decreasing the need for residential care and admission to hospital [10] and in allowing earlier discharge from hospital [11].

Although day hospitals are thought to provide a method of decreasing hospital costs [12] there are then additional costs for the community services and family [13]. There have been several small studies comparing the cost effectiveness of day hospital against inpatient care [4, 8, 14, 15]. They have been unable to provide a clear-cut confirmation of the cost effectiveness, probably because the alternative to day hospitals for some patients may not be inpatient care but social day centres or domiciliary rehabilitation.

There are a large number of day hospitals, but there is a 'paucity of any serious attempts to critical evaluation' [16]. it is difficult to judge the effectiveness of day hospitals unless the goals for individual patients are defined. For instance, in day hospitals predominantly managed by nursing staff with a custodial attitude, there were longer stays and fewer patients reached the original objectives than in smaller units staffed by therapists with a rehabilitation approach [17]. Nevertheless, in one controlled study there was no essential difference between those treated in hospital and those managed in the day hospital for physical or functional outcome, although the day hospital care was less expensive [2].

One controlled trial of demented 'social' cases, randomly allocated to day hospitals or to the type of care they would have received before the day hospital opened, found that there was early improvement in the activities of daily living of the patients attending the day hospital and that the day hospital patients showed continuing improvement in mental function and depression [18]. It was concluded that rehabilitation could be provided more economically by inpatient and domiciliary services and that it would be more productive to develop these services than day hospitals. This rather begs the question of what 'rehabilitation' is, implying that it is purely based on physical recovery.

Patients do tend to become dependent on the day hospital [19], as much psychologically as physically. This can usually be accomodated in less expensive forms of support, although where there is a lack of social day centres there will inevitably be a large number of long-term attenders.

The siting of the day hospital is probably important. Although there are advantages, especially in large catchment areas, of having local day hospitals near to the patient's home, there are major advantages in having the day hospital as part of the main geriatric unit where there is easier continuity of management between inpatient and outpatient care, good access to investigational facilities, and better communications, and education for staff. However, this model can only be applicable where there is a formal geriatric unit and cannot be translated to other countries [20]. Nevertheless day hospitals have been shown to have a role in management of the elderly in other countries, including the United States [21–26], Australia [27], Sweden [28], Israel [29] and Hong Kong.

The advantages of the day hospital might be summarized as follows:

- It provides full hospital skills and resources while the patient is experiencing the problems of living at home. Actual problems of daily living can therefore be assessed and managed.
- It provides a social outlet for disabled people. Although this is not a

primary role, and there are other ways of providing this, most patients and relatives regard it as an important part of the attendance [5].

- It is an efficient use of scarce resources. For instance, one trained nurse can treat as many as ten times more patients in a day hospital than would be possible on a ward [30], although the levels of need are likely to be different.

The importance of day hospitals can be seen in the number of patients who deteriorate [31] or require admission to hospital [32] when the ambulance service is disrupted.

However, there are several problems with day hospitals, the commonest being that of transport [5]. In general ambulances used for the emergency service are unsuitable both in design and in reliability – they may be called away for an emergency. Several authors have emphasized the need for special ambulances designed for day patient attendance [5, 33, 34]. This is important to overcome the problems of the patient's timed arrived. Many day hospitals are, in fact, half-day hospitals, since the patient may not arrive until 11 a.m. and leave shortly after 2 p.m., with obvious limitations on the amount of time available for treatment. Patients may also be waiting several hours for the ambulance to arrive, which increases anxiety and fatigue [35]. Since there can be no guaranteed time for the ambulance to arrive some patients do not get undressed the night before, or get up very early, in order to be ready for the arrival of the ambulance. Many patients, especially men, do not like travelling in the ambulance [36], though some of this can be improved [37] by having the same ambulance crew bring the patient on each occasion.

A day hospital ambulance should ideally have [5]:

- front-facing or angled permanent seating with arm supports;
- room to manoeuvre within the vehicle and space for one or two wheelchairs; access by a side entrance, with steps for fairly ambulant patients; a tail-lift at the rear for the more disabled patients; large, clear windows to give patients a good view; and a two man crew of assist the more heavily disabled patients.

The ambulance ride itself can be quite distressing for some patients. As many as 20 per cent of patients attending day hospitals have travel sickness at some time [38]. Spasticity seems to be made worse by the ambulance journey – the therapist then spends valuable time releasing the spasticity just for it to be further induced by the return journey! Other conditions which are sometimes not conducive to an ambulance journey are pain (especially of the spine), dyspnoea, gross deformities, severe balance problems, vertigo, nausea and anxiety states; and the journey can be unpleasant for those who are very frail, acutely ill or easily fatigued. Probably because of these problems as many as 10 per cent of booked attendances to day hospitals are cancelled by the patient, resulting in many wasted ambulance journeys [39]. This is important because transport accounts for about one-third of the cost of the day hospital [5, 8, 30, 40]. It is probably too cynical to suggest that if the patient is fit enough to attend the day hospital then he is too fit to require it, but there are many conditions for which alternative forms of management would be more appropriate.

The day hospital, as for inpatient management, is an artificial setting and bears little relationship to what the patient can actually do at home. In one study of day hospital attenders, the functional ability of stroke patients was measured in the day hospital and then the activities patients actually carried out were assessed at home [41]. There were major differences between what the patient *could do* and what he or she *did do* – largely related to what the chief carer knew about the patient's ability and whether the carer regarded it as safer, quicker or easier to assist the patient than to encourage independence. Thus many of the skills learnt in the day hospital were not being used, emphasizing the importance of training the relatives and continually assessing the real needs.

Non-attendance at day hospitals is often higher than 10 per cent [42–44], most of which is due to the patient being too ill to attend [44] (although failure of ambulances to collect the patient is also quite common).

Domiciliary management

In view of the problems associated with day hospital management, interest has been shown in providing the treatment at home. The advantages of this include the following:

1. The patient does not have to travel and so avoids the need to rise early, is not tired by the journey and does not suffer the complications of travelling.
2. The home is a more realistic environment in which to train the patient.
3. The relatives can be trained in the appropriate levels of assistance required.
4. Goals are easier to decide.
5. The environment can be adjusted to the needs of the patient and the family.

The disadvantages are the following:

1. The full range of skills of an integrated team is not available.

2. There is a limit to the amount of specialist equipment that can be transported to the patient.
3. There is very little social outlet for the patient.
4. It does not provide relief to the carer.

Home care as an alternative to hospital management for all types of disorders has been pioneered in France [45], and it is claimed that the cost of this approach is about 40 per cent of the inpatient costs in the Basque region and one-third those in Paris. Opit [46], on the other hand, has shown that there is little economic advantage in the home care of severely disabled people since the revenue costs of domiciliary care may be equal to or greater than the average residential, hospital or custodial care whilst providing inadequate levels of care. There are difficulties in this costing [47], since many of the costs of the home would still have to be met even if the patient were in hospital and the capital cost of the institutions had not been taken into account.

Most of the publishes research on domiciliary rehabilitation has been descriptive rather than controlled trials [48–51]. Frazer [52] did attempt a controlled study of domicilliary physiotherapy with day hospital management and found that the outcome was similar but that home treatment required less time to achieve similar results than did the day hospital. It is generally felt that it must be more expensive for a therapist to be spending time travelling and seeing fewer patients. It did seem from Frazer's study that home treatment was cheaper because fewer total staff were required and there was not the need for the very expensive ambulance service. It can also be argued that providing rehabilitation to people who will not use their skills on returning home is not a cost-effective way of running a service.

The great advantage of an integrated geriatric service is the armamentarium that the geriatrician has at his disposal. It is difficult to compare the costs of each type of facility since ideally each provides different specialized management for the needs of individual patients.

References

1. Do, C.O. and Kibat, W.H. (1975) Evaluation of multidisciplinary care programme for stroke patients in a day center. *Journal of the American Geriatrics Society* 22: 63–9.
2. Cummings, V., Kerner, J.F., Arones, S. and Steinbock, C. (1985) Day hospital service in rehabilitation medicine: an evaluation. *Archives of Physical Medicine and Rehabilitation* 66: 86–91.
3. McComb, S.G. and Powell-David, J.D. (1961) A geriatric day hospital. *Gerontologia Clinica* 3: 146–51.
4. Pathy, M.S. (1969) Day hospitals for geriatric patients. *Lancet* 2: 533–4.
5. Brocklehurst, J.C. and Tucker, J.S. (1980) *Progress in Geriatric Day Care.* King Edward's Hospital fund for London, London.

6. Hildick-Smith, M. (1980) Geriatric day hospitals: practice and planning *Age and Ageing* **9**: 38–46.
7. Andrews, J., Fairley, A. and Hyland, M. (1970) A geriatric day ward in an English hospital. *Journal of the American Geriatrics Society* **18**: 378–86.
8. MacFarlane, J.P.R. Collings, T., Graham, K. and MacIntosh, J.C. (1979) Day hospitals in modern clinical practice – cost benefit. *Age and Ageing* **8** (Suppl.): 80–6.
9. Victor, C.R. and Vetter, N.J. (1985) Use of community services by the elderly 3 and 12 months after discharge from hospital. *International Rehabilitation Medicine* **7**: 56–9.
10. Woodford-Williams, E., McKeon, J.A., Trotter, I.S. *et al.* (1962) The day hospital in the community care of the elderly. *Gerontologia Clinica* **4**: 241–56.
11. Brocklehurst, J.C. (1964) The work of a geriatric day hospital. *Gerontologia Clinica* **6**: 151–66.
12. Deparment of Health and Social Security (1981) *Growing Older*. HMSO London.
13. Donaldson, C., Wright, K. and Maynard, A. (1986) Determining value for money in day hospital care for the elderly. *Age and Ageing* **15**: 1–7.
14. Rose, D.N. (1976) Geriatric day hospitals: counting the cost compared with other methods of support. *Age and Ageing* **5**: 171–5.
15. Anand, K.B., Thomas, J.H., Osborne, K.C. and Osmolski, R. (1982) Cost effectiveness of a geriatric day hospital. *Journal of the Royal College of Physicians* **16**: 53–6.
16. Hodkinson, H.M. (1980) A need for evaluation. *British Medical Journal* **281**: 1000.
17. Martin, A. and Millard, P.H. (1976) Effect of size on the function of three day hospitals: the case for the small unit. *Journal of the American Geriatrics Society.* **24**: 506–10.
18. Tucker, M.A., Davison, J.G. and Ogle, S.J. (1974) Day hospital rehabilitation – effectiveness and cost in the elderly: randomised controlled trial. *British Medical Journal* **289**: 1209–12.
19. Wadsworth, M.E.J., Sinclair, S. and Wirz, H.M. (1972) A geriatric day hospital and its system of care. *Social Sciences and Medicine* **6**: 507–25.
20. Gustafson, E. (1974) Day care for the elderly. *Gerotologist* **14**: 46–9.
21. Kostick, A. (1974) Levindale day-care program. *Gerontologist* **14**: 31–2.
22. Turbow, S.R. (1975) Geriatric group day care and its effect on independent living. *Gerontologist* **15**: 508–10.
23. Lorenze, E.J., Hamill, C.M. and Oliver, R.C. (1974) The day hospital: an alternative to institutional care. *Journal of the American Geriatrics Society* **22**: 316–20.
24. Kennedy, R. (1975) The day hospital as a rehabilitation resource in the United States. *Rehabilitation* **92**: 44–50.
25. Mehta, N.H. and Mack, C.M. (1975) Day care services: an alternative to institutional care. *Journal of the American Geriatrics Society* **23**: 280–3.
26. Koff, T.H. (1974) Rationale for services: day care, allied care and coordination. *Gerontologist* **14**: 26–9.
27. Blake, D.H. (1968) A day hospital for geriatric patients: the first twelve months. *Medical Journal of Australia* **2**: 802–4.
28. Hagvall, K. and Suurkala, J. (1975) Geriatric day hospital care – experience from a three year study. *Lakavtidningen* **72**: 1091–4.
29. Robins, E.G. (1975) *Report on Day Hospitals in Israel and Great Britain.* National Centre for Health Services Research, Department of Health, Education and Welfare, Washington, DC.

30. Hildick-Smith, M. (1984) Geriatric day hospitals: changing emphasis and costs. *Age and Ageing* **13**: 95–100.
31. Prinsley, D.M. (1971) Effect of industrial action by the ambulance service on day hospital patients. *British Medical Journal* **3**: 170–1.
32. Berrey, P.N.E. (1986) Increase in acute admissions and deaths after closing a geriatric day hospital. *British Medical Journal* **292**: 176–8.
33. Brocklehurst, J.C. (1970) *The Geriatric Day Hospital.* King Edward's Hospital Fund for London, London.
34. Hildick-Smith, M. (1974) A typical journey to and from the day hospital. *Gerontologia Clinica* **16**: 263–9.
35. Beer, T.C., Goldenberg, E., Smith, D.S. and Mason, A.S. (1974) Can I have and ambulance, doctor? *British Medical Journal* **1**: 276–8.
36. Peach, H. and Pathy, M.S. (1977) Evaluation of patient's assessment of day hospital care. *British Journal of Preventative and Social Medicine* **31**: 209–10.
37. Simpson, R.G. and Shaw, M.J.M. (1971) The geriatric clinic – a fifteen year experience. *Health Bulletin* **29**: 30–2.
38. Stokoe, D. and Zuccollo, G. (1985) Travel sickness in patients attending a geriatric day hospital. *Age and Ageing* **14**: 308–11.
39. Peach, H. and Pathy, M.S. (1981) Role of non-attendance statistics in assessing the efficiency of geriatric day hospitals. *Community Medicine* **3**: 123–30.
40. Irvine, R.E. (1980) Geriatric day hospitals: present trends. *Health Trends* **12**: 68–71.
41. Andrews, K. and Stewart, J. (1978) Stroke recovery: He can but does he? *Rheumatology and Rehabilitation* **18**: 43–8.
42. Farquhar, M. and Earle, V.E.R. (1981) Day hospital: a program development perspective. *Dimensions of Health Service* **58**: 16–8.
43. Tyndall, R.H. (1979) Day hospital dilemma: when patients refuse. *Modern Geriatrics* **8**: 34–7.
44. Rai, G.S. and Murphy, P. (1985) Analysis of a geriatric day hospital. *Age and Ageing 14*: 139–42.
45. Clarke, F. (1977) Hospital at home. *Concord* **8**: 21–5.
46. Opit, L.J. (1977) Domiciliary care of the elderly sick – economy or neglect? *British Medical Journal* **i**: 30–3.
47. Brocklehurst, J.C. (1977) Domiciliary care of the elderly sick. *British Medical Journal* **1**: 374.
48. Borhani, N.O. (1974) Stroke surveillance: the concept of the stroke team in diagnosis, treatment and prevention. *Stroke* **5**: 78–80.
49. Compton, A. (1973) The physiotherapist in the community. *Physiothrapy* **59**: 75–9.
50. Holgate, B. (1977) Report of a pilot scheme for domiciliary physiotherapy service. *Chest, Heart and Stroke Association Journal* **2**: 238–42.
51. Partridge, C.J. and Warren, M.D. (1977) *Physiotherapy in the Community.* Health Service Research Unit, University of Kent.
52. Frazer, F.W. (1980) Domiciliary physiotherapy – cost and benefit. *Physiotherapy* **66**: 2–7.

Index

Index